Bolt Attachment changes Partial Denture Prosthodontics

Suginaka "Riegel"(Bolt)® System with
various applications to prosthodontic rehabilitation

Koh-ichi Suginaka

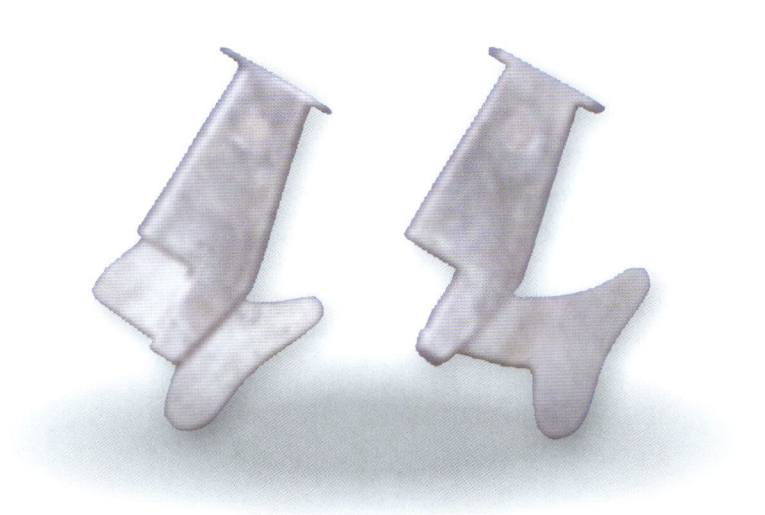

Nagasue Shoten

Bolt Attachment changes Partial Denture Prosthodontics
— Suginaka "Riegel"(Bolt)® System with various applications to prosthodontic rehabilitation —
By Koh-ichi Suginaka

Copyright © 2015 by Koh-ichi Suginaka
All rights reserved.

ISBN: 978-4-8160-1295-2
Printed in Japan

Published by Nagasue Shoten,Ltd.
69-2 Itsutsujicho Kamigyo-ku
Kyoto 602-8446 Japan
TEL+81-75-415-7280
FAX+81-75-415-7290
http://www.nagasueshoten.co.jp

Author's Profile

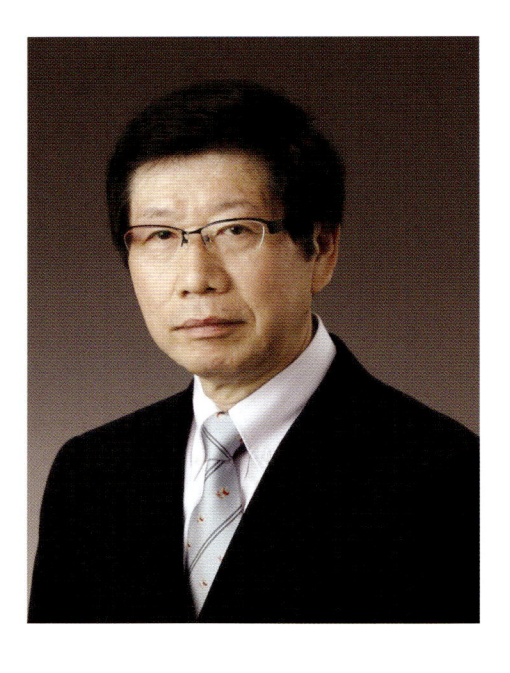

Koh–ichi Suginaka

Born in Nara, Japan in 1942
Graduated from Osaka Dental University
A practitioner in Nara, Japan, DMD
Invented and patented a bolt (Riegel) re-
tainer for retaining the denture
A member of Japan Prosthodontic Society
A member of Nippon Academy of Dental
Technology

Recommendation

Practicing dentist Dr. Koh-ichi Suginaka recently published "Bolt Attachment changes Partial Denture Prosthodontics — Suginaka "Riegel"(Bolt)® System with various applications to prosthodontic rehabilitation — ." (The term "Riegel" is German by origin, that corresponds to "Bolt" in English).

He had been interested in bolt attachments from around 1990. However, their use required a high level of technical accuracy in laboratory procedure. Thus, he designed and developed the prefabricated Suginaka bolt device through trial and error for easier fabrication of bolt attachment dentures.

The conventional bolt attachments included the vertical rotating and horizontal rotating types: the former one was consisted of the rotating section with locking latch placed on the outer telescopic crown into slots or depressions created on the axial wall of the inner telescopic crown, the latter one was consisted of inserted or latched bar in the lower part of a projection to the proximal surface adjacent to the edentulous area of a abutment crown of removable partial denture. The Suginaka bolt attachment are contained in a removable parts with standardized prefabricated kit consisting of the rotating part made of a precious alloy and the housing. The use of this kit allowed wider application of a bolt attachment to a prosthesis than before.

The use of this bolt attachment device in conventional partial dentures allows to eliminate a visible clasp arm in appearance. Application of the Suginaka bolt attachment can also be indicated in removable bridges with conceivable excess retentive forces during removal of the structure. In addition, using it as a device for fixing an implant superstructure with a removable section to the inner crown would be effective. The clinical and technical application of this bolt attachment will be discussed about in the following chapters.

Of course, although it goes without saying that there are "indications and limitations" in any system, I believe that the use of the Suginaka bolt attachment allows an increase of clinical flexibility to select the retainers for partial dentures and removable bridges.

January, 2012
Yoshimasa Igarashi: professor of Graduate School, Tokyo Medical and Dental University

Introduction

Do you know the Riegel attachment? This is a retainer used in partial dentures and was introduced into Japan about 30 years ago (The term "Riegel" is German by origin that corresponds to "Bolt" in English). The Cone-crown telescopic system (Konuskronen Teleskop in German corresponds to Cone-crown telescope in English) was almost fashionable when it was introduced in Japan. The author was also totally absorbed in it and knew nothing of dental prosthesis with Bolt attachment. The Cone-crown telescopic system with less denture breakage as well as good oral feeling, better functions, including phonation and mastication, and excellent esthetics were highly evaluated and widely used as a central part of partial dentures.

However, this system has many advantages, dynamic troubles, such as difficult denture insertion and removal due to an excessive interlocking force between the cone inner and outer crowns, fall-out of the cone inner crown (or with the post core) or tooth fracture, were often caused. Particularly, because of a tight fit between the inner and outer crowns, it is an important problem that the occlusal load exerted on the denture was directly-transmitted from the cone outer crown to the cone inner crown, thus suggesting that the abutment tooth may be affected with occlusal trauma. So, the author thought that this problem would be solved by loosely-fitting telescopic crown without applying friction to the cone inner and outer crowns, but this would lead to loss of denture retention. Therefore, there rose a need to resolve a problem with occlusal trauma as well as a new retentive method.

The author of this book found a book titled, "The world of Riegel Attachment" translated into Japanese from German (Quintessence Publishing Co., Ltd., 1988). When I tried to use this new retainer and first knew the existence of a retentive method with the bolt attachment. At the same time, I then knew that this was the retainer that I was trying to design.

The precision bolt retainer described in this book is all made by hand and the lever acting as a retentive function is incorporated into the prosthesis, allowing for smooth rotation. Therefore, a high degree of skill equal to precision machining is required during laboratory work. The difficulty and complex laboratory procedures seem to have prohibited the progress of the precision bolt retainer.

According to the trends of recent RPD design, a dentist need less retentive force if the function of support and bracing are adequately-fulfilled. The riegel (bolt) retainer uses the latch mechanism (effect) for securement (stabilizing) of mechanical retention of locking, unlike clasps, precision attachments or the Cone-crown telescopic system using friction. Thus, the use of the precision bolt attachment allows realization of no friction between the abutment tooth and the retainer even during denture insertion and removal, resulting no adverse effects of retention due to friction on the abutment tooth. Thus, the use of the precision bolt attachment promotes to avoid frictional retention between the abutment and the retainer, which may cause the loosening of the abutments.

The most difficult prosthetic laboratory procedure in the bolt precision retainer used widely around Germany is to allow smooth rotation of the lever incorporated into the prosthesis, for which a high degree of skill and the high laboratory cost are required, and thus it did not come into popular use. In addition, in the precision bolt retainer, because of a retentive projection adjacent to the denture basal surface and the rotating lever is tightly-fitted into a slot prepared into the retentive projection, the function forces applied to the denture base are directly-transmitted to the abutment tooth, suggesting the potential occlusal trauma to the abutment.

The Suginaka bolt attachment designed by the author consists of a prefablicated kit of smoothly rotating lever housed in advance. Since this device is only to be embedded in the denture base without soldering, the laboratory process becomes markedly easier and a significant cost reduction can be achieved. In addition, since there is no contact between the retentive projection and the denture basal surface. On the other hand, the bolt lever contacts the retentive projection at rest, while this lever is free from the retentive projection during function, no functional force is directly-transmitted to the projection. Thus, the abutment tooth is not affected with occlusal trauma.

In preventive dentistry, minimal intervention (MI), i.e. minimally invasive to the healthy tooth conserving the tooth structure, has become the dominant consideration in modern dentistry. The precision bolt retainer is originally combined with telescopic crowns with a great volume of tooth preparation. The Suginaka bolt attachment can also be combined with clasps as well as telescopic crowns. Among the various retainers used in partial dentures, clasps exhibits the least tooth preparation. The lock retainer is introduced in this book, with which only a rest and a guide plane preparation is required matching to the modern concept. Thus, the application of the Suginaka bolt device can further be extended to many cases.

In these days, prosthodontic oriented dentists have not so much selected the cone-crown telescope system as retainers with RPD and removable bridge as before, cause of increase of troubles in dental laboratory technical problems as well as clinical problems due to occlusal dynamics while mastication.

Nowadays, dental implant therapy has become prevailing but on the other hand, there are many patients whose prosthetic interventions have to be performed with removable dentures. The author believes that the use of the Suginaka bolt attachment do contribute to various dental patient's needs without use of dental implants in many situations. Of course, this Suginaka bolt attachments is also applicable to implant dentures retained by dental implants.

The author of this book feels it grateful if the readers of this textbook will choose the Suginaka bolt attachment as a retainer options in the prosthetic treatments.

It passed about seven-year since I first decided the publication of the text book on my Suginaka bolt attachment. I felt much frustration without publishing my home-task to the public.

I got acquainted to meet Dr. Yoshimasa Igarashi, who gave much influence to the author of this book.

He was a professor of graduate School of Tokyo Medical and Dental University. The author is deeply grateful to Prof. Igarashi for his recommendation as well as peer review, revision, and helpful advice.

In addition, the author is grateful to dental technician Yamamoto Nobuyoshi and Ogura Kazuhiro for trial production, productization and popularizationof the Suginaka riegel, respectively.

January, 2012
Koh-ichi Suginaka

INDEX

*Some images used in Chapter 7: Clinical cases with Suginaka riegel system are not handsomely printed because of low resolution. However, we decided to publish their images as they are for unifying the lay-out design with consideration for easy searching by readers. Please be forewarned.

Chapter 1

Requirements for retainers used in removable partial dentures (RPD's)

The purpose of RPD's is to replace the missing teeth and associated structures by the artificial teeth with denture plates to restore the occlusal contacts as close to the natural dentition as possible; this is accomplished to restore the occlusal stops in the centric position of mandible. The remaining teeth and residual alveolar ridge mucosa contribute to the achievement of this purpose among various intraoral tissues, mainly in the RPD's. Among them, the abutment teeth play a main role in stabilizing the dentures. Therefore, it is necessary to prevent overloads on the abutment teeth from various functional movements.

When a functional load is imposed on a healthy tooth, the periodontal ligament tissue can bear the maximum occlusal force because of its highly-resistant nature to a vertically exerted load. However, because of the structure of periodontal ligament tissue, its resistance to lateral forces at right angles to the tooth axis is extremely reduced compared to a vertically exerted load. In addition, the progression of alveolar bone resorption leads to a significant decrease in resistance to lateral forces, resulting in periodontal tissue destruction (break down). Therefore, it must be firmly noted in the design of retainers to be exerted a small lateral forces as possible on the abutment tooth with little resistance from the viewpoint of tooth preservation.

The denture mobility must be reduced to restore the occlusal support and maintain the oral function, including phonation and mastication through the removable partial dentures. This is markedly influenced by the contact relationship between the artificial teeth set-up and the opposing teeth, adaptation of the denture basal surface to the residual ridge mucosa, and the connecting mechanism between the denture base and the abutment tooth. Three-dimensional forces are exerted on dentures during chewing, leading to denture mobility. To control this mobility, it is necessary to minimize the displacement of soft tissues during occlusal contact between the artificial dentition on the denture base placed on the edentulous ridge and the opposing teeth, and to maximize the supporting area of the denture basal surface. In addition, since the connecting mechanism is to be designed so that the functional force is exerted as vertically as possible on the denture base and the abutment tooth without resulting in excessive forces on them. It is necessary to understand throughly about the dynamic properties of retainers as the component about their connecting mechanism.

To maintain stability of dentures, retainers must be constructed so that they can achieve the following three functions that means, support, bracing and retention.

Vertical force includes the occlusal and retentive forces. Support against occlusal load in clasp dentures is established by an exact fit between a rest seat prepared on the abutment tooth and an occlusal rest provided with the partial denture, in telescopic dentures by an adequate fit between the inner and outer crowns, and in the edentulous area by a close fit between the residual ridge mucosa and the denture base. The occlusal load exerted on the abutment tooth is transmitted in occluso-apical (longitudinal) direction and at the same time on the residual ridge mucosa is also loaded vertically under the denture base. This is the best direction for dentures to obtain support, thereby allowing achievement of vertical stabilization.

Bracing against lateral forces is established together with components of removable partial dentures, including the denture base, major and minor connectors as well as retainers and can stabilize the horizontal mobility of dentures. In addition, the minor connector and proximal

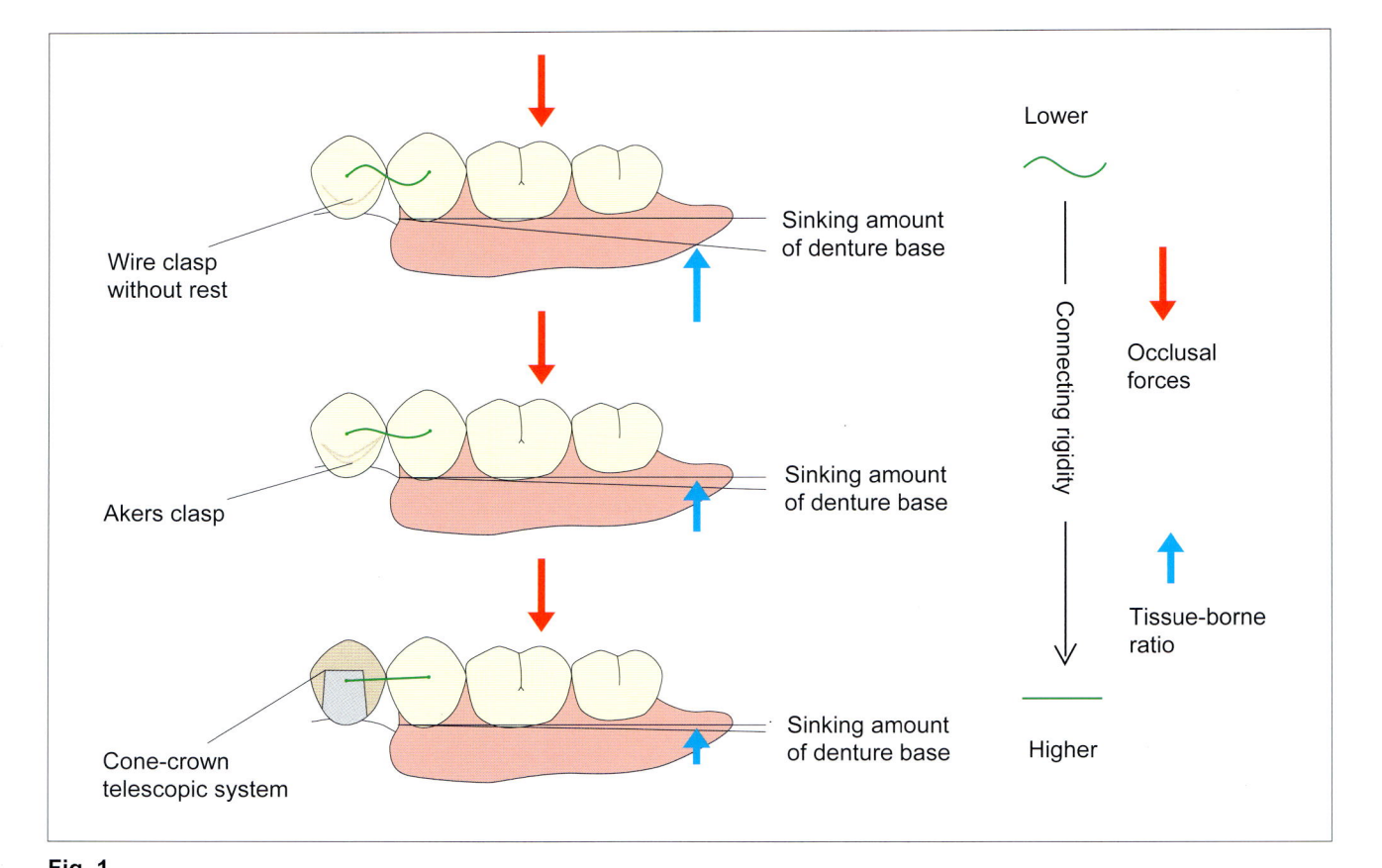

Fig. 1
Differences in tissue-borne load ratio against to the total occlusal forces exerted influenced by the connecting rigidity of retainers (modified from the report by Ogata and Igarashi [20, 21]). Under the same denture base conditions, the lower the connecting rigidity of the retainer against to the total occlusal forces is, the higher the tissue-borne ratio is, or the higher the connecting rigidity is, the lower the tissue-borne ratio is.

plate are designed to make contact with the guide plane prepared on the abutment tooth to enhance the bracing function securely. Reinforcement of the bracing function of the abutment tooth results in centralization of retention while displacement of dentures in the vertical direction, controling the path of denture insertion and removal, and increasing frictional resistance of the guide plate, thus less need for strong retention against displacement of dentures.

Man can recognize the problems in the denture design that there is a difference between the abutment tooth and the residual ridge mucosa in occlusal load bearing capacity. Since there is a significant difference in the amount of tissue displacement under pressure between the abutment tooth (periodontal ligament) and the residual ridge mucosa under denture base, in distal extension dentures particularly, the mobile connection at a junction between the abutment tooth and the denture base was performed as the denture design in former times. This is the thought of stress-breaking support modality called as "flexible support."

Many of the stress-breaking retainers were designed in former time. However, they did not result to protect the abutment tooth and residual ridge because of an increase of mobility in dentures as well as an increase of load on the edentulous ridge, resulting in residual ridge resorption and mobility of the abutment tooth.

In contrast, the non-resilient support modality called as "rigid support" was introduced. This idea is based on obtaining the maximal support from the abutment and the denture base through rigid connection between the abutment tooth and the denture base. The reason why this non-resilient support modality was attracted among dentists was because of good results have been achieved [18] from a long-term follow-up and experimental outcomes of the Cone-crown telescopic dentures with rigid conection to the abutment tooth. Commonly, a discrepancy exists in between the abutment tooth and the retainer dynamics, the retainer is displaced on the abutment tooth when exerting a load on it. This discrepancy/displacement

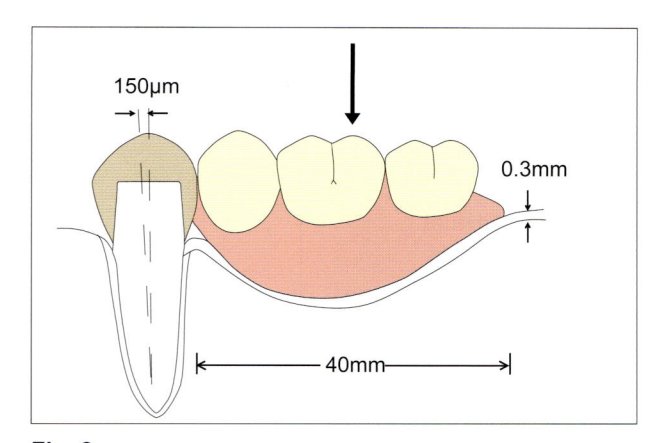

Fig. 2
Rehm's chart[1] shows that even if the denture base and the abutment tooth are rigidly connected in a long-saddle distal extension denture base, an inclination of the abutment tooth due to sinking at the distal end of the denture base is in an acceptable range of physiological mobility of the abutment tooth.

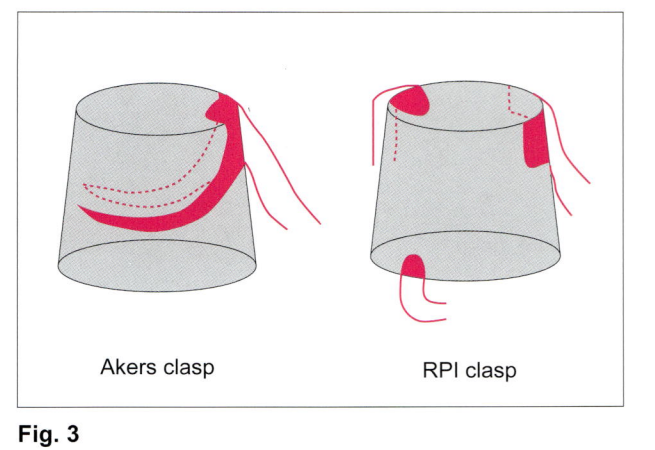

Akers clasp   RPI clasp

Fig. 3
Comparison of supporting and bracing components of the Akers clasp, RPI clasp, and Cone-crown telescope. In the Cone-crown telescope, the ceiling and axial surfaces of the inner crown act as the support function and its surrounding axial surface serves as the bracing function, thus the Cone-crown telescopic system has overwhelmingly broader functional area compared to clasps. This leads to a stronger connecting rigidity.

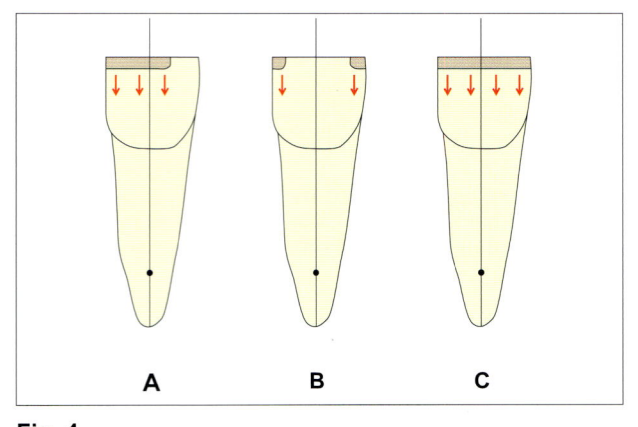

A   B   C

Fig. 4
To direct the occlusal forces in tooth longitudinal direction, there seems to be considered three options (quoted from the report by Goto[17] modified):
A: rest preparation to the area more than half of the mesiodistal width on the occlusal surface;
B: rest preparation on both mesial and distal marginal ridges on the occlusal surface;
C: rest preparation across the entire occlusal surface, sometimes called as a continuous occlusal rest preparation, or channel rest preparation.

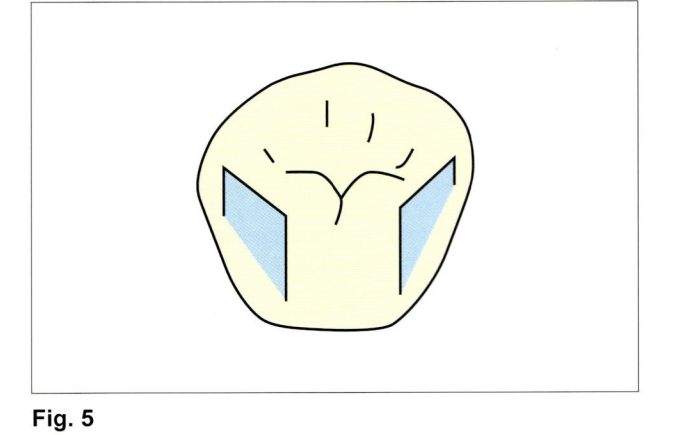

Fig. 5
The preparation of the wide guide planes parallel to both proximal surfaces allows achievement of a strong bracing effect.

on the abutment tooth is referred to as the connecting rigidity, which has been recognized as an important key to distal extension dentures.

Figure 1 shows the occlusal load distribution on the abutment tooth and the residual ridge mucosa under the same denture base with different retainers of connecting rigidity in distal extension dentures. It has been demonstrated[20,21] that the higher the connecting rigidity against the total occlusal forces is, the lower the tissue-borne ratio is or the lower the connecting rigidity is, the higher the tissue-borne ratio is. Also, it has been shown that when a certain level of connecting rigidity is established, there is almost no change in the tissue-borne ratio. The fact that the higher the connecting rigidity is, the lower the tissue-borne ratio against occlusal load is, means that the denture mobility is also reduced, resulting in the advantage to controling it. A decrease in occlusal force exerted on the denture base places a burden on the abutment tooth. Of the occlusal forces imposed on the abutment tooth, the vertical load can be supported by it, but the horizontal

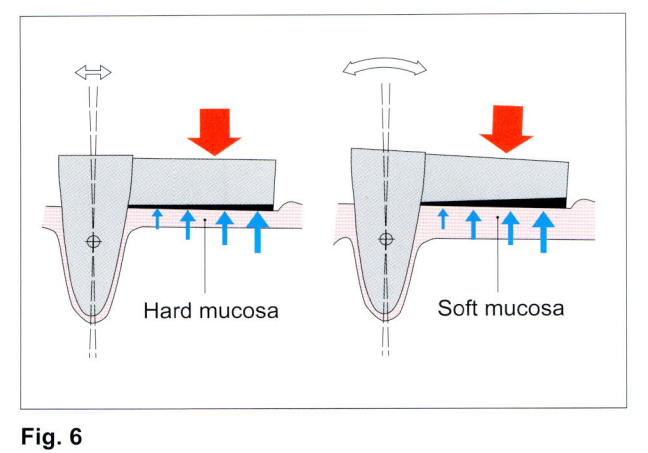

Fig. 6
Relationship between the displacement of oral mucosa and the rotation angle of abutment tooth (quoted from the modified report by Sekine et al.[8]).

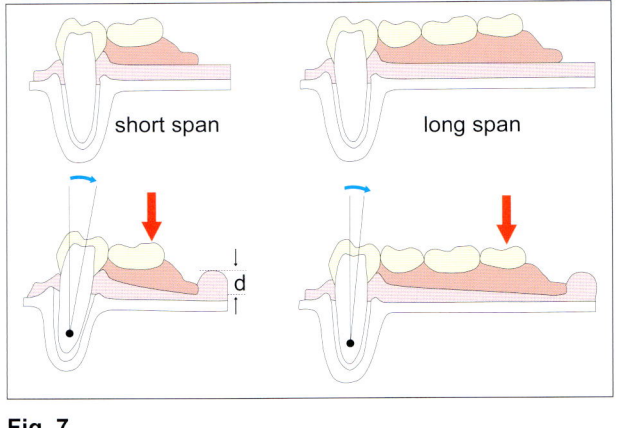

Fig. 7
Differences in the rotation angle of abutment tooth with distal extension denture base in long-saddle and short-saddle (quoted from the report by Nokubi & Igarashi.[27] modified).

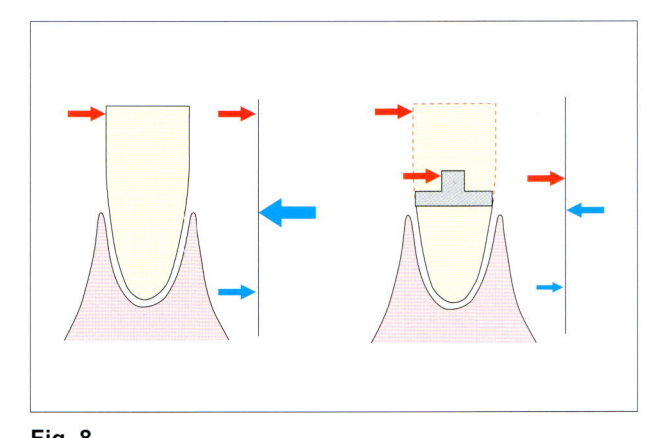

Fig. 8
The lower working point of occlusal forces (lateral forces) on the abutment tooth reduces the burden on periodontal tissue (modified from the report quoted by Sekine et al.[5]).
Left: An increase in coronal length due to alveolar bone resorption results the lateral force transmission from the denture to a higher position of the crown, resulting in heavy load on periodontal tissue.
Right: Cutting the crown to lower the position to the apical, the lateral force exerted on it leads to reduce a load to the periodontal tissue.
This can also be applied to a normal abutment tooth that the lateral force bearing allows reduction of a load on periodontal tissue at a lower coronal position than at a higher coronal position.

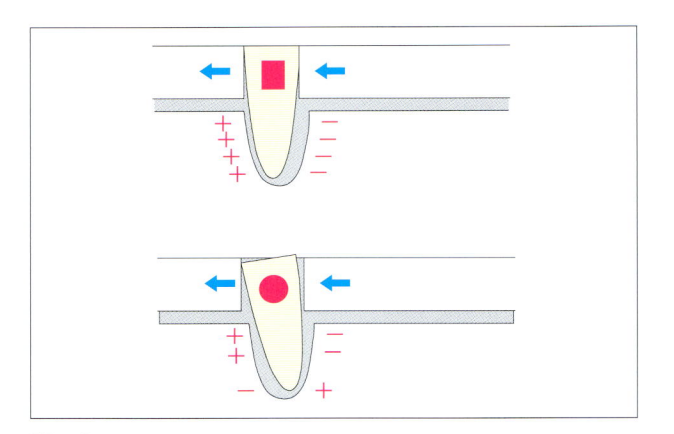

Fig. 9
Differences of functional burden on the abutment tooth with different connecting rigidity (quoted from the report by Sekine et al.[8] modified)
Top: a higher connecting rigidity leads to horizontal movement (bodily tooth movement) of the abutment tooth;
Bottom: a lower connecting rigidity leads to rotation of it.

load is adverse against the periodontal ligament.

However, Rehm gave a theoretical analysis to the problem to this matter. According to Rehm, in the distal extension situation, an inclination of the abutment tooth due to sinking at the distal end of the denture base is in an acceptable range of physiological mobility, if connected rigidly between a long saddle denture base and the abutment tooth [1] (Fig. 2).

In other word, even if the denture base is rigidly-connected to the abutment tooth , the abutment tooth is within an acceptable range of physiological mobility while denture sinking. A factor that influences the connecting rigidity depends on the functional area for support and bracing. When compared to Akers clasps, the cone-crown telescopic system has overwhelmingly wider functional area of bracing function (Fig. 3). The ceiling surface of the Cone inner crown acts as the support function and its axial surface acts as support and bracing in

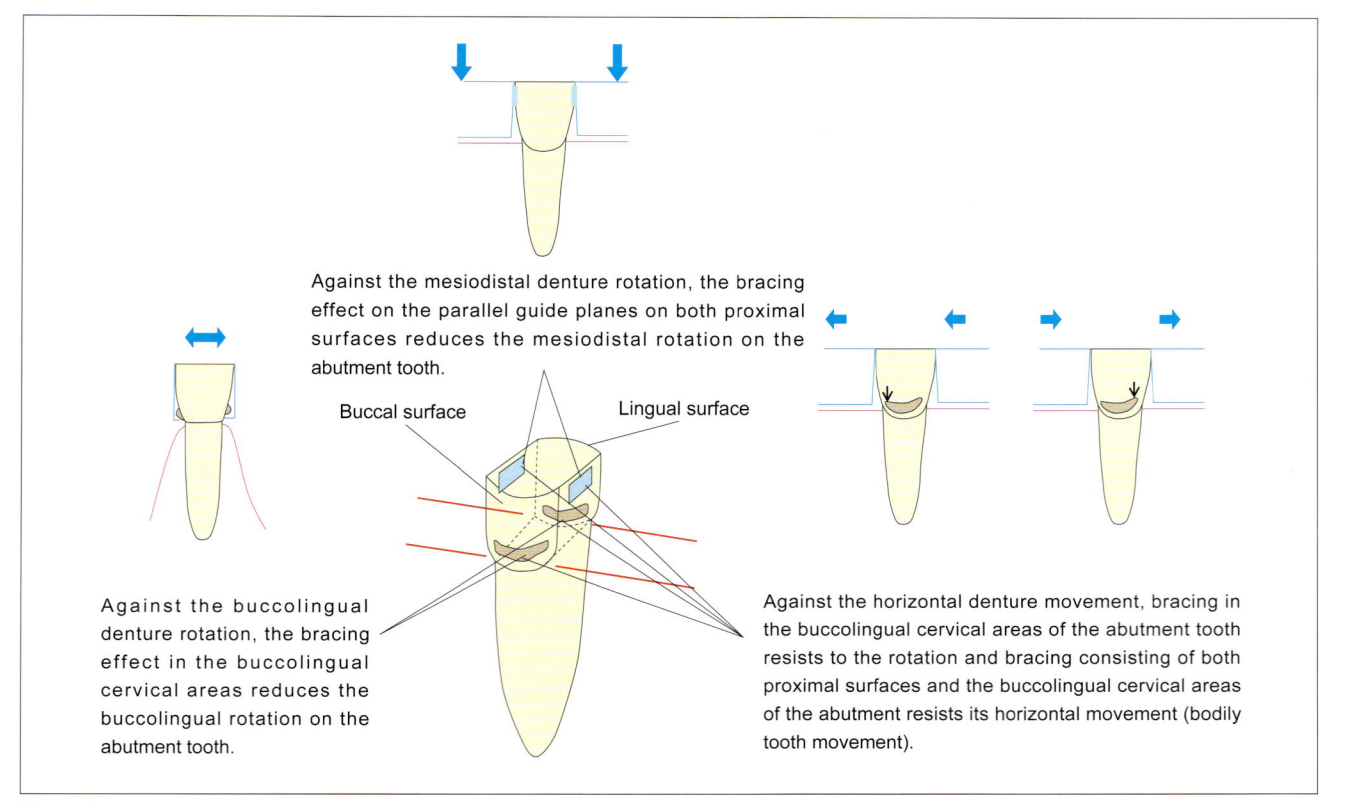

Fig. 10
Bracing forms for reduction of burden on the abutment tooth against mesiodistal and buccolingual rotation or horizontal movement of the denture.

function. In Akers clasps, a small occlusal rest and thin arm act as the function of support and bracing, respectively. Also, the axial surface of the Cone inner crown has an angle near-parallel to the tooth axis, leading to strong bracing function and enhancement of the connecting rigidity. Thus, enhancing the connecting rigidity leads to realize the function of bracing as well as support.

To enhance support function in clasps, a close fit between a rest and rest seat, and the positioning of rest is key to require and then it is important for the occlusal rest to guide the occlusal forces effectively in the axial direction of the abutment tooth. For this purpose, three options are considered; first, rest preparation to the area more than half of the mesiodistal width of the occlusal surface. secondly rest preparation on both mesial and distal marginal ridges of the occlusal surface ,or third rest preparation across the entire occlusal surface,that means they are called as continuous occlusal rest preparation, or channel rest preparation[17] (**Fig. 4**). On the other hand, the ceiling and axial surfaces of the Cone inner crown guide and support the occlusal forces along with the longitudinal direction of the abutment.

To enhance bracing function, there is a way to increase the contact area (frictional area) between the retainer and the abutment tooth, which acts as a bracing function and directing the contact surface parallell or almost parallell to the long axis of the abutment tooth. In clasps, the preparation of the wide guide planes parallel to each other on both proximal surfaces of the clasped tooth allows enhancement of the bracing function and the connecting rigidity (**Fig. 5**).

In the Cone-crown telescopic system, the strong bracing is acquired through the surface contact between the axial wall of outer and inner crowns.

However, the rigid connection between the abutment tooth and denture base derived from the ridgid support can only be achieved in long-saddle distal extension dentures with the excellent residual ridge mucosa and healthy periodontal tissue of the abutment tooth. Even in long-saddle denture bases, the rotation angle of the abutment tooth with hard residual ridge mucosa is smaller than in soft one[8] (**Fig. 6**). Also, even in hard ridge mucosa, the rotation angle of the abutment tooth in short-saddle denture base is larger than that of the long-saddle[27] (**Fig. 7**).

The fact that with larger rotation angle, it means that lateral forces on the abutment tooth is also larger, resulting in overestimated range of physiological mobility. Therefore, it is not allowed to use retainers with rigid connection to the short-saddle distal extension denture base with the poor residual ridge mucosa.

Although Rehm's theory is applicable to the cases with teeth loss of posterior to the canine or first premolar, the amount of mucosa displacement under pressure of the residual ridge mucosa or the length of denture bases varies in each case of distal extension denture. Therefore, even if the abutment tooth is connected rigidly to the denture base, two different cases may be conceivable; the case where the occlusal forces on the denture base can be supported on the abutment tooth as well as the residual ridge mucosa, and the other case where a reduction of the connecting rigidity of the retainer results to impose the occlusal forces on the residual ridge mucosa (mucosa-borne denture) because the occlusal forces on the denture base becomes overloaded to the abutment tooth[1].

If the abutment tooth is overloaded however, it is necessary to joint every abutment tooth in form of splinting.

Effects of the mesiodistal abutment tooth movement by sagittal denture rotation was already described, but dentures also rotate buccolingually. In bilateral designed dentures, there is almost no problem with less buccolingual rotation, but in unilateral distal extension dentures, the abutment tooth is affected by the buccolingual connecting rigidity. When the connecting rigidity is low, the buccolingual rotation angle of the abutment tooth is small and the abutment tooth is subject only to a small lateral force, but when the connecting rigidity is high, that of the abutment tooth is large and may be subject to a larger lateral force. Therefore, resistance to the lateral forces at a lower coronal position of the abutment tooth seems to be effective than at a higher coronal position thus reducing a transmitted force on the abutment tooth[5] (Fig. 8). However, even so, when the abutment tooth becomes overloaded, it is necessary to add an abutment tooth for splinting of stable abutment teeth.

It is said that the horizontal denture movement may occur. In this situation, the horizontal denture movement might result in additional horizontal stresses to the abutment tooth. Retainers with higher connecting rigidity might lead to horizontal movement (bodily tooth movement) of the abutment tooth and a lower connecting rigidity might lead to rotation of it[8] (Fig. 9).

Thus, in case the denture movements, including mesiodistal and buccolingual rotations or horizontal movement, are exerted to the abutment tooth, no rotational forces should affect to the abutment tooth beyond the acceptable physiological range of the tooth movement.

The ideal bracing mechanism for retainer to prevent rotational forces on the abutment tooth is considered as follows: against the mesiodistal denture rotation, it is necessary to control the connecting rigidity on the parallel guide planes prepared on both proximal surfaces of the abutment tooth; then to resist the buccolingual denture rotation through the bracing effect in the buccolingual cervical areas of the abutment tooth. Against to the horizontal denture movement, it is also necessary to support the horizontal movement (bodily tooth movement) of the abutment tooth through the bracing effects consisting of the parallel guide planes prepared on both proximal surfaces and the buccolingual cervical areas of the abutment tooth (Fig. 10).

Requirements of support and bracing mechanisms for abutment teeth were described as above. However, a retentive mechanism is required to prevent denture displacement during phonation, mouth opening especially in mastication. In the support mechanism for retainers, supporting force component should be directed the occlusal forces in vertical direction along the tooth axis. Even if the bracing function allowing less pressure with rotational load on the abutment tooth, the retentive force should not exert a load on the abutment tooth.

In the next chapter, the retentive mechanism of retainers and its adverse effects will be described.

Even with the complete dentures, with scarce support, bracing, and retention

Oftenly patients demand to increase more retention after felt their RPD's with insufficient retention. This is judged as unreliable from a professional design by the doctor with adequate retention. To the contrary, some denture wearers with both partial or complete ones use his/her denture throughly with good masticatory efficiency; where the denture support, bracing, and retention are clearly lost in such cases with removable partial dentures without bracing, support functions, deformed or fractured clasps and abutment tooth loss, or with complete dentures with significant occlusal wear as well as a poor retention between the denture base and mucosal surface due to absence of adaptation to the mucosa. Denture wearers with such poor partial or complete dentures, do masticate throughly with masticatory forces at the most stabilized position without feeling pain through stabilizing his/her denture with oral peripheral muscles, even if support, bracing, and retention are insufficient (**Fig. 11**) .

It is often appreciated to replace such poor old dentures with new dentures by wearers. However, almost of all wearers, who have been ever satisfied extremely with their old dentures give claims during replacement. Since the new dentures are scanned through the muscular sensation, which was already established by old dentures, including a slight discrepancy of occlusal position, a difference in occlusal vertical dimension, overlapping of anterior teeth, a difference in base border, and the thickness of denture base.

Thus, "Please be careful" when you replace the wearer's favorite old denture to a new one !

Fig. 11
Patient's intraoral appearance, who used ill-fitted dentures over a long period of time, with the both upper and lower dentures.
A: Edentulous maxilla after loss of tooth #17.
B: Edentulous mandible.

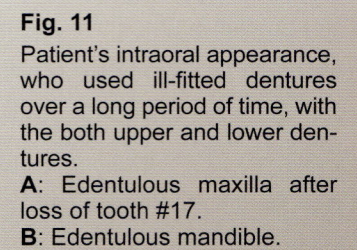
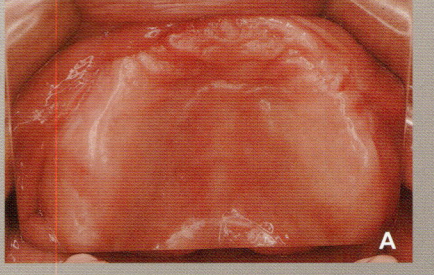
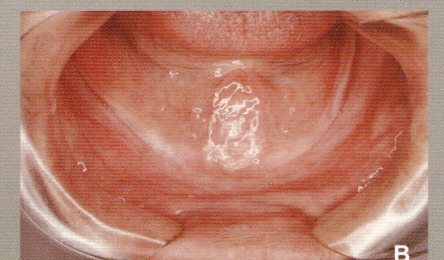

C: Occlusal view both of upper and lower dentures with significant occlusal wear.
D: Mucosal view of mandibular complete denture. No adaptation of denture base to the residual ridge mucosa.

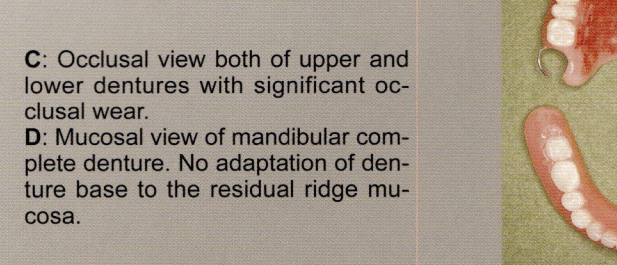
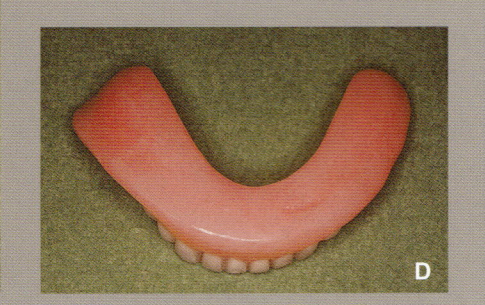

Chapter 2

Problems with the retentive mechanism for RPD retainers

Retainers used in the removable partial dentures require the retentive mechanism to resist denture dislocation and fall-out during mouth opening, phonation, and mastication as well as the support and bracing mechanisms. With the exception of the retentive mechanism using magnetic force, most of retainers utilize the elastic and frictional force. In clasps using the undercut area just beneath the survey line and in precision attachments using the undercut area under a projection placed on the abutment tooth, elastic forces arise as a retentive source in the process of placing at the retentive section in the undercut area; then frictional forces are obtained as the elastic force by the clasp arm and that of the interlocking regulatory section in precision attachments. Besides, there is a retentive mechanism using friction resulted from the vertical surface contact with the abutment tooth parallel to the path of denture insertion and removal between the inner and outer crowns like the Cone-crown telescopic system; it is necessary to prevent the frictional force from exerting a load to the abutment tooth during insertion or function of the denture.

Although the best maintenance for denture wearers are to remove and clean their denture, their removal force might exert excess removal force on the abutment tooth during denture removal, which may cause a problem. The removal force on the abutment excessively over the genuine retention results in exerting traction to the abutment tooth. Since the longitudinal periodontal ligament resistant to the traction force exists only a little in the cervical and apical region, the excessive retention should be avoided. Also, during removal of the denture with clasps exerting stronger retention, the clasped tooth is swayed by removing forces, making a movement like a pestle in a mortar (Fig.1-A). Retainers using frictional contact with the tooth surface parallel to the path of denture insertion and removal, no strong retention is required during denture removal. However, stronger tractive and lateral forces are exerted on the abutment tooth for detecting

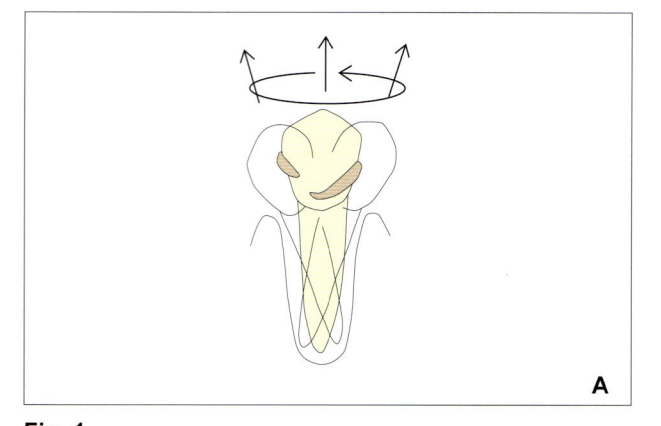

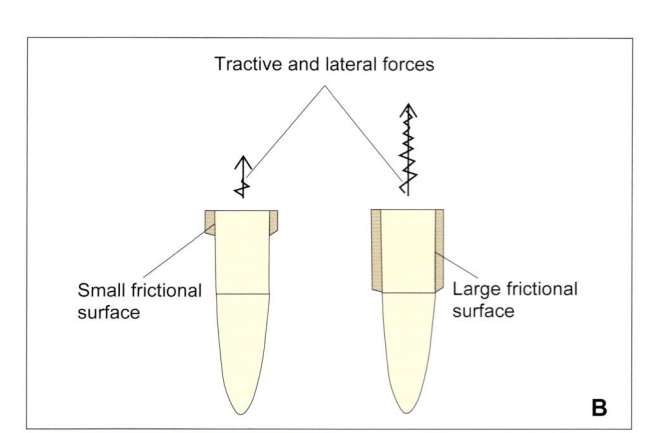

Fig. 1
Effect of friction between retainer and abutment tooth on its removal force
A: In clasp retainer with exess retentive force, abutment tooth plays a movement like a pestle in a mortar during denture removal.

B: For retainers depending on friction, if the parallel mesiodistal proximal plates prepared on the abutment tooth are short and narrow, the denture can be smoothly removed. However, if they are long and wide, tractive and lateral forces become stronger on the abutment tooth as a process while detecting the path of denture removal even if he predetermined retention is small.

the path of denture removal (Fig.1-B). Since the removal force of the denture is further increased by addition of the retentive or tractive force of the retainer, the retentive and removal forces should be reduced as small as possible.

So, several retainers are chosen for example to describe their features and problems with the retentive mechanism.

Fig. 2
When a rest, body, and shoulder of an Akers clasp are designed on the missing side, the abutment tooth tilts toward to the distal missing side.

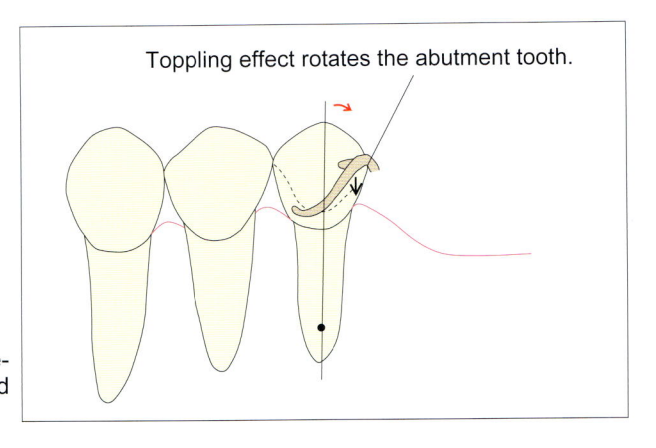
Toppling effect rotates the abutment tooth.

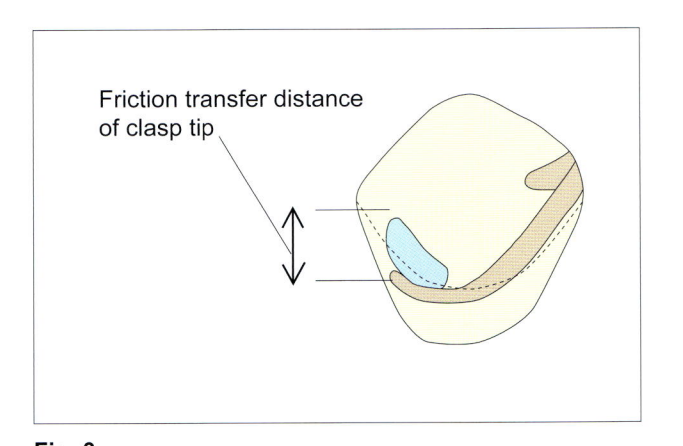
Friction transfer distance of clasp tip

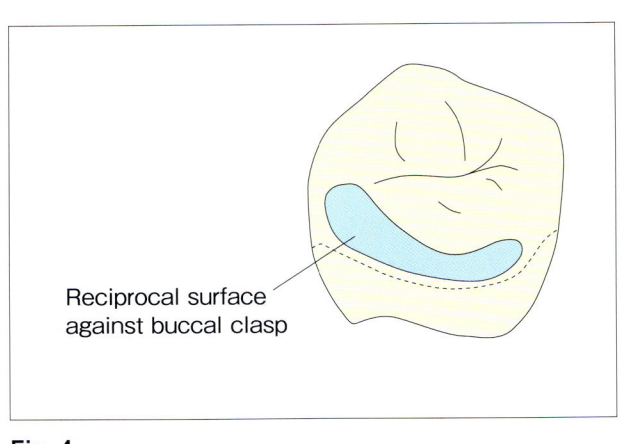
Reciprocal surface against buccal clasp

Fig. 3
The creeping distance of clasp tip from the stable and non-activated posision into the undercut area below the survey line is determined by the degree of tooth contour. It is difficult to design the lingual reciprocal arm against a lateral force from the buccal arm onto the curved lingual surface.

Fig. 4
To make a lingual clasp arm reciprocation against a buccal clasp, a guide plane must be prepared on lingual surface from just beneath the rest seat to the center of the crown on the surveyed line at height of contour.

1. Akers clasp

1) Akers clasp

The Akers clasp is the first choiced easy-to-use direct retainer with support, bracing, and retention for removable partial dentures, and is most commonly used in practice. However, because the clasp arm crosses the survey line, there are some unreasonable problems.

When an Akers clasp is selected as a retainer on the abutment tooth in distal extension denture, if an occlusal rest is placed on the disto-occlusal proximal missing side and a clasp shoulder lies on the survey line, the abutment tooth rotates to the missing direction through occlusal forces with lateral forces (toppling effect) (Fig. 2). Also, if the distance of frictional transfer is so long from the clasp tip making static contact to the tooth surface till the undercut area beneath the survey line, designing the lingual arm against a lateral force from the buccal arm

onto the curved lingual surface becomes difficult (Fig. 3). It is nessesarry to overcome this phenomenon that a guide plane must be correspondingly prepared to the lingual surface from just beneath the rest seat to the center of the crown restoration on the abutment tooth prepared (Fig. 4).

When the Akers clasp is used as a direct retainer in distal extension RPD's, the position of the clasp tip causes a problem. When the denture base is rotated and sunk with a rest as a fulcrum, the clasp tip which is placed in the undercut area in the mesial surface on the abutment tooth, acts to extract the abutment tooth (nail extracting effect) (Fig. 5). In addition, if a lifting force acts to the posterior border of denture base due to sticky food, the clasp tip rotates the denture base as a fulcrum (Fig. 6). However, an increase of retentive force to prevent this

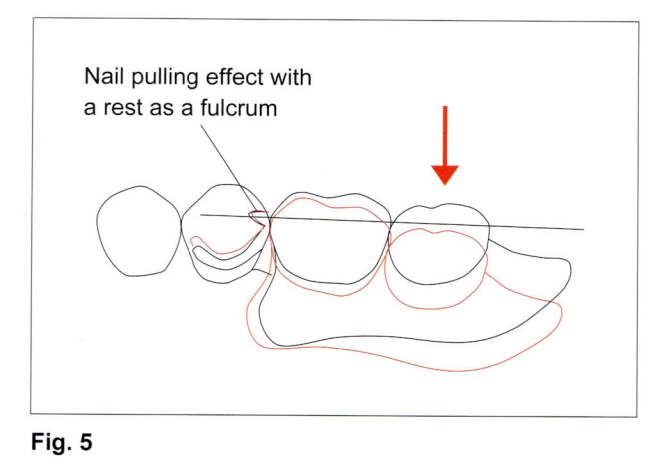

Fig. 5
When the distal extension denture base rotates around the distal rest as a fulcrum, the clasp tip acts to extract the abutment tooth (nail pulling effect).

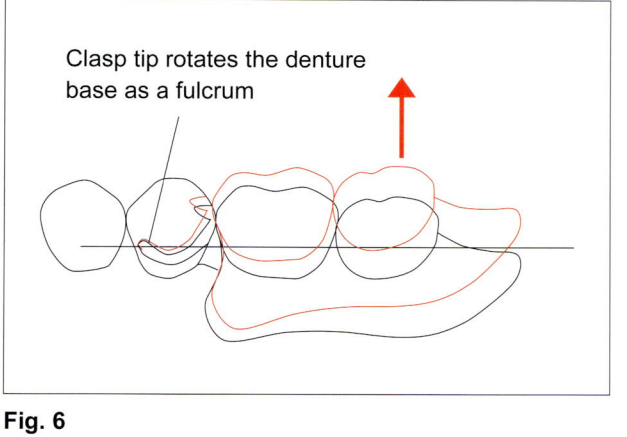

Fig. 6
If a force is exerted to float the posterior border of distal extension denture base, the clasp tip rotates the denture base as a fulcrum.

movement leads to an increase in denture removal force as well as the nail extracting effect, resulting overload. Therefore, Akers clasps with distal rest on the terminal abutment are inadequate as a retainer in case of distal extension dentures.

2) Half and half clasp

The half-and-half clasp consists of a buccal arm arising from one direction and a lingual arm arising from the other direction which is suitable for both a retentive and a reciprocal arms. Because the occlusal rests are placed both on the mesial and distal marginal ridges, the occlusal force can be directed along with the longitudinal direction of the tooth but this clasp can only be indicated only to a free standing tooth (Fig. 7).

3) Ring clasp

The ring clasp has the following disadvantages; because with a longer retentive arm, a deeper undercut is indicated, it is difficult to provide the adequate reciprocal surface against the retentive arm, and a lateral force during denture insertion and removal gives overload to the abutment tooth. In addition, a reinforcement arm leads to uncomfortable tongue sensation (Fig. 8).

4) Extended arm clasp

The extended arm clasp has the form of extending the buccal and lingual arm in an Akers clasp to the adjacent tooth and an effect of splinting the abutment teeth, thus reducing the toppling effect of the abutment tooth with

the distal rest as a fulcrum. However, a deeper undercut is required in the area where the clasp tip runs due to a longer clasp arm. The nail pulling effect and rotation of the denture with the distal rest as a fulcrum occur like as the Akers clasp (Fig. 9).

5) Twin arm clasp (Double Akers)

The twin arm clasp is used as a direct or indirect retainer described as double Akers clasps jointed at the body and is excellent in support, bracing, and retention. However, sufficient space must be provided between the abutment teeth in their occlusal third to make room for the common body of the twin arm clasp, and yet the contact area should not be eliminated entirely. This clasp often demonstrates a high percentage of fracture and separation of both abutment teeth caused by inadequate tooth preparation in the contact area. The twin arm clasp should always be used with double occlusal rests (Fig. 10).

6) RPI (mesial Rest, proximal Plate, I-bar) clasp

The RPI clasp includes the Krol's stress-breaking and Kratochvil's less-stress-breaking types (Figs. 11, 12) and is mostly used in distal extension dentures, in which the mesial rest is often placed to prevent mesial rotation of the abutment tooth (Fig. 13). There is also the advantage that the functional stress transmitted from the denture base which is exerted on the distal marginal gingival area can be more vertically directed in the mesial rest than in the distal rest (Fig. 14).

The Krol's stress-breaking RPI system consists of a

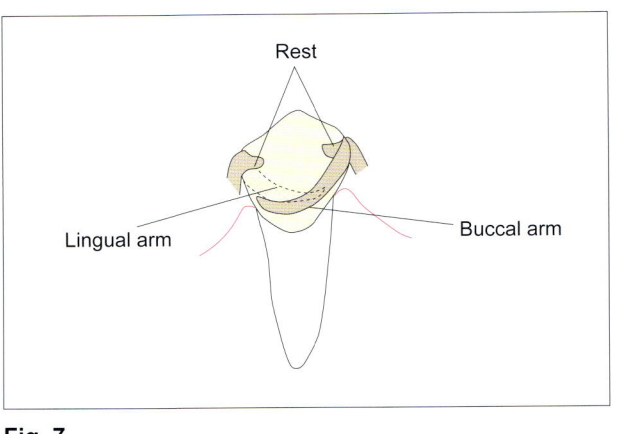

Fig. 7
Half and half clasp has a good balance of support and bracing.

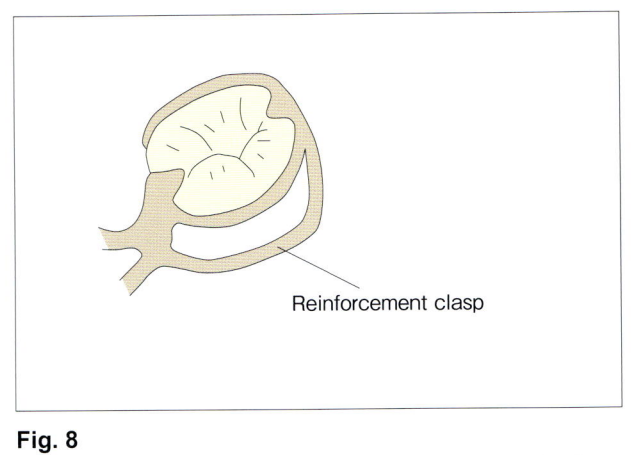

Fig. 8
An reinforcement clasp placed on a ring clasp leads to uncomfortable tongue sensation. Also, it is difficult to position a lingual arm against a buccal clasp.

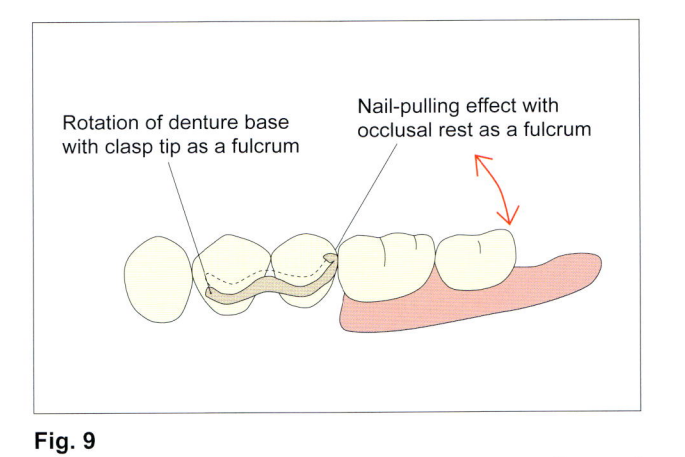

Fig. 9
The extended arm clasp causes the nail pulling effect and rotation of the denture like as the Akers clasp.

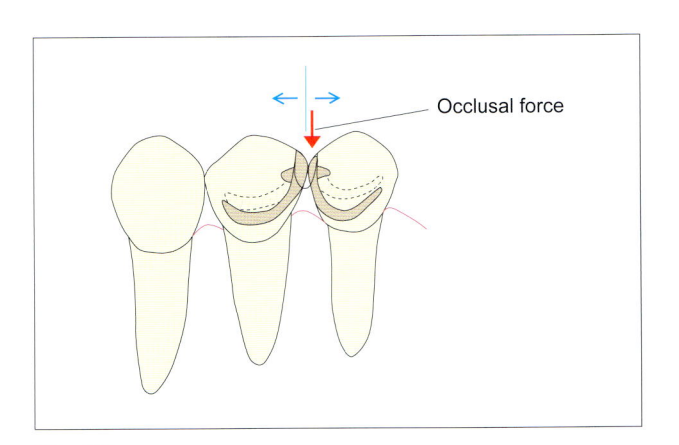

Fig. 10
Inadequate interproximal preparation leads to separation of both mesial and distal abutment teeth due to an occlusal force. Rest seat preparation must always be required. More tooth preparation is required for the adequate thickness for mechanical rigidity of the clasp.

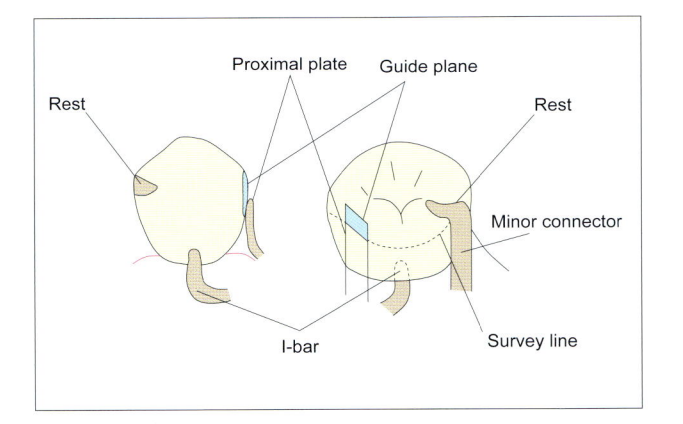

Fig. 11
Stress-breaking RPI clasp by Krol with less bracing.

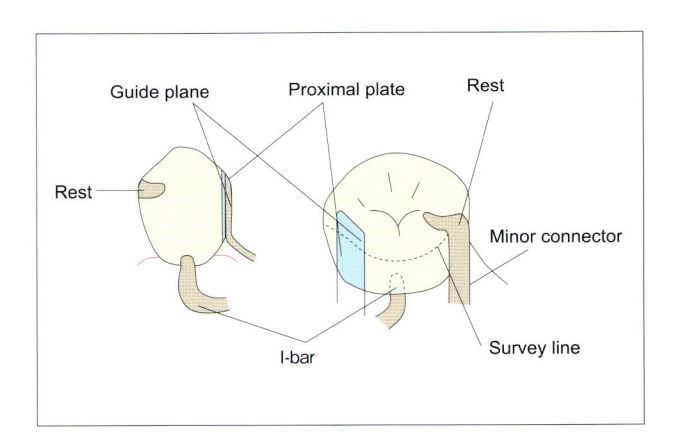

Fig. 12
Less-stress-breaking RPI clasp by Kratochvil with much bracing.
It needs more tooth reduction for a guide plane preparation to prevent denture displacement compared to Krol's RPI clasp.

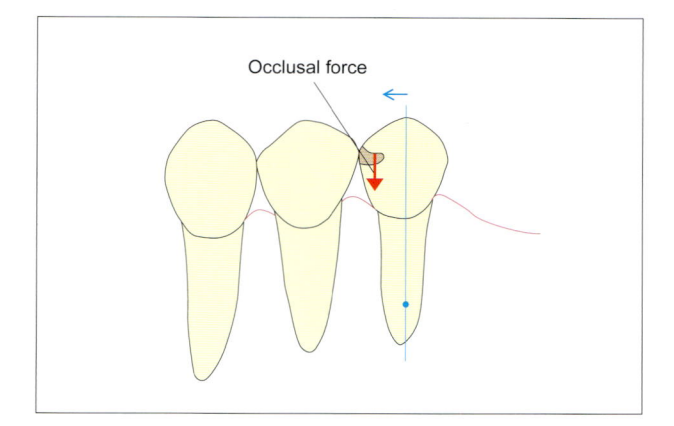

Fig. 13
Rotation of the abutment tooth is prevented by the adjacent tooth due to the mesial rest in the RPI system.

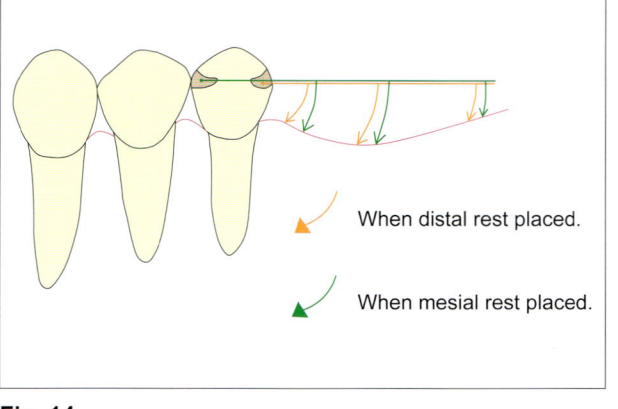

When distal rest placed.

When mesial rest placed.

Fig. 14
A difference in the direction of force exerted on the distal gingiva compared with the mesial and distal rests placed on the abutment tooth.

mesioocclusal rest with the minor connector placed into the mesio-lingual embrasure, a distal proximal plate with occlusal third of the tooth surface, and a buccal I bar, and therefore the abutment tooth tends to horizontally rotate, the bracing effect is less, and the connecting rigidity is lower depending on the form of the abutment tooth. Because the Kratochvil's nonstress-breaking RPI system has a wide proximal plate extending to the marginal gingival sulcus, the connecting rigidity becomes significantly stronger, but more tooth reduction is required and the indication is limited to a restored tooth with contouring.

If there is a deeper undercut around the abutment tooth or a patient with high frenulum position, the I-bar clasp arm cannot be indicated. In addition, since the I-bar retainer placed at the maximal prominence of contour with upper canines/first premolars to the gingival third aesthetics is usually undesirable.

7) RPA (mesial Rest, proximal Plate, Akers) clasp

The RPA clasp is a retainer that replaced an I-bar, one component of a RPI clasp with an Akers arm (Fig. 15). This clasp has a higher bracing effect and does not limit an undercut in the mucosa around the abutment tooth and anomaly of the frenum compared to the RPI clasp, thus applied to many cases. Of course, its proximal plate has the same requirements as the RPI clasp.

However, the body of an Akers clasp runs on the survey line from the origin and its clasp tip must run within the undercut area below the survey line. If the clasp arm other

than the clasp tip is placed over the survey line, an occlusal force is exerted on the distal side of the abutment tooth, resulting in the toppling effect.

8) RPPI (mesial Rest, bi-Proximal Plate, I-bar) clasp (Igarashi: 1990)

Igarashi (1990) intended to modify the RPI clasp design by Kratochvil and to realize the nonstress-breaking retainer, which consists of wide and parallel both mesio/distal bi-proximal plates, a mesial rest with the minor connector placed into the mesio-lingual embrasure, and I-bar. This retainer intended to realize the connection between the abutment and the retainer as telescopic retainer in the distal extension saddle RPD in simplified clasp design.

An increase in bracing through the parallel mesio-distal guide plates can decrease in retention. However, since the path of denture insertion and removal is extremely limited, stronger tractive and lateral forces might result to the abutment tooth while detecting the path of denture insertion/removal. This shows the same condition as removal of a parallel telescopic crown (Fig. 16). However, the connecting rigidity may be modified by changing the area of the guide plane.

9) RPPA (mesial Rest, bi-Proximal Plate, Akers) clasp (Igarashi: 1990)

The RPPA clasp is a retainer that replaced an I-bar, one component of a RPPI clasp with an Akers arm (Fig. 17). This clasp is such a nonstress-breaking retainer as the

RPPI clasp system and has a stronger bracing effect than the RPPI clasp, so that both tractive and lateral forces exerted on the abutment tooth during denture removal become stronger. That is, the connecting rigidity may be modified by changing the area of the guide plane.

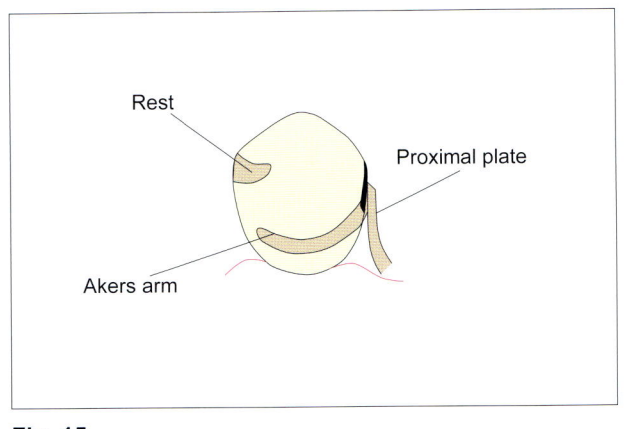

Fig. 15
RPA clasp, which replaced an I-bar, one component of a RPI clasp with an Akers arm.

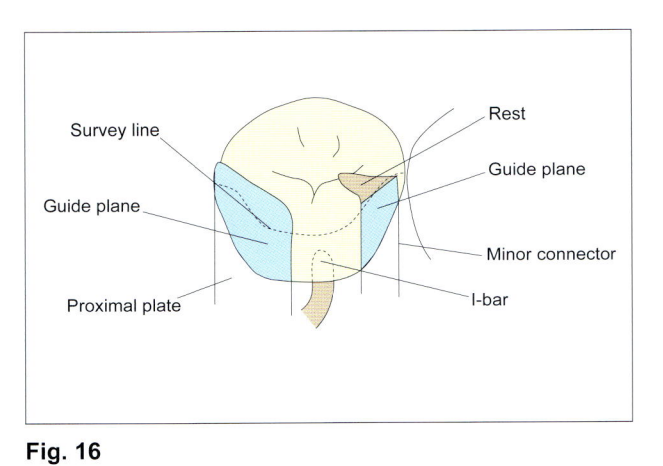

Fig. 16
RPPI clasp, which aligns the wide minor connector with a mesial rest and proximal plate parallel to each other to make contact with the proximal tooth surface.

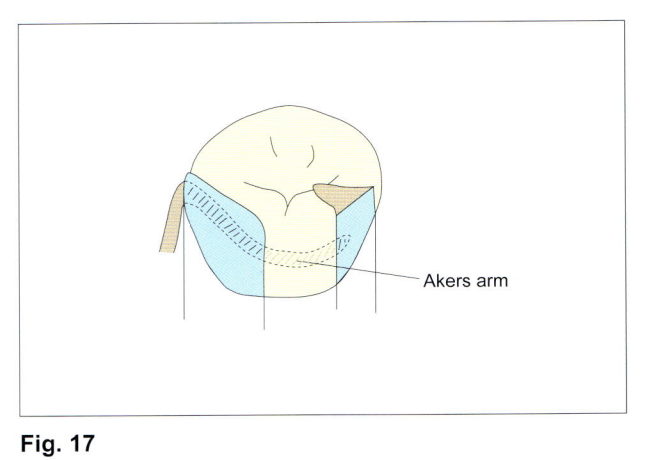

Fig. 17
RPPA clasp, which replaced an I-bar, one component of a RPPI clasp with an Akers arm.

2. Precision attachments

1) Dalbo 667

The Dalbo 667 system consists of a female part, a coil spring, and an L-shaped male part with a ball placed at the base. The male part placed on the missing side of the abutment tooth can be combined frictionally to the female part with a coil spring placed in the denture base. This is a stress-breaking extracoronal attachment which can move only vertically through a coil spring placed in the female part (Fig. 18).

The connecting rigidity between this attachment and the abutment tooth becomes reduced and the denture mobility increases due to the stress-breaking action. Because the ball male part is placed extracoronally, to prevent rotation of the abutment tooth, it is necessary to add

an abutment tooth for splinting of the abutment teeth. Because of this device is small and has weak bracing, retention tends to be enhanced, resulting an increase of removal force. In addition, the coil spring is subject to breakage due to an increase in denture mobility.

A broken coil spring can be replaced with a new one, but a broken interlocking section is not possible to repair.

2) Mini Dalbo

The Mini Dalbo system consists of a female part and an L-shaped male part with a ball placed at the base. The male part placed on the missing side of the abutment tooth can be combined frictionally to the female part without a coil spring placed in the denture base. This

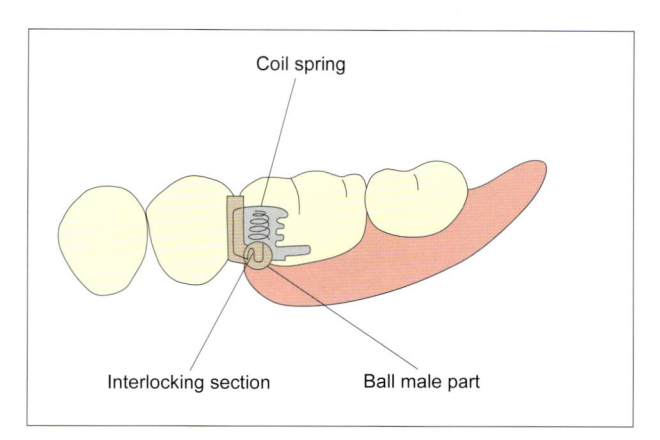

Fig. 18
Dalbo 667, which is a stress-breaking attachment that allows only a vertical movement.

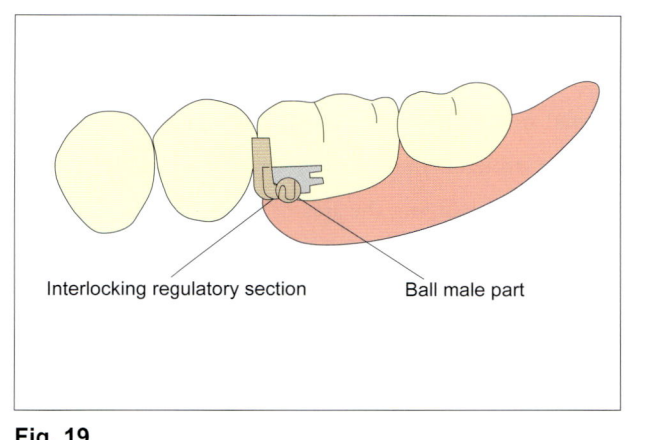

Fig. 19
Mini Dalbo, which is a stress-breaking attachment that allows only a hinge movement.

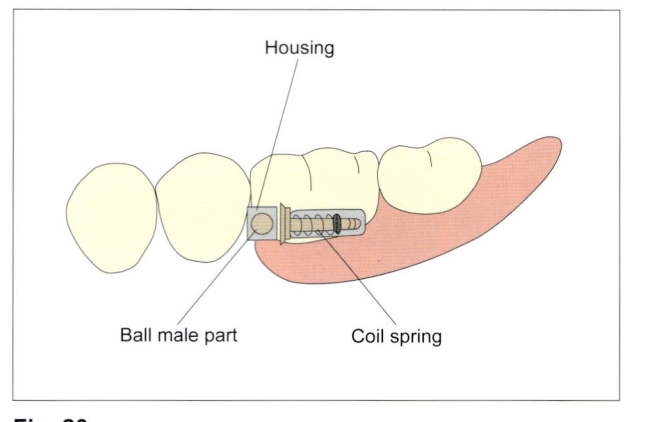

Fig. 20
ASC 52, which is a free movable stress-breaking attachment.

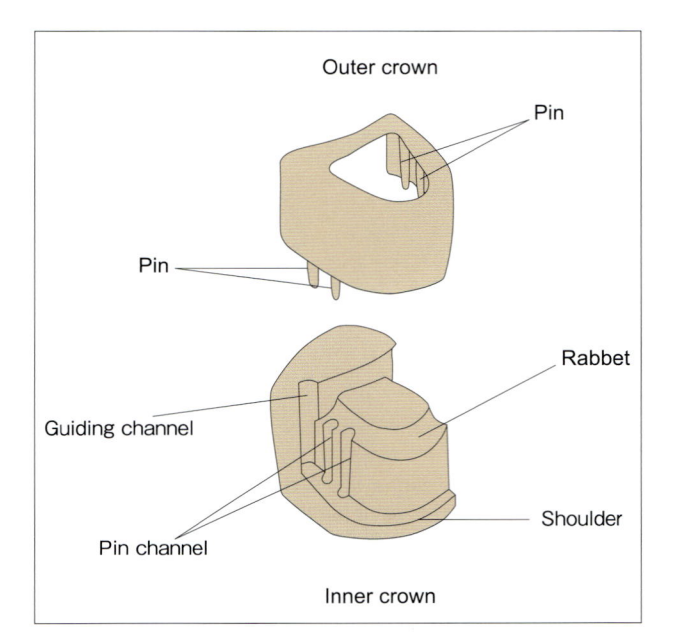

Fig. 21
CSP attachment, which can obtain retention through inserting the pins prepared on the inner surface on the outer crown into the pin channels formed on the axial surface of the inner crown.

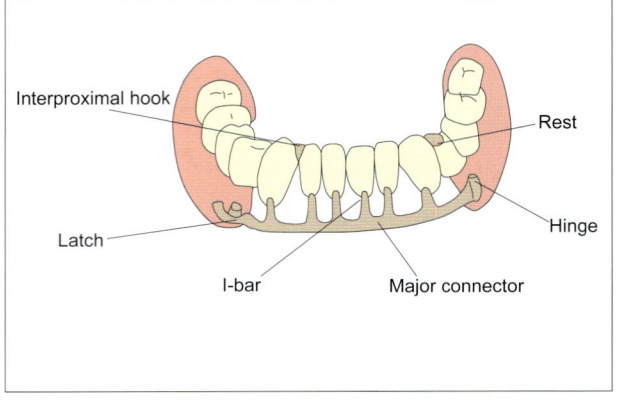

Fig. 22
Swing-lock attachment, which contacts the I-bars jointed to a major connector with labio-buccal rotation within the undercut area below the survey line for latching it through pinching in the residual anterior teeth between the I-bars and the lingual base.

is a stress-breaking extracoronal attachment which allows only a hinge movement (Fig. 19).

Because of this device is small and has weak bracing, retention tends to be lost. Functional force on the denture rotates the abutment tooth since the ball male part is placed extracoronally. It is necessary to splint the abutment teeth. Since the functional force applied to the denture base is directly-transmitted to the ball male part, the interlocking section in the female part is not only broken frequently, but the male part may be also broken, which are fatal damages.

3) ASC52

The ASC 52 system is a stress breaking resilient joint

16

extracoronal attachment and the denture base can be easily inserted and removed without any risk for the abutment teeth. It allows for both vertical and hinge movements.

The ball male part with a coil spring placed in the denture base is inserted to the housing (female part) on the abutment tooth (Fig. 20).

It is necessary to connect and splint the abutment tooth with the adjacent tooth to prevent the abutment tooth from rotational movement because the ball male part is extracoronally placed. As denture mobility is higher due to weaker bracing, a coil spring is often broken.

4) CSP (Channel Shoulder Pin) system by A.Steiger

The CSP system designed by A.Steiger consists of an inner crown and outer crown. On the axial surface of inner crown, guiding channels, pin channels, shoulders, and rabbets are formed. On the outer crown, pins with separated end are prepared at the inner surface. The axial surface of the inner crown is parallel for strong retention, and the outer crown is retained auxilliary by parallel pins on its axial surface. The outer crown is inserted onto the inner crown guided the pins into the pin channels (Fig. 21).

The parallel axial surface and friction pins lead to higher connecting rigidity and stronger retention, thus exerting stronger tractive and lateral forces on the abutment tooth during denture removal. Therefore, this retainers should be used very carefully in distal extension dentures. The highest level of laboratory procedures and delicate adjustment of retention are required. The damaged pin is irreparable.

5) Swing-lock retainer

The retentive mechanism used in most partial dentures is friction, but alternatively, the swing-lock mechanism can be used. This attachment can secure retention by latching I-bars within the undercut area below the survey line. The minor connectors (I-bars) are jointed to a major connector with one end being a hinge and the other end being a latch to contact these I-bars with the labial mar-

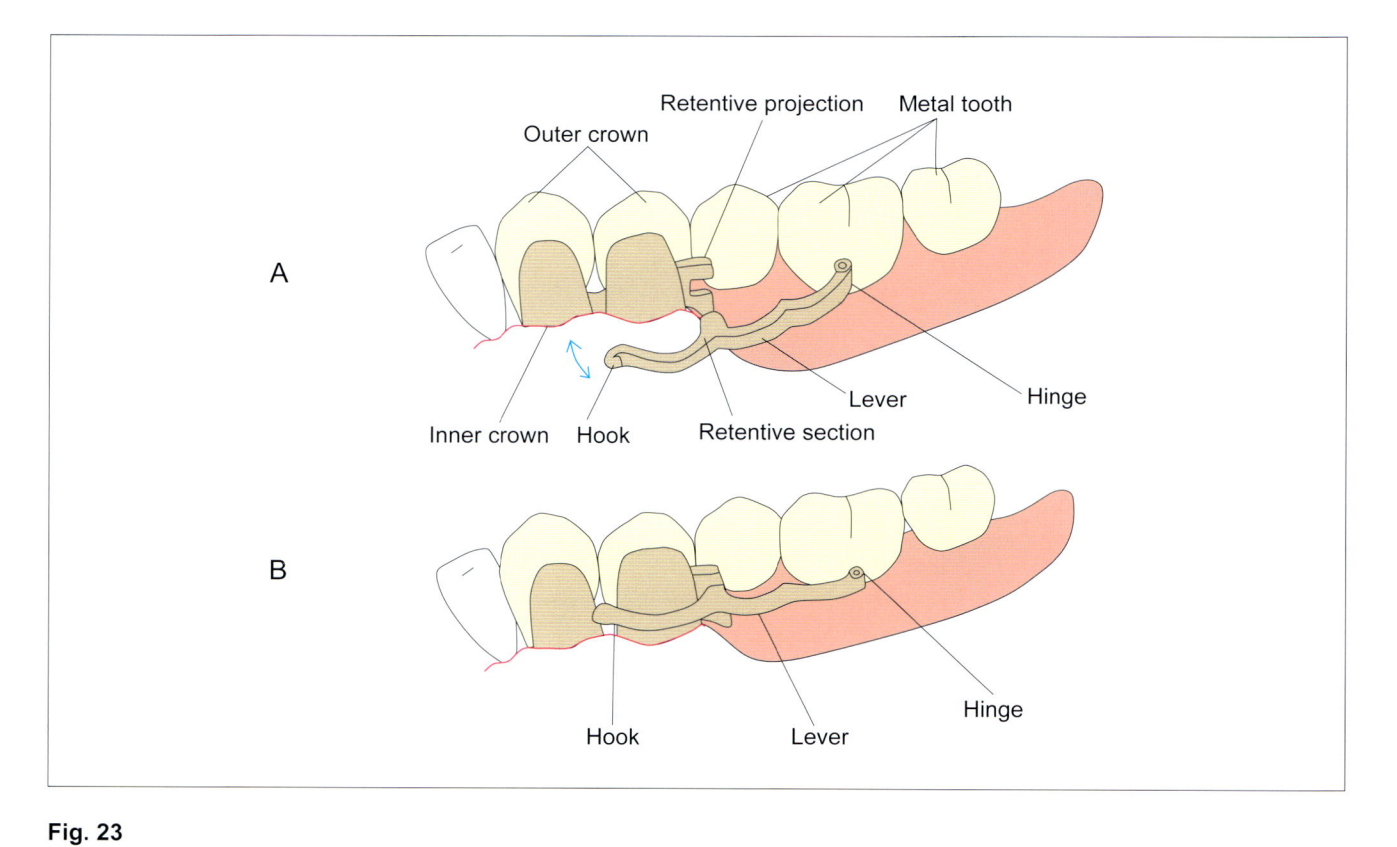

Fig. 23
Bolt attachment, which inserts a horizontally both opening and closing lever into a slot prepared on intracoronal surface of the abutment tooth or a retentive projection placed extracoronally for providing retention between the retainer and the denture base.
A: Lingual view with horizontal lever opened.
B: Lingual view with horizontal lever closed.

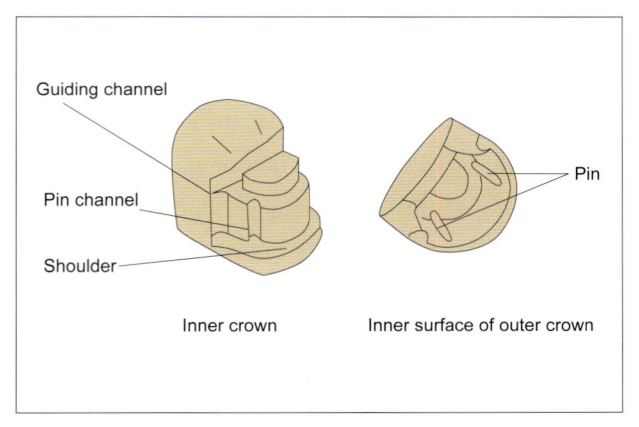

Fig. 24
Parallel telescopic crown by Böttger modified from the CSP system.

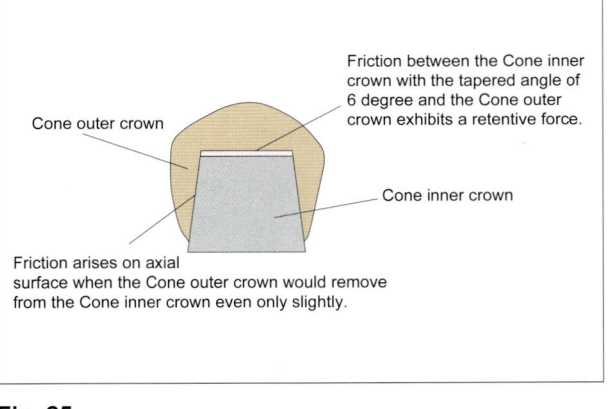

Fig. 25
Cone-crown telescopic system, with the tapered angle of Cone inner crown as 6 degree.
The relationship between the inner and outer crowns corresponds to that between a wedge and a hoop, so it is difficult to provide an adequate retentive force.

gin of the abutment teeth by turning the major connector; the mechanism of pinching in the residual anterior teeth between the I-bars and the lingual base labio-lingually (Fig. 22).

Therefore, this attachment has many advantages of allowing achievement of secure retention, reduction of the denture mobility, and less denture breakage. However, when using the swing-lock attachment in distal extension denture cases, because the position of rest and rest seat is far located posterior to the I-bar position, it presents a problem of tooth wear due to vibration of the I-bar through the lever action during denture function and also results an aesthetic disadvantage of exsisting many I-bars.

6) Bolt (Riegel) Precision retainer

In bolt attachment retained dentures, the latch mechanism locking the denture into place consists of a rotating lever or a rotating axis providing a retentive projection into a deep slot on the restoration with the abutment tooth. The application of bolt attachments includes both the vertical and horizontal methods. A horizontal bolt attachment is suitable for the people like Japanese with small teeth. This is the mechanism of inserting a horizontally-rotating lever into a slot prepared into a projection placed on the inner crown on the abutment tooth with a hinge as a fulcrum placed in the denture base for providing retention between the outer crown and the denture base (Fig. 23).

Thus, the use of a bolt attachment realizes no frictional retention between the abutment tooth and the retainer during denture insertion and removal, resulting in no tractive and lateral forces exerted on the abutment tooth. However, on the other hand, because the retentive lever is tightly-fitted into the slot, there is a major disadvantage that the functional force is transmitted directly to the denture to the abutment tooth. In addition, more complicated and advanced laboratory techniques are required for fabricating bolt dentures.

3. Telescopic crown

1) Parallel telescopic crown by H.Böttger

This is a telescopic crown developed the CSP system (Steiger). Laboratory procedures require highly complicated and advanced techniques (Fig. 24). The adjustment of retention is to be done through pin activation , but a slight bend of a pin causes a large change of the retention. If a pin breaks, it is impossible to repair in this retainer.

The formation of the parallel axial wall of the inner crown allows an increase in connecting rigidity, a limitation of the path of denture insertion and removal, and an increase in retention through pins, thus exerting significantly stronger tractive and lateral forces on the abutment tooth. Therefore, the indications are limited.

2) Cone-crown telescopic system (Konuskronen Teleskop by K.H.Körber)

The Cone-crown telescope is a retainer, which uses frictional forces derived from the wedge effect as retention (Fig. 25). The Cone-crown telescopic system has broader contact area between the Cone inner crown and the Cone outer crown, which acts so effective as to the support and bracing functions than any other retainers. Cone-crowns made by gold alloy exhibits the most stabilized bracing and retentive forces only when completely seated and when the tapered inner crown is 6 degrees, giving the greater connecting rigidity. However, an adequate bracing force between the Cone inner and outer crowns allows provision of the desirable retentive and removal forces, but even a slight increase in bracing force leads to an increase in retentive and removal forces.

In contrast, a decrease in bracing force leads to a decrease in retentive and removal forces, then consequently no denture retention will be gained.

Because it is very difficult to provide the accurate friction between the Cone inner and outer crowns, many problems, including an excessive interlocking force between the Cone inner and outer crowns, it happens so often such as difficult denture insertion and removal, and fall-out of the Cone inner crown (or with post core).

From the point of view of the dental laboratory, it is difficult to provide an adequate frictional force (retentive force, about 600 g) for Cone-crowns based on a difference in crown size, an error in the laboratory procedures, and the contact surface characteristics between the inner and outer crowns. Even if the accurate frictional force is provided, addition of retentive forces with an increase in the number of abutment teeth for Cone-crowns leads to a further increase in removal force of the denture.

The Cone-crown telescopic system with the greater connecting rigidity allows a reduction in denture mobility. However, if the abutment tooth is subject to functional force beyond physiological tooth mobility from the denture base, the large lateral force is exerted on it and consequently fracture or mobility of the abutment tooth due to occlusal trauma occurs. The Cone-crown telescopic system is contraindicated to the short-span distal extension denture base.

However, even in the long-span denture base, the use of this telescopic system involves taking risks in such cases with an abutment tooth of its physiological mobility lower than average, and poor alveolar ridge mucosa in the missing area.

Summary

In retainers utilizing friction, the retentive and bracing mechanisms may overlap to each other. Therefore reinforcing of bracing force also leads to frictional force only in a given direction, but retentive force can be decreased. However, this result is that the stronger tractive and lateral forces will be exerted on the abutment tooth for detecting the path of denture removal by limiting the path of denture insertion and removal. As the number of abutment teeth increased, this tendency becomes stronger. Also, because retainers with weak bracing increase denture mobility, an increase in retentive force for decreasing this mobility leads to an increase in removal force. Thus, an increase in bracing and retentive forces in retainers, of course, leads to a further increase in removal force.

Like this, in bracing and retentive mechanisms, retainers with friction extreamlly affects to bracing and retentive forces. Therefore, the retentive mechanism is requested to provide retentive and removal forces as zero or near zero without the influence to the bracing mechanism. Thus, the method based on the mechanical retention of locking based on the latch principle like swing-lock and bolt attachments can be desirable.

Conical-shaped commodities around us

Many of the conical-shaped commodities are observed around us. Among them, the first thing come into mind are flowerpots and cups. Even if flowerpots are stacked, they can easily be separated. This is because the frictional force between flowerpots is reduced through increasing the flange width, raising the bottom or increasing the rim of the bottom to prevent flowerpots from being unseparated to an excessive frictional force. In cups, friction between cups is reduced through step formation on the wall surface in the same manner (**Fig. 26**).

The relationship between the Cone inner and outer crowns corresponds to that between a wedge and a hoop; the Cone inner crown acts as a wedge to the Cone outer crown and the Cone outer crown as a hoop to the Cone inner crown, thus it may be difficult to separate the Cone outer crown from the Cone inner crown due to excessive friction (**Fig. 27**). This seems to more commonly occur also in the mechanical engineering field.

To prevent it, it is necessary to finish the Cone-crown telescope with the interlocking relationship between the Cone inner and outer crowns just before the wedge or hoop effect acts on them, but the laboratory procedures are difficult to get to that state.

Fig. 26 Conical-shaped flowerpots and metal cups

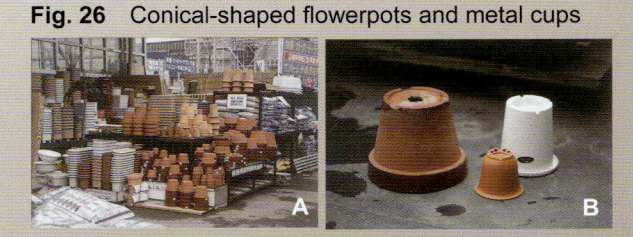

A: Flowerpots which are stacked on sale can easily be separated.
B: A frictional force is reduced through increasing the flange width, raising the bottom or increasing the rim of the bottom to prevent flowerpots from being unseparated due to significant friction.

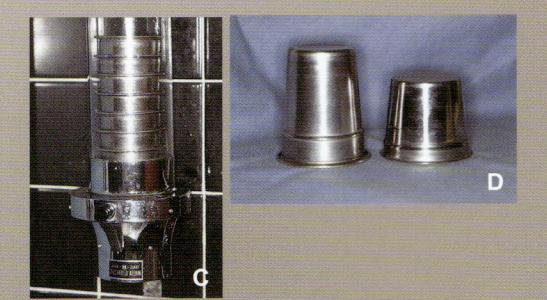

C: Stacked cups can also be separated easily.
D: Steps are formed on the wall surface to reduce friction between cups.

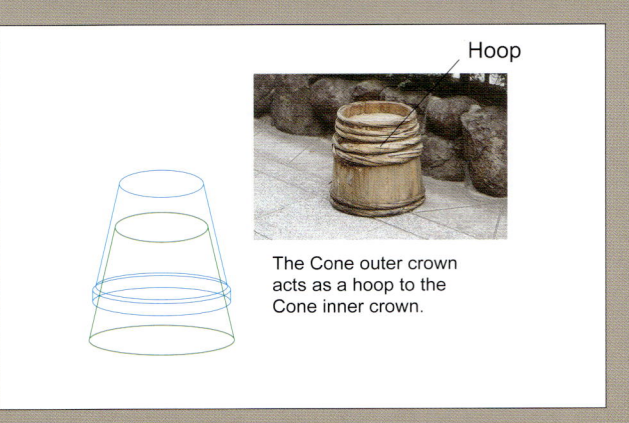

Wedge

The Cone inner crown acts as a wedge to the Cone outer crown.

Hoop

The Cone outer crown acts as a hoop to the Cone inner crown.

Fig. 27 Relationship between the Cone inner and outer crowns.

Chapter 3

Superiority of the retentive mechanism with Bolt (Riegel) Attachment

Most retentive mechanisms for retainers used in partial dentures are based on the undercut retention utilizing the area below the survey line or in a retentive projection placed on the abutment tooth. There are two methods to utilize the undercut area for retention: One method is to use the frictional forces, and the other is the latch principle of locking (**Fig. 1**). However, because the retentive mechanism for retainers to provide retention by friction overlapping the abutment for bracing mechanism at the same time, the connecting rigidity and the bracing strength result in exerting an effect on retentive and removal forces. Therefore, an independent retentive mechanism without exerting this damaging effect is required. For this purpose, the retentive method with locking principle with latch mechanism seems as most suitable.

Retainers utilizing the retentive method of locking include swing-lock system and bolt attachments. In swing-lock dentures, the I-bars act as not only locking function but also bracing function, resulting in tooth wear on the labiobuccal surface due to vibration of I-bars and less aesthetics with many I-bars (**Fig. 2**). Also, bolt dentures, in which latching a lever is tightly-fitted into a slot prepared into a retentive projection, have a serious disadvantage, causing damage to the abutment tooth particularly in distal extension dentures since the functional forces applied to the denture base is directly-transmitted to it (**Fig. 3**).

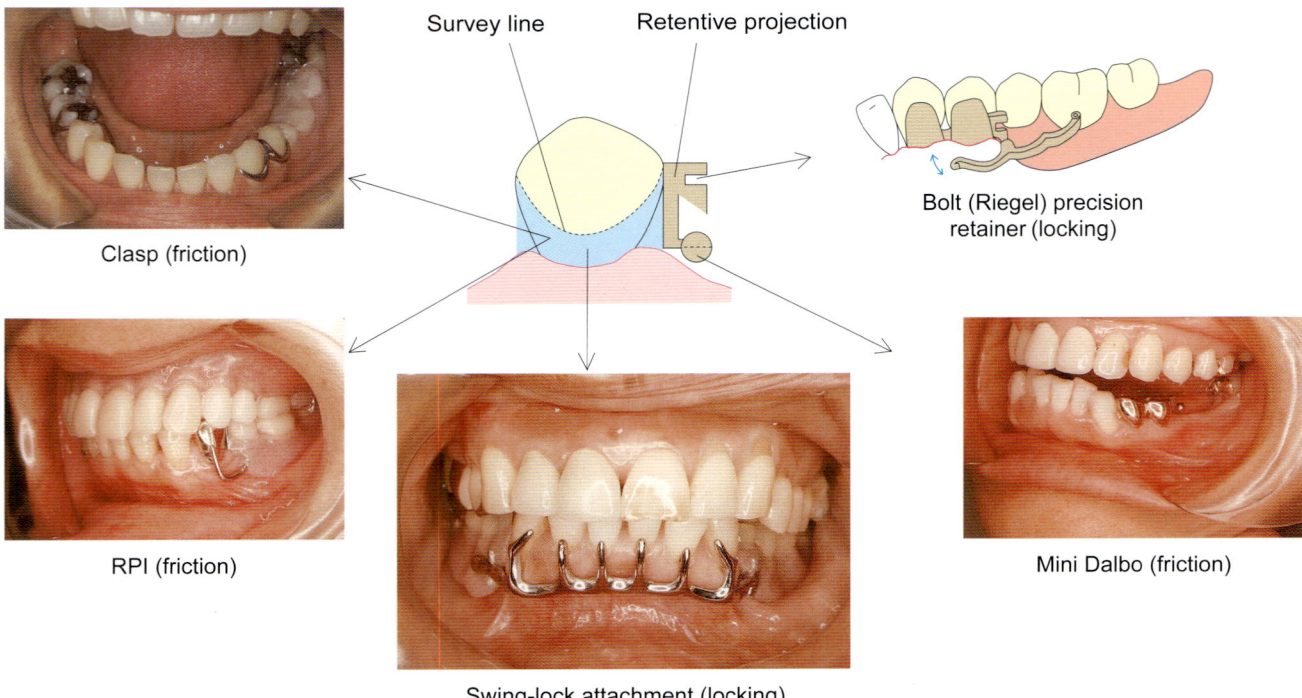

Clasp (friction)

Survey line   Retentive projection

Bolt (Riegel) precision retainer (locking)

RPI (friction)

Swing-lock attachment (locking)

Mini Dalbo (friction)

Fig. 1
Most retainers used in the partial dentures obtain their retentive mechanism through friction or locking based on the latch principle, utilizing the undercut area below the survey line or in a retentive projection placed on the abutment tooth.

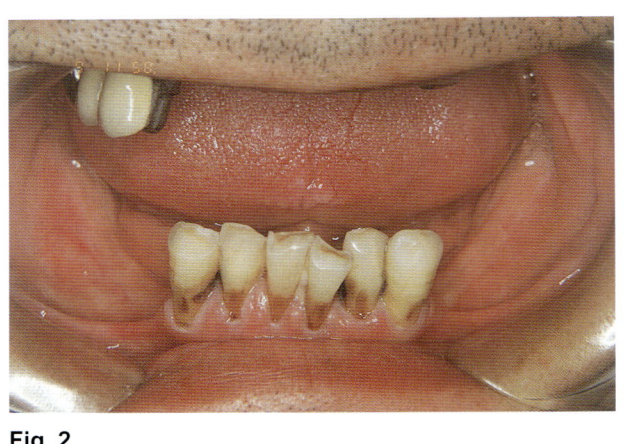

Fig. 2
Teeth wear on the labial surfaces of the mandibular anteriors of the patient treated with a swing-lock partial denture.

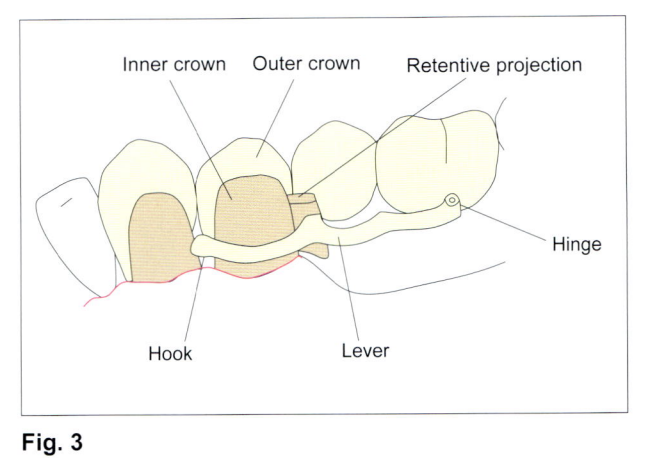

Fig. 3
Since the lever of the bolt precision retainer is tightly-fitted into a slot prepared in the retentive projection, the functional force applied to the denture base are directly transmitted to the abutment tooth.

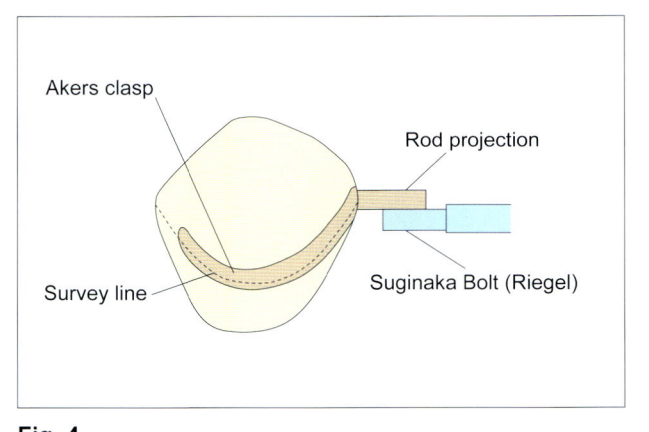

Fig. 4
Advantage for incorporating the bolt retentive mechanism into an Akers clasp.
As the clasp arm acts as only bracing function through placing the clasp tip on the survey line, there is no need to use the lingual arm as the reciprocal arm. bolt retentive mechanism is not affected by the bracing and supporting mechanism.

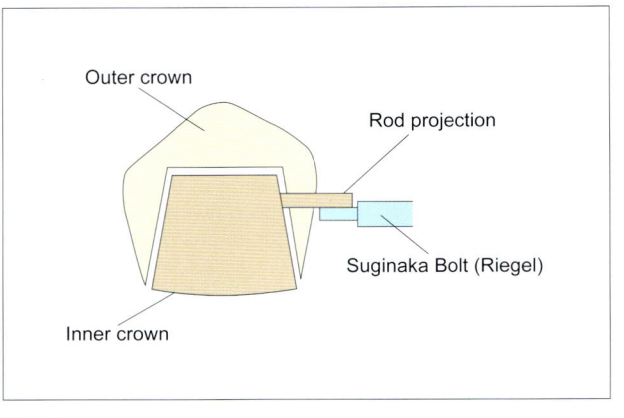

Fig. 5
Advantage for incorporating the bolt retentive mechanism into the Cone-crown telescopic system.
In a Cone-crown-type double crown fitted loosely between the inner and outer crowns, the ceiling of the inner crown can be made as bulky with the inner surface of the outer crown and no frictional force is exerted on the axial surface of the inner crown. By incorporating the bolt retentive mechanism into it, various troubles in practice can be solved.

So, during denture sinking, the retentive section of the bolt attachment is separated from a retentive projection, thus resulting in the separation of mucosal surface from the denture base, no functional force is applied to the denture base without transmitting to the abutment tooth. In addition, both in function and rest, secure denture retention can also be obtained through the latch effect and the denture insertion or removal from the mouth can be done simply by opening or closing the lever. Then no retentive and removal forces derived from the frictional force, are exerted on the abutment tooth. In other words, disadvantages of the retentive mechanism for each retainer can be eliminated converting the retentive mechanism to the bolt retentive mechanism.

23

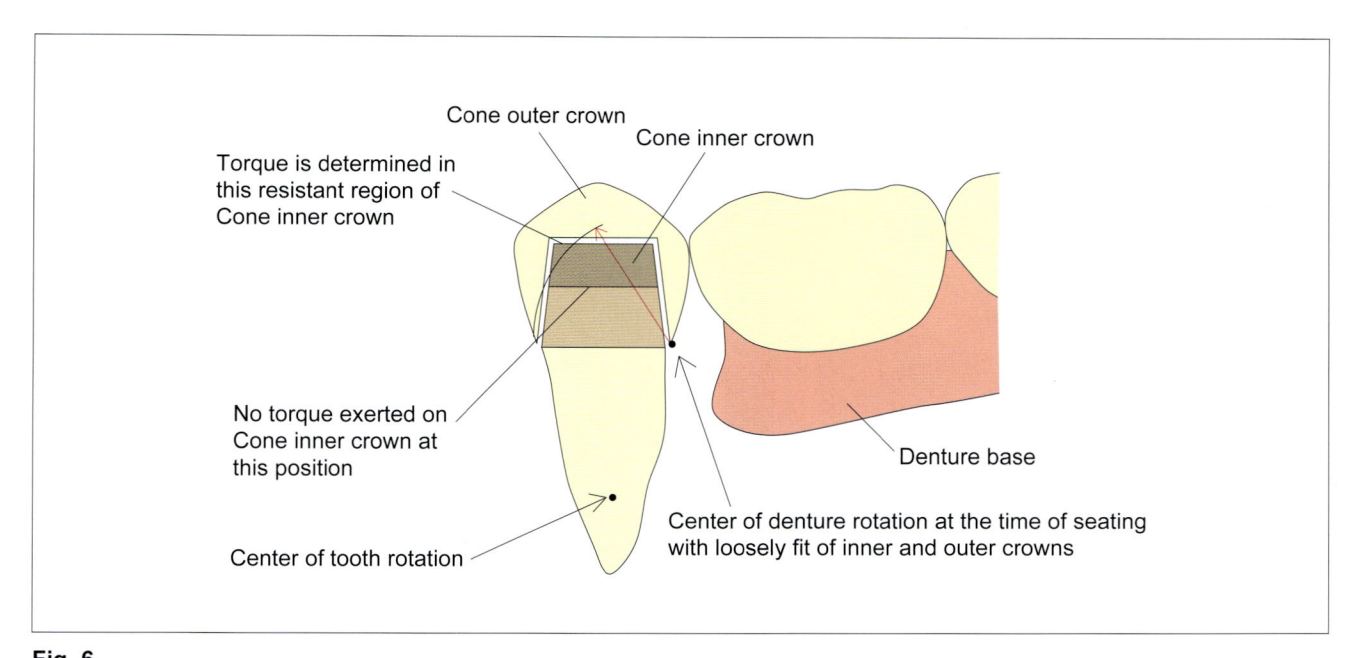

Cone outer crown

Cone inner crown

Torque is determined in this resistant region of Cone inner crown

No torque exerted on Cone inner crown at this position

Center of tooth rotation

Denture base

Center of denture rotation at the time of seating with loosely fit of inner and outer crowns

Fig. 6
In the Cone-crown telescopic retainer in distal extension removable partial denture, while the denture base is sunk by occlusal force, rotational force is applied to the abutment tooth. Although the center of the tooth rotation is located in the root region of the abutment tooth at first, once an acceptable range of physiological mobility is exceeded, the center of rotation will shift to the cervical region of the outer crown adjacent to the edentulous area, and thus a torque is thought to be exerted on the inner crown. While shortening of the Cone inner crown in length might lead to a decrease in torque, it becomes difficult to obtain adequate retention between the inner and outer crowns. So, incorporation of the bolt retentive mechanism into Cone-telescopic-crown distal extension dentures allows achievement of secure retention even any changes in bracing.

C O L U M N

What is "Bolt (Riegel) ?"

The term "Bolt" means "Riegel" in German and the reason why it is used as a retentive device is based on its latch principle. The bolt dental prosthesis has developed around Germany and is delicate enough to be included as an assignment also in a dental technician master certification exams in Germany.

To fabricate a bolt precision retainer, as highly-accurate laboratory techniques with such as milling machine technique, you could also just say "bolt," the bolt prosthesis refers to a bolt precision retainer (**Fig. 7**).

Riegel ⎯ ⌈ Riegel or Riegelprothese in German
⎯ Bolt attachment in English
⎣ Riegel or Riegel attachment in Japanese

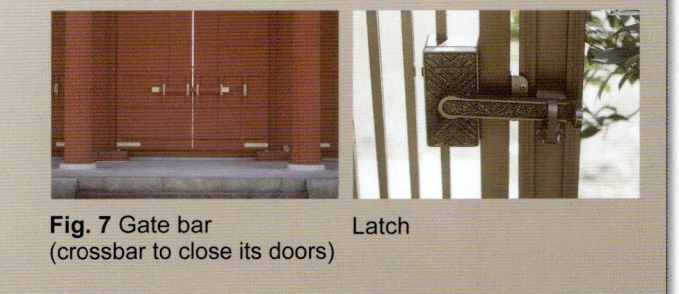

Fig. 7 Gate bar (crossbar to close its doors)   Latch

Chapter 4

Suginaka Bolt (Riegel) Attachment can simplify the dental prosthetic laboratory procedure

Among the components of Removable Partial Dentures (RPD's), retainers play the most important role in producing the stability and the function of dentures. Therefore, it can say that the choice of retainer dictates over them without exaggeration.

Laboratory procedures of retainers lies also from the range of simple one to the elaborated one.

Above all, because the laboratory procedures of bolt precision retainers not only require high technological skills and time but also high treatment cost, they have been little used in general practice. The most difficult process in the laboratory procedures of bolt prosthesis is to fabricate a smooth-rotating lever section. Thus, the author of this book considered that if a smoothly-rotating lever kit prefablicated is placed in the denture base, the laboratory work could be so easy to be done, so the author developed the Suginaka bolt system (Fig. 1). This might lead a greater ease in laboratory procedures and a decrease in cost, resulting in extending the range of application of bolt attachments.

The Suginaka Bolt made of Au-Pt alloy (ADA Type IV Gold Aloy) consists of a housing, in which a 0.8 mm-thick L-shaped lever with a rotation axis at its one end and a hook for opening or closing at the other end capable to rotate within the range of 20° with its hook exposed (Fig. 2 and 3). The retentive section (angle region) serves the retentive function of locking. However, because the 1.7 mm wide lever lacks slightly in retention, its width is increased up to 2.0 mm. The lever with the retentive section is designed to fit in the housing (Fig. 4).

The protruding knobs of the housing near the rotating axis act as retention for embedding and fixing the Suginaka bolt device in the denture base plastic without soldering.

In addition, a wing-shaped hook can prevent poor tongue sensation due to a groove-like depression on the denture polished surface during opening/closing of a lever (Fig. 5).

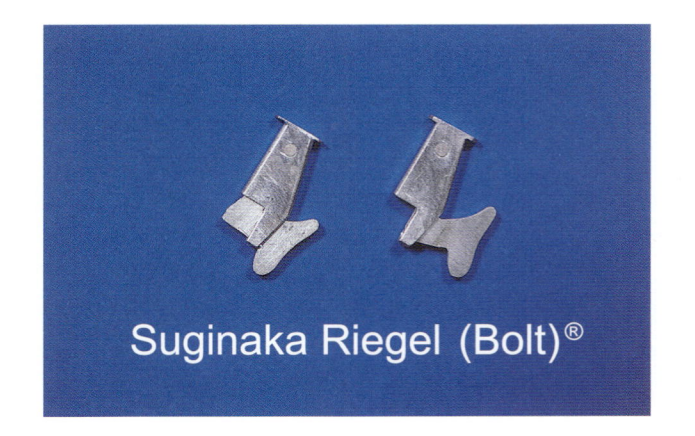

Fig. 1
Suginaka Riegel (Bolt)® (In 2014, the company's name was changed to DENKEN-HIGHDENTAL Co., Ltd.)

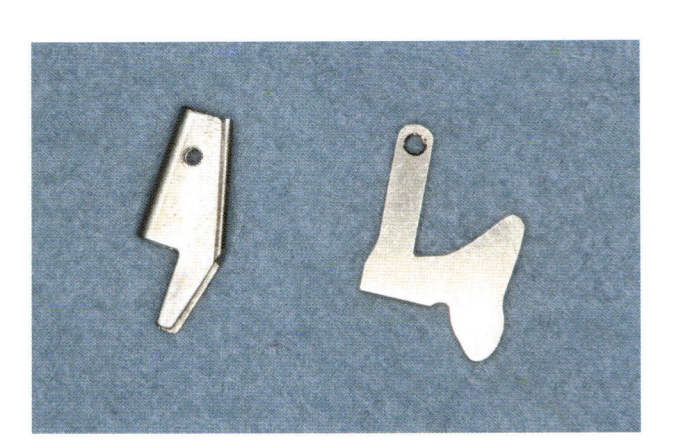

Fig. 2
Dismounted Suginaka Riegel (Bolt)®

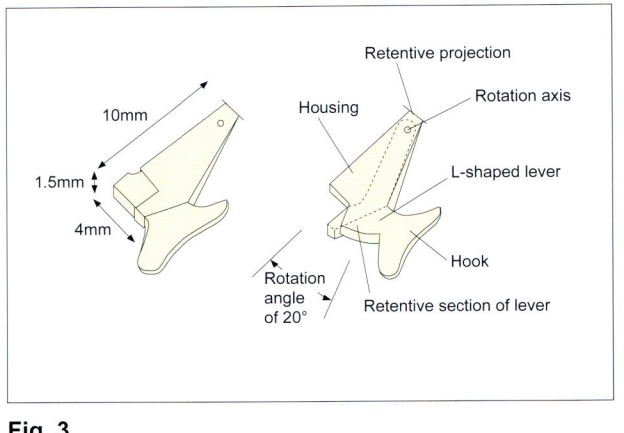

Fig. 3
Dimensions and structure of Suginaka Riegel (Bolt)®

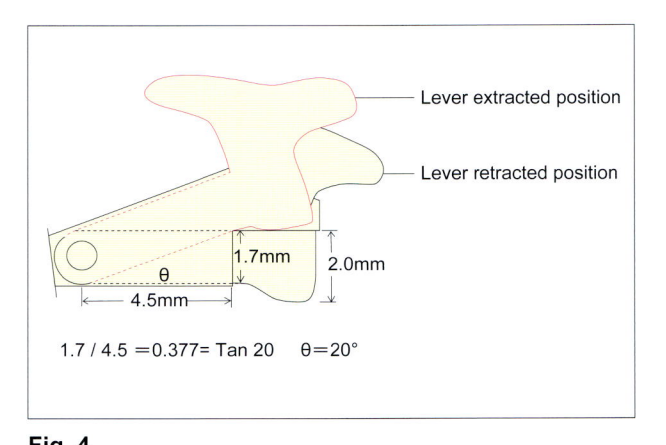

1.7 / 4.5 ＝0.377＝ Tan 20 θ＝20°

Fig. 4
Figure of retentive section of Suginaka Riegel (Bolt) ® and rotation angle of lever.

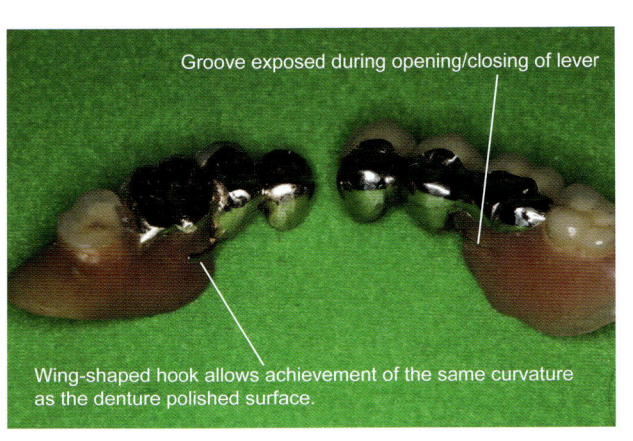

Fig. 5   Hook, reacts well to the tongue sensation
Wing-shaped hook preventing poor tongue sensation owing to a groove-like depression on the denture polished surface during opening/closing of a lever.

C O L U M N

In fact, "Inoue attachment" was a bolt attachment.

The author of this book had used previously "Inoue attachment" for providing the latch retentive mechanism to Cone-crown-type double crowns fitted loosely between the outer and inner crowns till the author designed the Suginaka bolt system (**Fig. 6**).

The Inoue attachment designed about 80 years ago seems out of production recently. This attachment resembles a bolt-type lock in general architecture with its form (**Fig. 7**).

The Inoue attachment is categorized to the hinge type, but the function is exactly the same as that of bolt attachment. In Germany, the bolt system was designed about in 1925 and the bolt attachment was born as the Inoue attachment around the same time also in Japan.

However, although this Inoue attachment can be used as an alternative to the bolt attachment, it has disadvantages of frequent falling off of a retentive pin, with too large in width, and aesthetic problems. Therefore, the need for designing a new bolt retainer was expected . This was one of the reasons for developping the Suginaka bolt system.

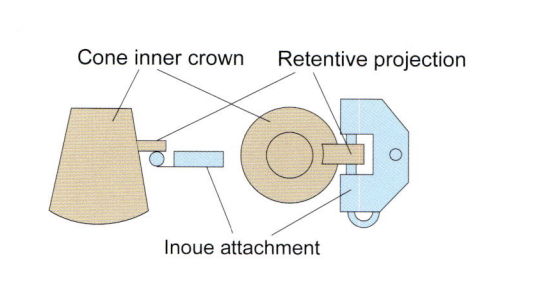

Cone inner crown   Retentive projection

Inoue attachment

Fig. 6
Telescopic denture, in which "Inoue attachment" is incorporated with a Cone-telescopic crown.

A: How to incorporate "Inoue attachment" into Cone-telescopic crown
A retentive plate projection is placed on the Cone inner crown, to which a pin of the Inoue attachment is locked and embedded in the denture base.

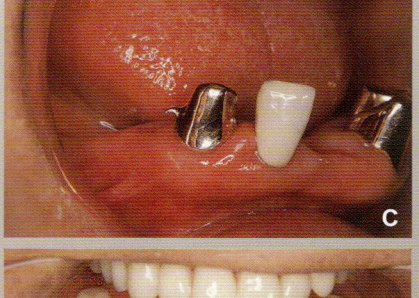

B: Inner crowns on the abutment teeth #43 and #33, #34, #35.

C: Retentive projection placed on the distal surface of the Cone inner crown on #43.

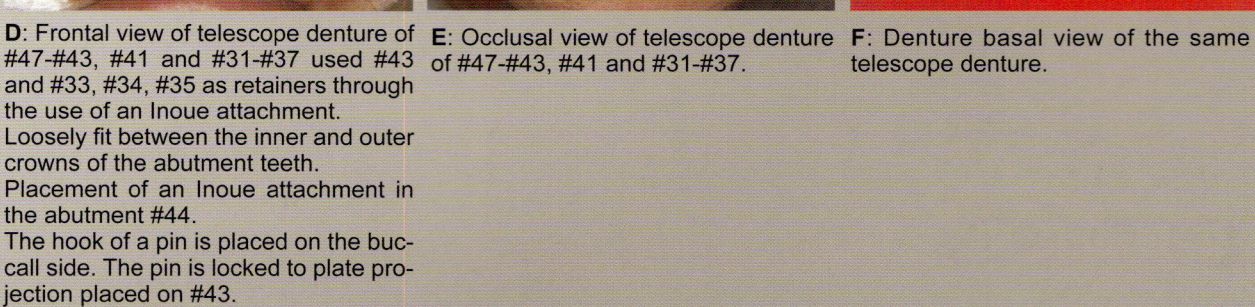

D: Frontal view of telescope denture of #47-#43, #41 and #31-#37 used #43 and #33, #34, #35 as retainers through the use of an Inoue attachment.
Loosely fit between the inner and outer crowns of the abutment teeth.
Placement of an Inoue attachment in the abutment #44.
The hook of a pin is placed on the buccall side. The pin is locked to plate projection placed on #43.

E: Occlusal view of telescope denture of #47-#43, #41 and #31-#37.

F: Denture basal view of the same telescope denture.

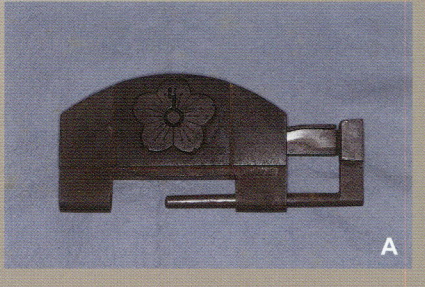
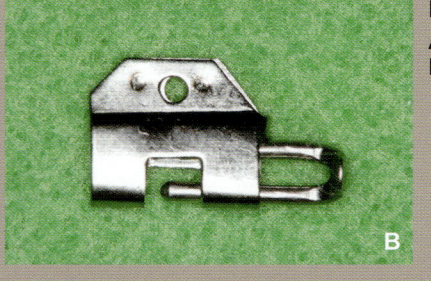

Fig. 7
A: Bolt-type lock
B: Inoue attachment

Chapter 5

Suginaka Bolt (Riegel) retainers

There are Two ways to realize the retention of locking; one is to use a retentive projection attached to the proximal surface adjacent to the edentulous area as a retainer, the other one is to use the undercut below the survey line of an abutment tooth. The Suginaka bolt system can be applied in these two ways.

There are two ways in use of the Suginaka bolt attachment; one is the attachment denture type incorporating it into clasps or Cone telescopic crowns, using a retentive projection attached to the proximal surface area adjacent to the edentulous area of a retainer, the other way is the lock denture type using a deep undercut area below the survey line on an abutment tooth (Fig. 1).

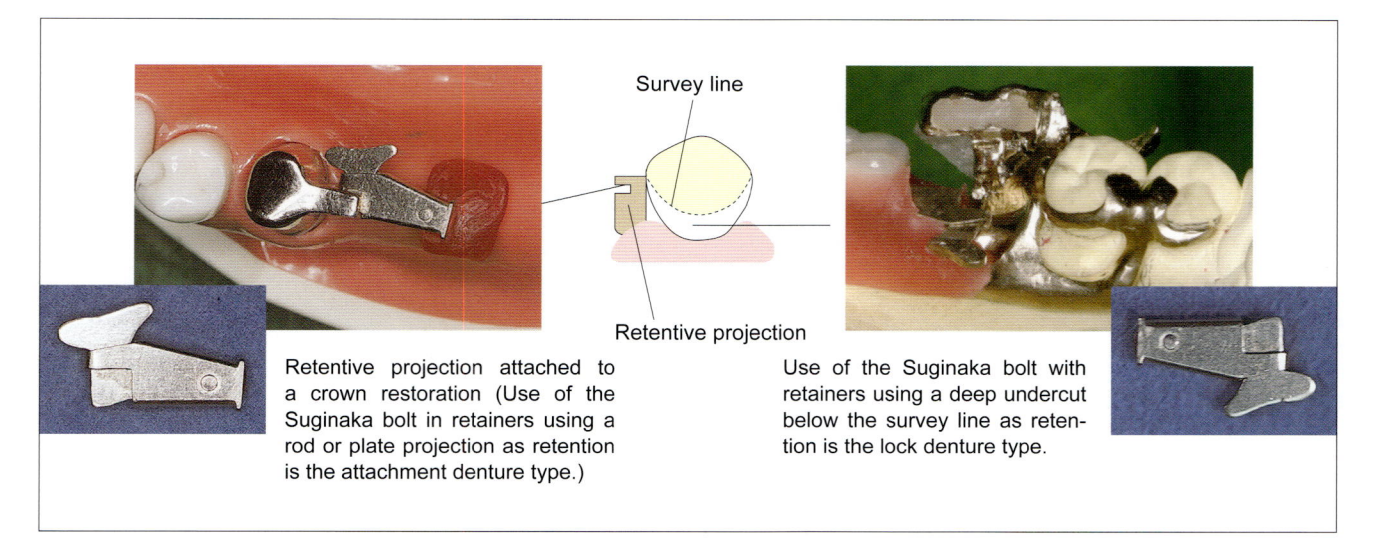

Survey line

Retentive projection

Retentive projection attached to a crown restoration (Use of the Suginaka bolt in retainers using a rod or plate projection as retention is the attachment denture type.)

Use of the Suginaka bolt with retainers using a deep undercut below the survey line as retention is the lock denture type.

Fig. 1 Two-type of Suginaka Bolt (Riegel)

1. Attachment denture type

To use the Suginaka bolt as an attachment, a retentive projection (rod or plate projection) should be attached to the proximal surface adjacent to the edentulous area of a retainer.

The Suginaka bolt can be applied to almost restorations used in clinical practice, including class 2 inlays, MOD inlays, 3/4 crowns, 4/5 crowns, full metal crowns, resin-facing crowns, metal ceramic crowns, CSC (Crown and Sleeve-coping) crowns, and double crowns (partial double crowns and Cone-crown-type double crowns fitted loosely between inner and outer crowns). A rod or plate projection can be attached to the proximal surface adjacent to the edentulous area of these restorations (Fig. 2). Particularly, because in class 2 inlays are easy to detach due to poor retention, it is necessary to prepare retentive pinholes (Fig. 3).

For a rod projection, the retentive section of the Suginaka bolt is brought into contact with the lower edge of a

Fig. 2 A retentive projection attached to crown restorations
A: Rod projection

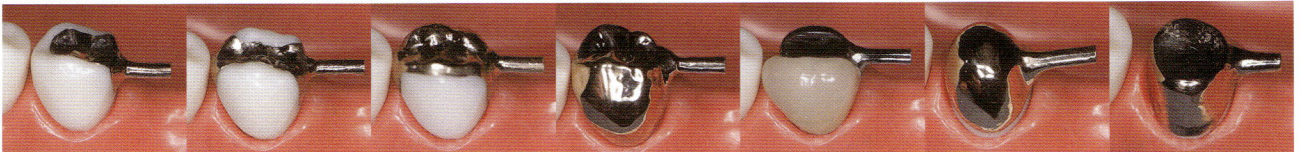

| Class 2 inlay | MOD inlay | 4/5 crown | Full metal crown | Resin facing crown or metal ceramic crown | CSC inner crown | Cone-crown-type inner crown |

B: Plate projection

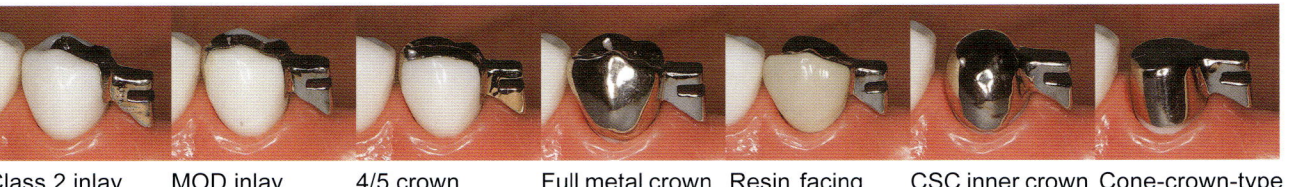

| Class 2 inlay | MOD inlay | 4/5 crown | Full metal crown | Resin facing crown or metal ceramic crown | CSC inner crown | Cone-crown-type inner crown |

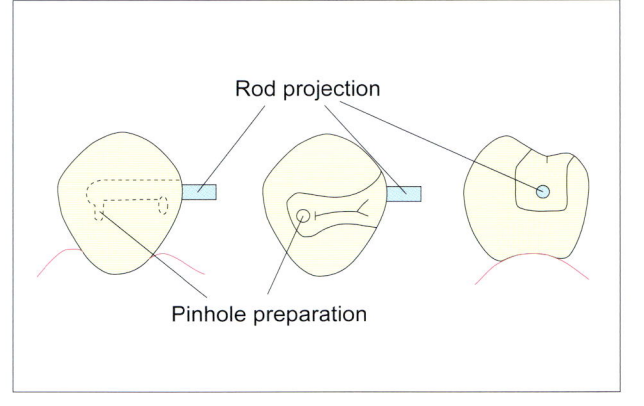

Rod projection

Pinhole preparation

Fig. 3
In class 2 inlays, it is necessary to prepare retentive pinholes for preventing their fall-out.

1.2-mm diameter rod projection (**Fig. 4**).

For a plate projection, a slit is prepared into a 1.5 mm thick projection for locking the retentive section of the Suginaka bolt, with the upper edge of which the retentive section of the Suginaka bolt is brought into contact (**Fig. 5**).

A space should always be left between the lower edge of the slit to prevent contact with each other in expectation of sinking of a denture base (**Fig. 6**).

In both projections, an important point of designing is to maintain a space of 0.5 mm between the retentive projection and the denture basal surface in order to prevent the occlusal/removal force applied to the rod/plate projection from transmitting directly to the abutment tooth. However, in the distal extension denture base in short span or the ridge mucosa with a poor condition, there is a need to maintain a space of 1.0 mm between the upper edge of the projection and the denture basal surface because of an increase in the accelerated sinking

of denture base,.

The position of a rod/plate projection to a retainer is as follows:

From above,

1) The thickness of a metal tooth should be over 1.5 mm,

2) A space of 0.5-1.0 mm between the basal surface of a metal tooth and the upper edge of a rod projection allows for preventing contact with one another during function .

3) A thick projection of 1.2 mm should be secured.

In the lower area, the 1.5 mm thick Suginaka bolt has to be housed within the denture base (**Fig. 7**).

With a rod projection, it needs only to bring the retentive section of the Suginaka bolt into contact with it. Also, the hook, which has a vertical/horizontal high degree of freedom, facilitates its placement in position (**Fig. 8**). Since a preformed slit prepared into plate projection, determining the opening/closing direction of the hook, attention must be given to positioning of the slit during

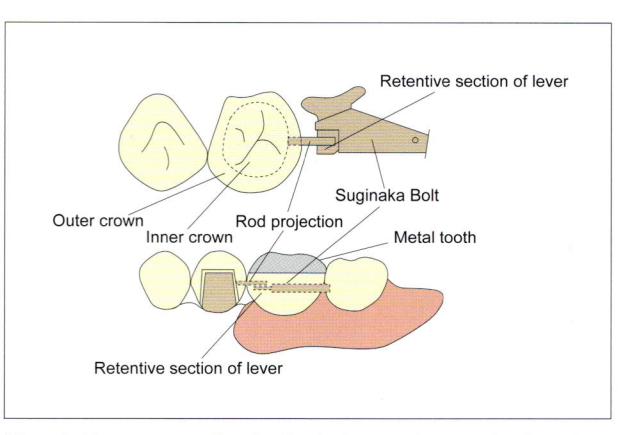

Fig. 4 How to use Suginaka bolt attachment (rod projection)

A rod projection of 1.2 mm in diameter is attached to the proximal surface adjacent to the edentulous area of a retainer (the figure shows Cone-crown-type inner crown), with the lower edge where the retentive section of the Suginaka bolt is brought into contact locating at the interdental space for covering by a metal tooth.

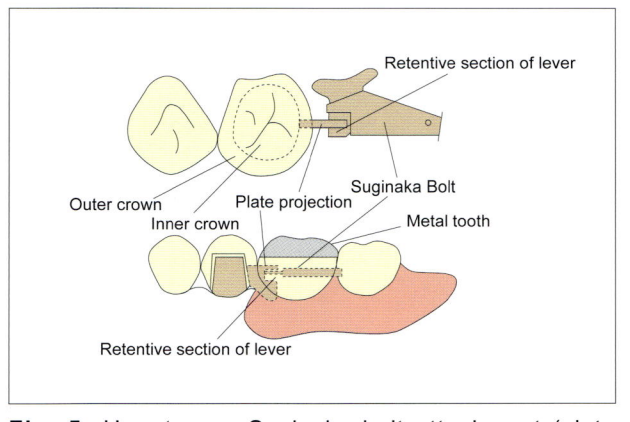

Fig. 5 How to use Suginaka bolt attachment (plate projection)

A plate projection of 1.5 mm in thickness is attached to the proximal surface adjacent to the edentulous area of a retainer (the figure shows Cone-crown-type inner crown), into which a slit is prepared.
The retentive section of the Suginaka bolt is brought into contact with the upper edge of the slit so that its hook is located at the interdental space for covering with a metal tooth.

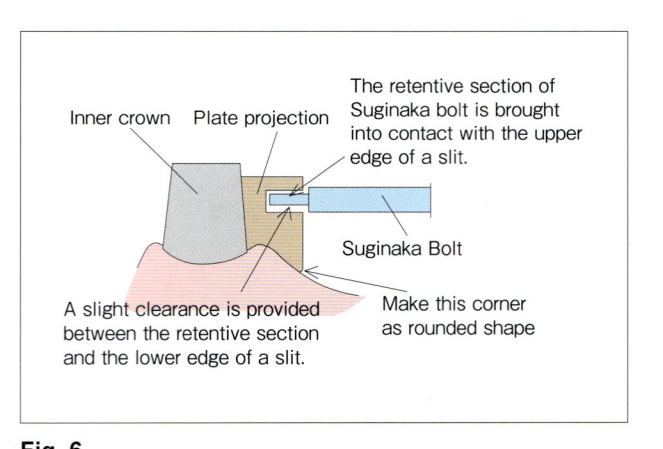

Fig. 6
Attention in use of plate projection.

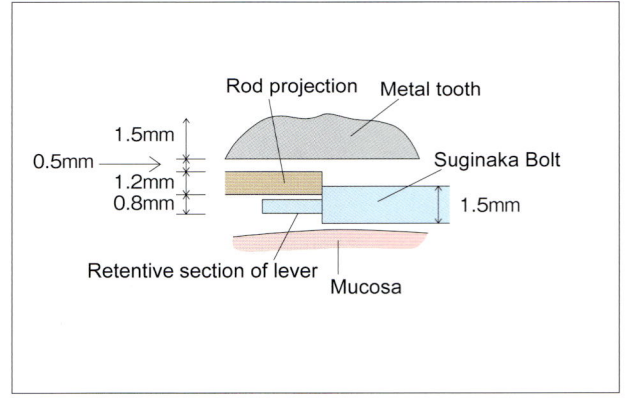

Fig. 7
Minimum occlusal vertical dimension needed to apply the Suginaka bolt.

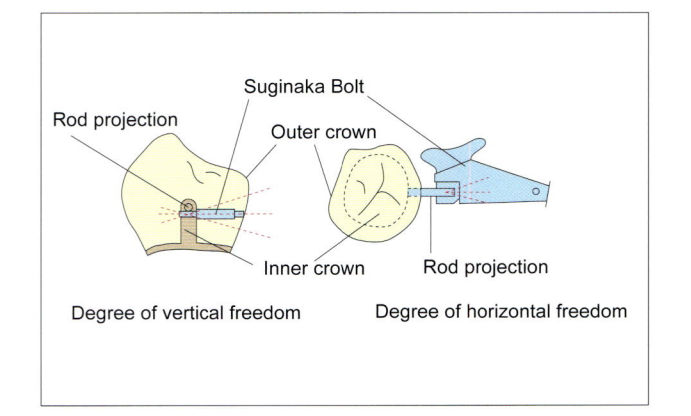

Fig. 8
Rod projection, which has a high degree of freedom in vertical/horizontal direction.

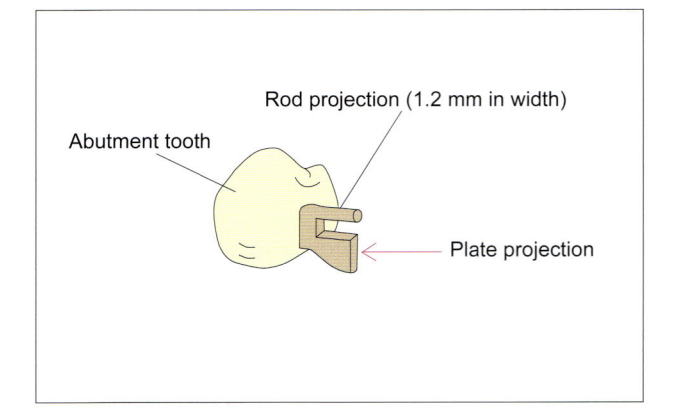

Fig. 9
Preventing a dead space emerging under the rod projection.

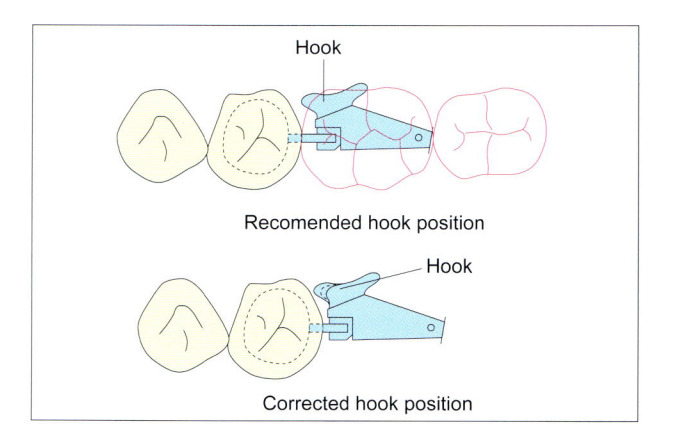

Recomended hook position

Corrected hook position

Fig. 10 Hook position in occlusal view
Although the edge of the hook should commonly be located at the interdental space, its edge can be corrected for ease of removal with patient's nail.

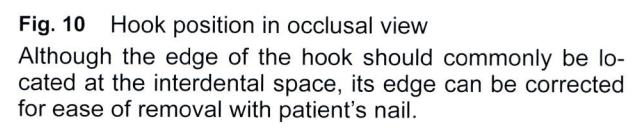

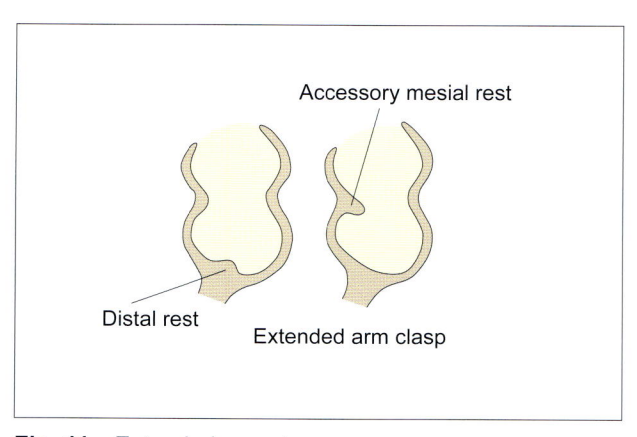

Fig. 11 Extended arm clasp
In short distal extension denture, or poor ridge mucosa, an accessary mesial rest is placed as shown in the right diagram rather than a distal rest in the left and the clasp arm should be placed on the survey line on the abutment near the edentulous area.

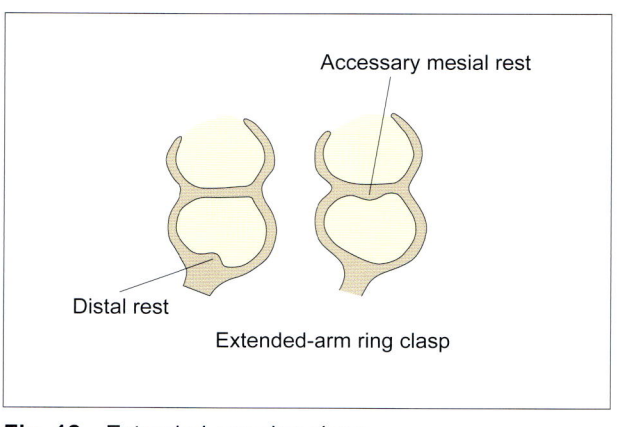

Fig. 12 Extended-arm ring clasp
In short distal extension denture, or poor ridge mucosa, an accessary mesial rest is placed as shown in the right diagram rather than a distal rest in the left and the clasp arm should be placed on the survey line on the abutment near the edentulous area.

waxing.

In addition, a dead space occurs under the rod projection. This can be avoided by placing a plate projection below the rod projection (Fig. 9).

Suginaka bolt with both projections are covered with a metal tooth or a facing-type metal tooth. In case with sufficient occlusal vertical dimension, a metal tooth fully covered with a hybrid resin or metal ceramic crown can be used.

Although this metal tooth and the retainer are commonly fabricated by one-piece casting, the metal tooth may be fabricated during artificial teeth set-up after soldering in cases with soldering the outer crown to a bar or a metal plate for double crown-type retainer.

The hook can be directed either buccally or lingually and its edge should be placed at the embrasure between the abutment tooth and the metal tooth. In addition, the edge of the hook may be modified for easy manipuration of the patient (Fig. 10).

The only thing to be done is to embed and fix the Suginaka bolt into a denture base, therefore there is no need of soldering even dentures with a casting bar or plate. Therefore, the Suginaka bolt can be removed easily from the denture base and is to reuse even when a need to remake of the denture is indicated.

As the Suginaka bolt has limited retentive function, when it might use as a retainer, there is a need to provide support and bracing functions with it.

Therefore, only retentive function is excluded from clasps or cone-crown telescopic retainers incorporating this function by Suginaka bolt into them. When incorporating the Suginaka bolt into clasps, the clasp tip should be placed on the survey line without placing under the survey line as bracing arms (see **Fig. 4** in Chapter 3). When incorporating the Suginaka bolt into the Cone-crown telescope retainer, it is necessary to use the Cone-crown-type double crown fitted loosely between the inner and outer crowns excluded of its retentive function (see

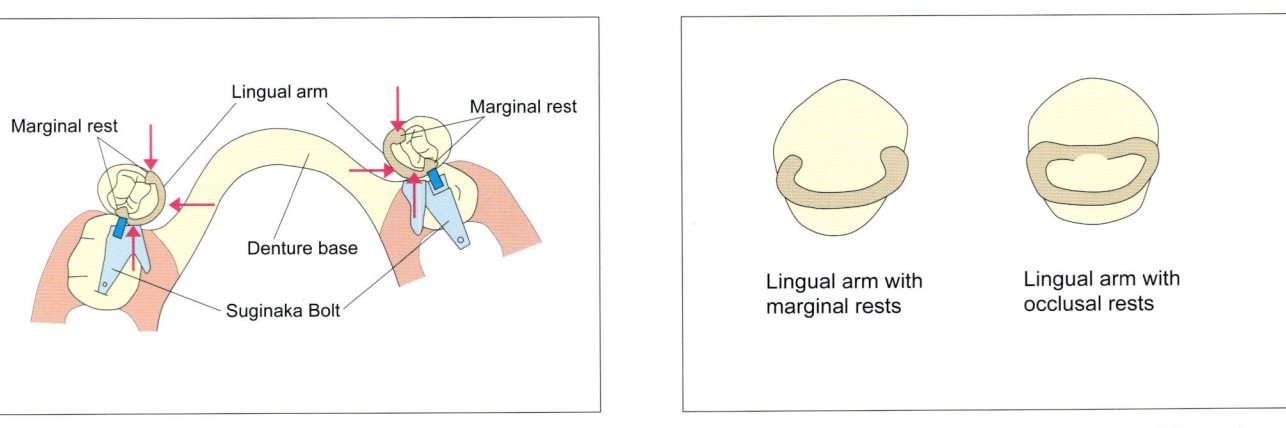

Fig. 13
In bilateral distal extension dentures, the lingual surfaces of both abutment teeth act as the reciprocal surface against horizontal forces (arrows).

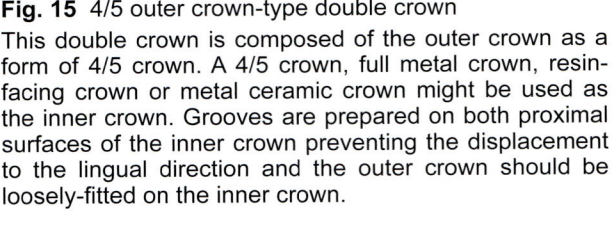

Fig. 14 Lingual arm with marginal rests and lingual arm with occlusal rests
Both lingual arms are primary placed on premolars, but it is applied to canines, a cingulum rest is placed.

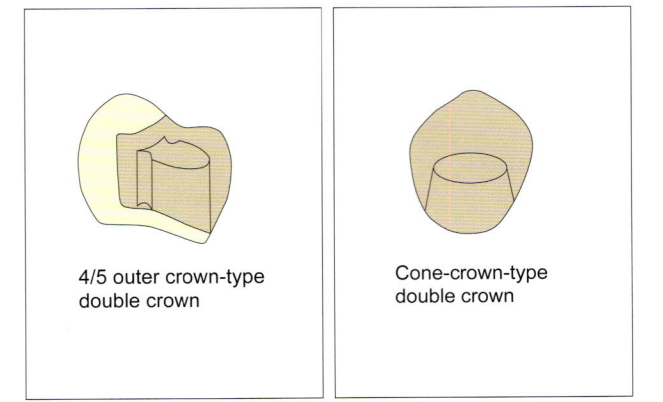

Fig. 15 4/5 outer crown-type double crown
This double crown is composed of the outer crown as a form of 4/5 crown. A 4/5 crown, full metal crown, resin-facing crown or metal ceramic crown might be used as the inner crown. Grooves are prepared on both proximal surfaces of the inner crown preventing the displacement to the lingual direction and the outer crown should be loosely-fitted on the inner crown.

Fig. 16 Cone-crown-type double crown
Cone-crown-type outer crown fit loosely to the inner crown.

Fig. 5 in Chapter 3). The extent of loose fit is that the inner crown is immobile when putting and shaking the inner crown into the outer crown with the occlusal surface side down and the inner crown smoothly drops out of the outer crown when the occlusal surface of the outer crown is upside down. The loose fit doesn't mean that the inner crown makes a rocking motion inside the outer crown.

Retainers commonly used in distal extension denture cases are as follows:

1) Extended arm clasp

Though this clasp is rarely used in general practice this can be used in unilateral resolution of distal extension cases with its high bracing effect.

The clasp arm is placed on the survey line of the abutment near the edentulous area and an accessary mesial rest may be placed rather than a distal rest in distal extension denture in cases with poor ridge mucosa with small number of tooth defects, such as missing molars (Fig. 11).

2) Extended-arm ring clasp

The use of an extended arm clasp may result in slightly opening of the clasp arm after the long usage. The extended- arm ring clasp was designed for preventing such a phenomenon and can also be used in unilateral restoration in distal extension cases. Similar to the extended arm clasp, the clasp arm is placed on the survey line and an accessary mesial rest should be placed rather than a distal rest in short distal extension denture with poor ridge mucosa with small number of tooth defects, such as missing molars (Fig. 12).

3) Lingual arm with marginal rests or lingual arm with occlusal rests

Concerning bracing function of bilateral retainers in bilateral distal extension dentures, the horizontal movement is restricted by a denture plate and a major/minor connector. In addition, since both lingual surfaces of the bilateral abutment teeth are designed as the reciprocal

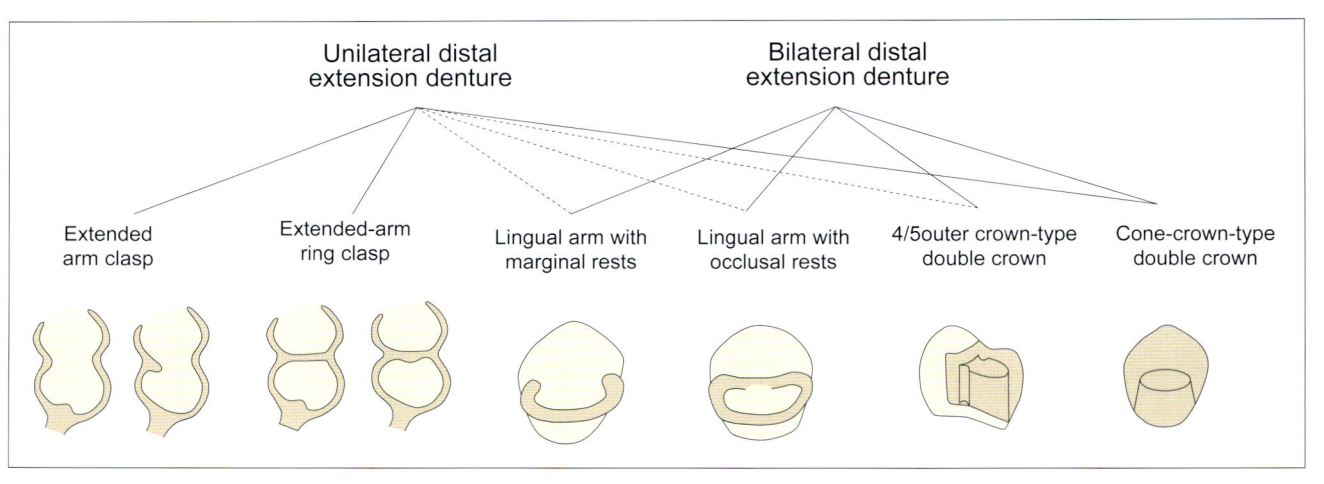

Fig. 17 Criteria for selecting retainers in distal extension dentures
The dotted lines show the choice for a cross-arch splint in unilateral distal extension dentures.

surface which diminishe the horizontal mobility of distal extension dentures, buccal bracing of the retainers can be omitted (Fig. 13). As the origin of the retentive projections is, braced by the metal tooth, bracing function is not always lost. Therefore, the lingual arm with marginal rests or occlusal rests can be used as a retainer in unilateral distal extension dentures with cross-arch stabilization as well as bilateral one (Fig. 14). Of course, both of these have the lingual arm running on the survey line.

4) 4/5 outer crown-type double crown (Horseshoe-type double crown)

Although the Böttger's telescopic crown is a high accurate-retainer, which exhibits greater retention, 4/5 outer crown-type double crown applying to the Suginaka bolt allows a loose fit between the inner and outer crowns with much a ease to laboratory operations (Fig. 15).

In 4/5 outer crown-type double crowns, grooves should be prepared on both proximal surfaces of the inner crown for preventing displacement in the lingual direction without the buccal bracing. Because of the lack in bracing, this retainer can be indicated in unilateral distal extension dentures with a cross-arch splint as well as bilateral ones, but cannot be used in unilateral distal extension denture cases. However, this can be used as a primary fixation auxiliary device for direct retainers.

5) Cone-crown-type double crown

The Cone-crown-type double crown refers to a Cone-crown telescope fitted loosely between the inner and out-er crowns. The use of the Suginaka bolt contributes for secure retention with avoidance of clinical troubles resulting from complicated laboratory techniques and errors in interlocking force between the fit of inner and outer crowns (Fig. 16).

The Cone-crown telescope is the most excellent retainer in support and bracing functions among the different retainers and a loose fit between inner and outer crowns exerts little influence on connecting rigidity. According to cases, to avoid excessive functional loads exerted on the abutment tooth, it is only necessary to connect and fix the inner crown to the adjacent tooth or to decrease the coronal length of the inner crown (see Fig. 6 in Chapter 3).

The Cone-crown-type double crown can be used in both unilateral and bilateral distal extension dentures.

As described above, the 6 different retainers are more commonly used as a retainer in distal extension dentures; among them, extended arm clasps, extended-arm ring clasps, and Cone-crown-type double crowns are used as a retainer in unilateral distal extension dentures. In bilateral distal extension dentures, the lingual arm with marginal rests or occlusal rests, and 4/5 outer crown-type double crowns and Cone-crown-type double crowns are most commonly used. In addition, the lingual arm with marginal rests or occlusal rests, and 4/5 outer crown-type double crowns can be used in unilateral distal extension dentures with a cross-arch splint (Fig. 17).

2. Lock denture type

For the Suginaka bolt lock type denture, the retainer form is similar to the RPPA-type clasp and its buccal arm should be placed within the deep undercut area below the survey line on the buccal surface of the abutment tooth for obtaining retention through the latch effect. To that end, a hinge is placed in the denture border corresponding to the position of a metal tooth which can be rotated around it while the buccal arm is joined together. Once the metal tooth with the buccal arm is put into place, the buccal arm extending from the metal tooth is placed within the deep undercut area below the survey line on the buccal surface of the abutment tooth, resulting secure retention through the latch effect.

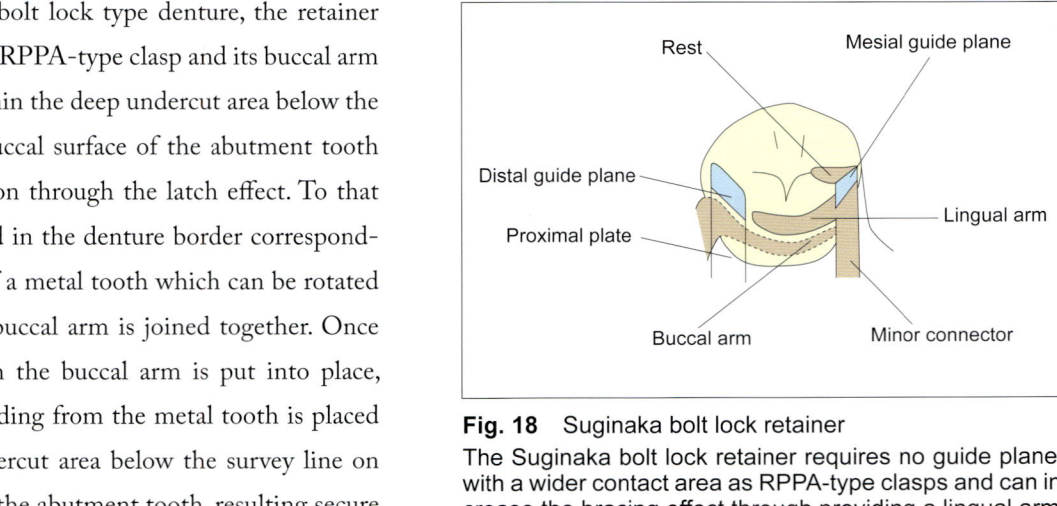

Fig. 18 Suginaka bolt lock retainer
The Suginaka bolt lock retainer requires no guide planes with a wider contact area as RPPA-type clasps and can increase the bracing effect through providing a lingual arm.

Fig. 19 Structure of Suginaka bolt lock retainer

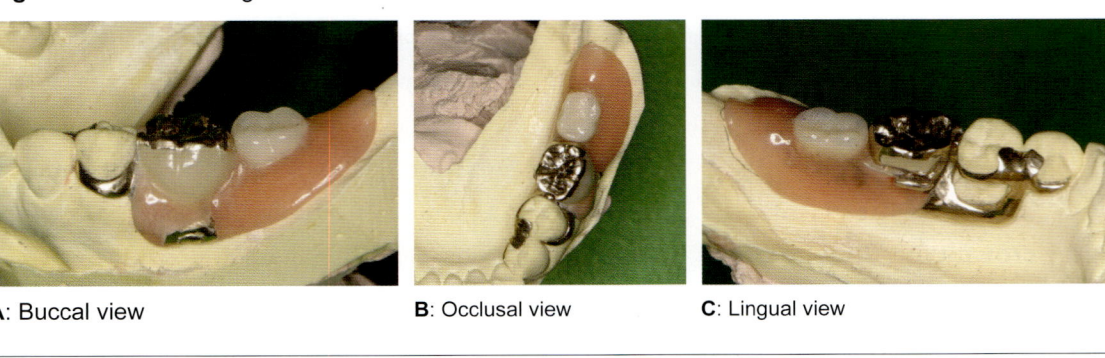

A: Buccal view **B**: Occlusal view **C**: Lingual view

D: Pattern diagram viewed from the lingual oblique above
The hook was pulled out, after which the metal tooth has been opened through buccally rotating it.

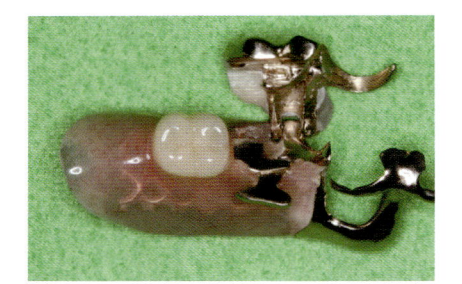

E: Lingual view, the metal tooth was rotated and opened. Denture insertion/removal is performed at this moment.

The RPPA clasp represents more rigid retainer because the guide plane on both proximal surfaces between the minor connector leading to the mesial rest and the proximal plate adjacent to the missing site is prepared as widely and parallel as possible. Therefore, the RPPA clasp is effective in decreasing the denture mobility, but its indications are limited. In addition, with this retainer, denture

insertion and removal seems difficult, causing greater tractive and lateral forces on the abutment tooth during denture removal.

If an abutment tooth is a sound tooth with a normal tooth contour, such wider and mesiodistally parallel guide planes can not be prepared. Therefore, even if the abutment tooth is non-vital and requires crown restoration, minimal tooth reduction is preferable.

The Suginaka bolt lock retainer has mesiodistally-paralleled guide planes for proving the minimal bracing function and a lingual arm leading to the mesial minor connector for increasing the bracing effect (**Fig. 18**).

Of course, the buccal arm is placed within the deep undercut area without contacting the gingival area on the buccal tooth enamel surface. At this moment, a Suginaka bolt device can be used for locking and retaining the

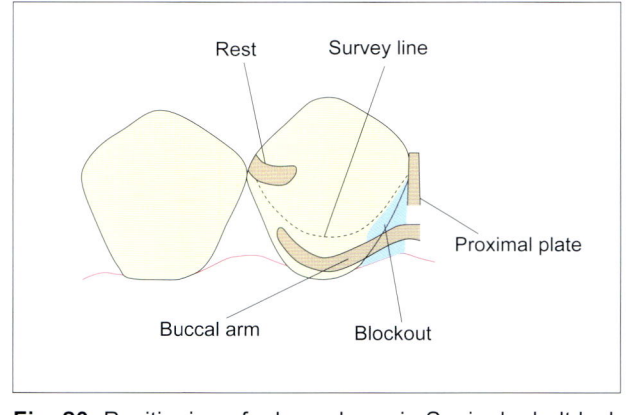

Fig. 20 Positioning of a buccal arm in Suginaka bolt lock retainer
The buccal arm should be placed within the deep undercut area without contact to the gingival tissue below the survey line. However, the area from the origin of the buccal arm to the buccal distal proximal corner tends to move forward and downward during denture sinking, resulting in compressing the tooth surface and preventing the denture base from sinking. Therefore, it is important to block out this area.

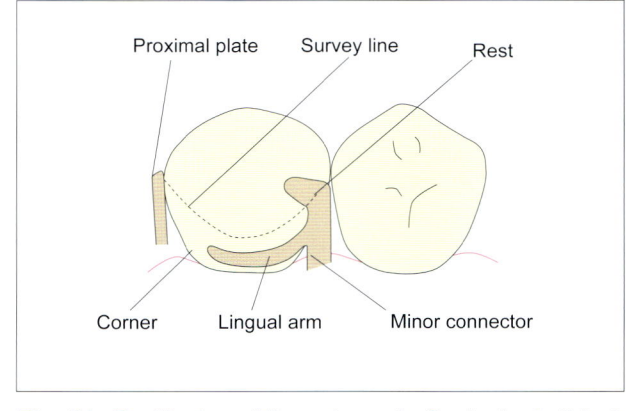

Fig. 21 Positioning of lingual arm in Suginaka bolt lock retainer
When restoring the unilateral distal extension case by unilateral design , the area from the origin of the lingual arm to its clasp tip should be placed within the deep undercut area under the survey line. In this situation, the clasp tip should be ended short before the lingual distal proximal corner. This is because the clasp tip tries to move forwards and downwards during denture sinking, resulting the compression of the tooth surface and preventing the denture base from sinking.

Fig. 22 Advice for hinge positioning
As the position of the hinge gets close to the area under the Suginaka bolt device, the tangent of the rotating circle in the metal tooth gets closer to the tangent of the hinge located below its retentive section, possibly resulting in spontaneously rotation of the metal tooth even if the lever is closed. Therefore, in case where the hinge gets close to the area under the Suginaka bolt device, it should be inclined between 5 to 10 degree toward the horizontal plane for preventing the metal tooth from rotating.

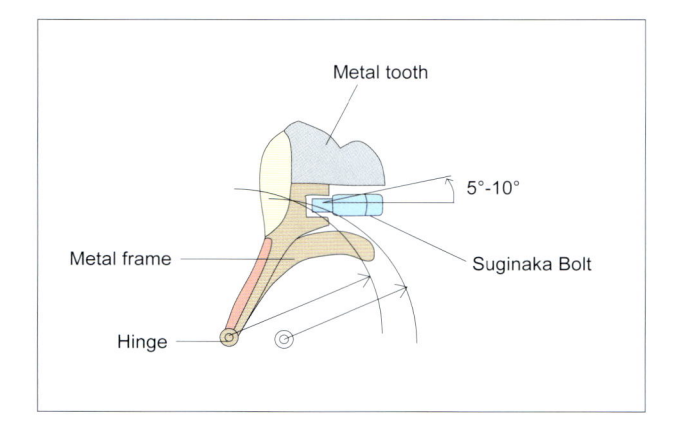

rotatable metal tooth with the buccal arm in place (Fig. 19). The Akers clasp can be assembled with both wrought wire (0.9 or 1.0 mm in diameter) and casting . Because the lock retainer uses the latch principle of locking for retention, it is not necessary to consider the elasticity of clasps.

Because the buccal arm is placed within the deep undercut area avoiding gingival contact, the clasp tip can be extended to the mesial proximal surface. However, attention should be taken to avoid contact with the tooth surface from its origin to the buccal distal proximal line angle. This area moves forwards and downwards during sinking or rotating of the denture base, exerted force may push the abutment tooth forward. To prevent this, it is necessary to relief out of the contact to this area (Fig. 20).

For unilateral distal extension dentures with a cross-arch splint or bilateral distal extension dentures, the lingual arm should be placed above the survey line. However, when the unilateral distal extension saddle is unilaterally restored, the lingual arm can be placed within the deep undercut area below the survey line.

It should be noted at this moment that the lingual arm should be extended within the deep undercut area from the origin of the mesial minor connector with the clasp tip just before the lingual distal proximal line angle (Fig. 21). The reason why is if the clasp tip of the lingual arm is extended to the distal proximal surface, it moves forwards and downwards and it exerts compression on the distal proximal surface during sinking or rotation of the denture base.

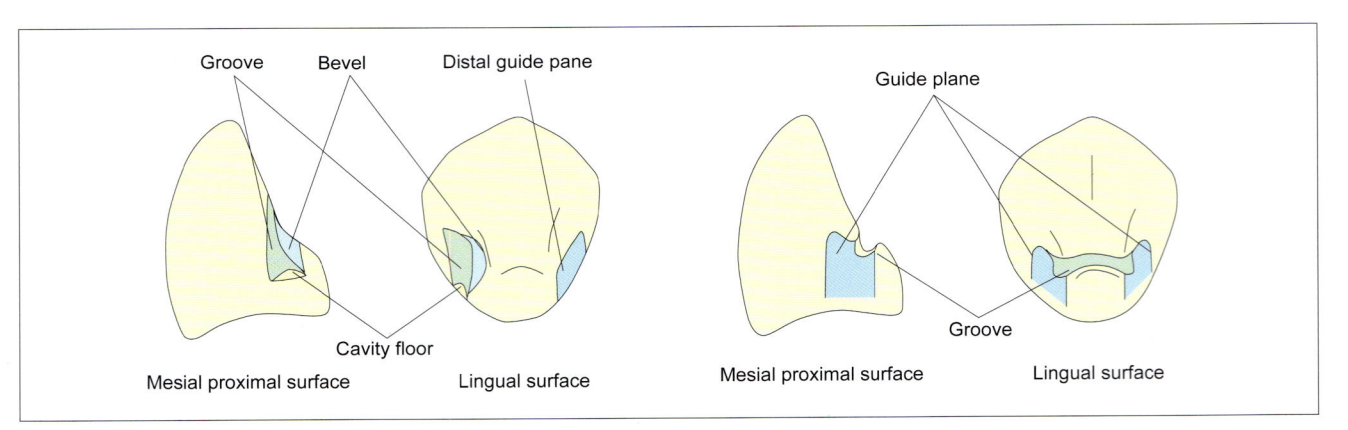

Fig. 23 Abutment preparation of canine

A: A 1.5-2.0 mm wide and 1.5 mm deep (cavity floor) semicircular groove is prepared parallel to the tooth axis on the mesial proximal surface of the canine and beveling while a wide dimple is performed along the ridge line between the cavity and the lingual surface for using it as a proximal marginal rest, in which the distal proximal guide plane should be lingually prepared.

B: The guide planes parallel to one another are prepared on both proximal surfaces of the canine and a 1.5 mm wide and 1.5 mm deep semicircular groove is prepared, in which both guide planes are connected across the cingulum for using it as a cingulum rest seat.

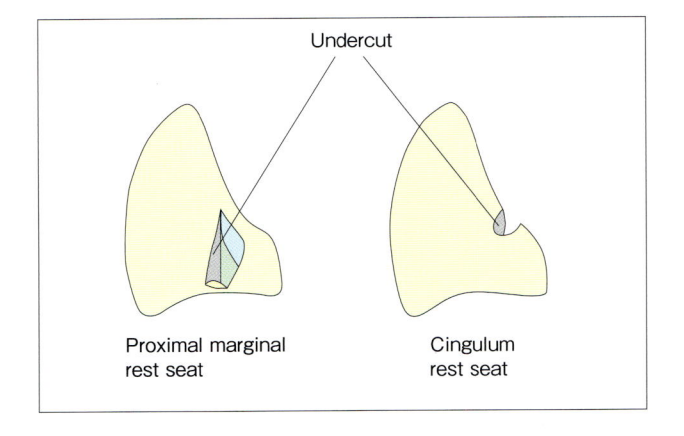

Fig. 24
When there is no undercut area on the labial surface of the canine, undercuts are prepared in the rest seat for increasing retention.

The Suginaka bolt lock retainer can increase the connecting rigidity structurally through preparing a parallel proximal plate on both proximal surfaces. However, when rotation of the denture base must be allowed, it is necessary to decrease the contact between the proximal plate and the abutment tooth. When the connecting rigidity on both proximal surfaces is greater, the abutment tooth can resist against the horizontal movement of the denture base through bodily movement. However, when the connecting rigidity becomes reduced, the horizontal movement of the denture base results in rotating the abutment tooth (see **Fig. 9** in Chapter 1). This poses an obstacle in tissue around the abutment tooth. The use of the Suginaka bolt lock retainer allows for buccolingual rotation of the denture base due to of a lower buccolingual connecting rigidity of buccal and lingual arm clasps placed near the cervical area, but which resist against rotation of the abutment tooth caused by a horizontal movement of the denture base, resulting in horizontal movement (bodily movement) of the abutment tooth and be capable of resisting against horizontal movement through all aspects of the root.

The Suginaka bolt lock retainer has advantages of no frictional force exerted on the abutment tooth during denture insertion/removal, allowing mesiodistal and buccolingual rotation of the denture base even during denture function, and avoiding rotation of the abutment tooth caused by horizontal movement of the denture base. This realized the ideal form of the bracing action with the Suginaka lock-retainer already shown in the figure10, chapter I.

It should be noted that a hinge cannot be placed when the alveolar ridge area where a hinge should be placed overhangs buccally or there is an undercut area on the alveolar ridge with existing root of a tooth. In addition, when the position of the hinge gets close to the area below the Suginaka bolt device, the tangent to the rotating circle of the metal tooth gets closer to the tangent to the hinge located below its retentive section, resulting in spontaneously rotating of the metal tooth possibly even if the lever is closed. Therefore, in case where the hinge gets close to the area below the Suginaka bolt device, it should be inclined between 5 and 10 degrees toward the horizontal plane for avoiding rotation of the metal tooth (Fig. 22).

To use a RPPA-type clasp in the canine in combination with the Suginaka bolt lock retainer, special preparations are required for the canine. There are two ways for this purpose: the first one is to give a 1.5-2.0 mm wide and 1.5 mm deep (cavity floor size) semicircular groove preparation on the mesial proximal surface of the canine and beveling a wide dimple performed along the ridge line between the cavity and the lingual surface for using it as a proximal marginal rest. In which the distal proximal guide plane should be lingually prepared; the another one is to give the guide planes parallel to each other prepared on both proximal surfaces of the canine and with a 1.5 mm wide and 1.5 mm deep semicircular groove preparation, with both guide planes connected across the cingulum for using it as a cingulum rest (**Fig. 23**). Some canines have no undercut area on the labial surface. In such cases, the labial arm is cervically placed and undercuts are created in the rest seat to increase retention (**Fig. 24**).

The abutment teeth, which are applicable to the Suginaka bolt lock retainer are both of the abutment tooth with sound tooth , or the treated tooth.

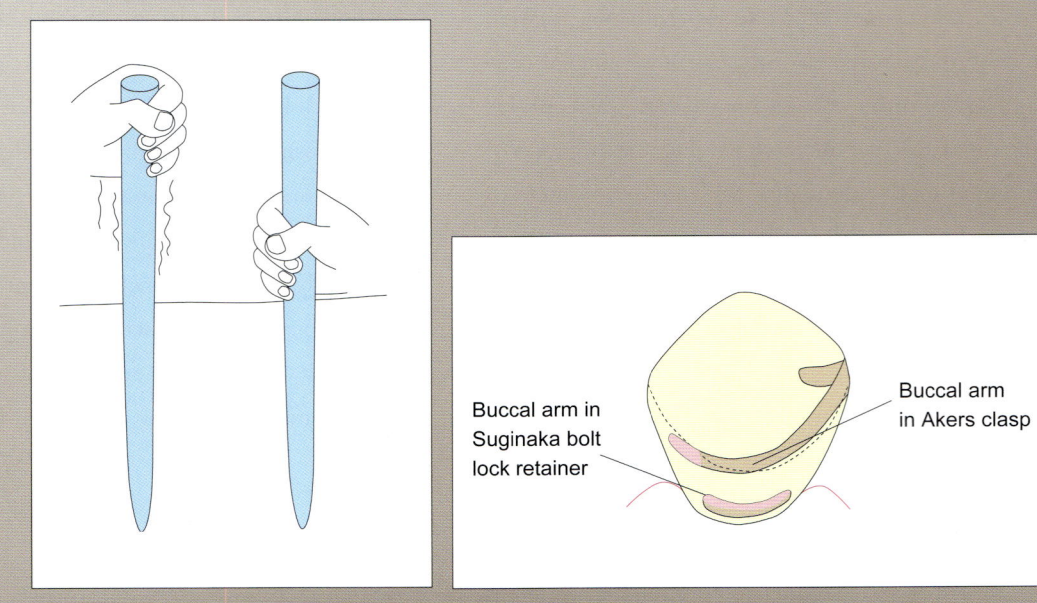

In case shaking the piled pillar

When shaking a plillar piled into the ground, do you know which part of the plillar is most effective emerging from the earth to swing immediately by shaking? , The answer is the plillar can be swung in easiest way by shaking it on its top. But in case,if the part near the level of earth is shaken with much power, it takes a lot of time to shaking the pillar (**Fig. 25**). The same phenomenon happens to Suginaka bolt lock retainers.

In the conventional clasps, since the exerting point of retention is decided based on the survey line, it tends to be situated nearer to the cusp from the center of the crown, facilitating mobility of the abutment tooth due to higher point of retentive action . However, in Suginaka bolt lock retainers, mobility of abutment tooth can be reduced because the action point of retention is cervically placed (**Fig. 26**).

Buccal arm in Suginaka bolt lock retainer

Buccal arm in Akers clasp

Fig. 25 A difference in power according to parts which shakes a pillar
To pull out a pillar piled into the ground with less power, it is better to shake it on its top than to the point just emerging from the earth.

Fig. 26
A difference in height of action point of retention through the buccal arm in clasps and a Suginaka bolt lock retainers.

Chapter 6

Suginaka bolt denture system

The Suginaka bolt denture system is categorized into 2 types: 1) attachment dentures using Suginaka bolt attachment-type retainers; 2) lock dentures using lock retainers.

In addition, the attachment dentures are categorized into 2 types: a) clasp dentures using retainers, in which the Suginaka bolt is combined with clasps; b) telescopic dentures using retainers, in which the Suginaka bolt is combined with 4/5 outer crown-type double crowns/Cone-crown-type double crowns (Fig. 1).

For attachment dentures, retention can be obtained

*The bolt dentures, which used the Suginaka riegel (bolt) should be originally referred to as "Suginaka riegel (bolt) bolt dentures," but they will be referred to as "Suginaka bolt dentures" for short in this book.

through the latch effect provided by locking the retentive section of the Suginaka bolt into a retentive projection placed on an abutment tooth. For lock dentures, retention can be obtained through the latch effect provided by locking a buccal arm in a lock retainer within the deep undercut area located cervically to the labial/buccal surface of the abutment tooth.

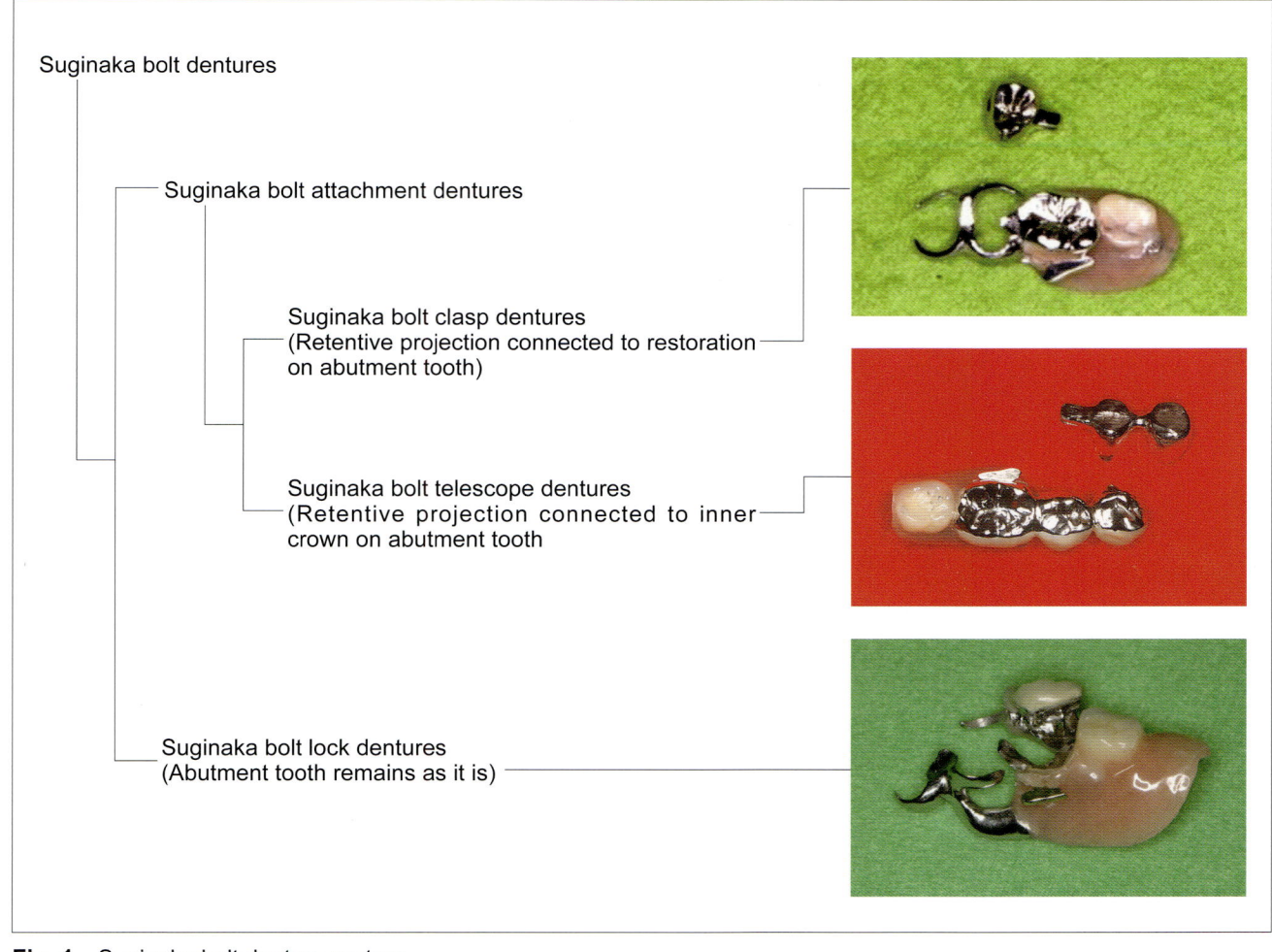

Suginaka bolt dentures

— Suginaka bolt attachment dentures

Suginaka bolt clasp dentures
(Retentive projection connected to restoration on abutment tooth)

Suginaka bolt telescope dentures
(Retentive projection connected to inner crown on abutment tooth

Suginaka bolt lock dentures
(Abutment tooth remains as it is)

Fig. 1 Suginaka bolt denture system

In addition, clasps, telescope crowns, and lock retainers used commonly as Suginaka bolt retainers can also be combined into a Suginaka bolt denture (Fig. 2).

Each of these is a retainer, which allows unilateral designing of unilateral distal extension tooth missing. In clinical situation, new distal extension missing often occurs on the opposite side after inserting a unilateral designed distal extension denture. When a dentist have to restore bilaterally, a unilateral distal extension denture utilizing any of them as a retainer is fabricated according to the conditions of an abutment tooth on newly missing side, after which a connection between the old and new unilateral distal extension dentures is performed with a bar or denture base for establishing a Suginaka bolt bilateral distal extension denture.

In other words, Suginaka bolt dentures have the advantage when a unilaterally-restored unilateral distal extension denture is comfortable to wear and the patient is also fully satisfied with the treatment, even if unilateral distal extension missing occurs also on the opposite side later, reforming to the bilateral distal extension denture.

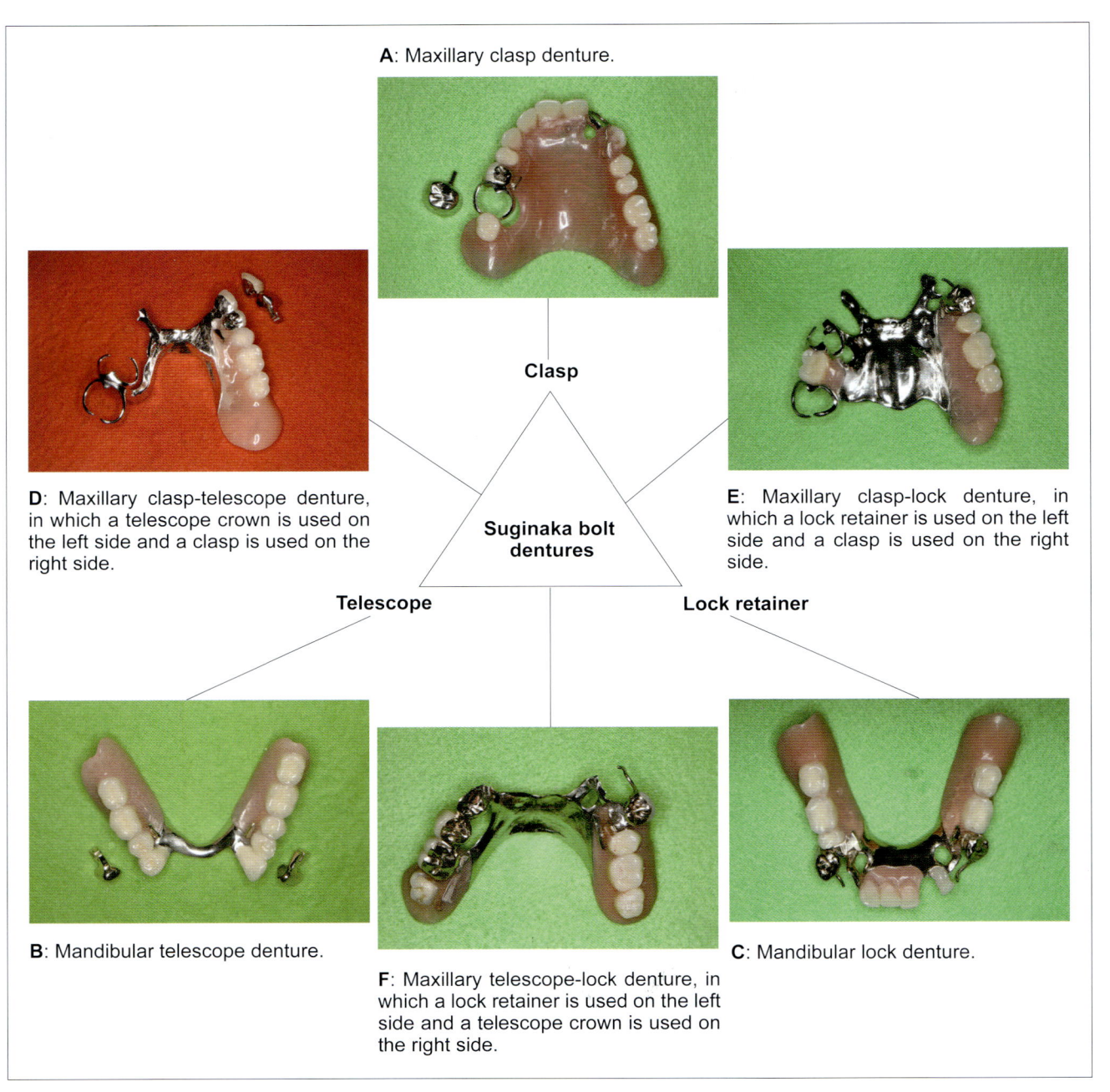

A: Maxillary clasp denture.

Clasp

Suginaka bolt dentures

Telescope

Lock retainer

D: Maxillary clasp-telescope denture, in which a telescope crown is used on the left side and a clasp is used on the right side.

E: Maxillary clasp-lock denture, in which a lock retainer is used on the left side and a clasp is used on the right side.

B: Mandibular telescope denture.

C: Mandibular lock denture.

F: Maxillary telescope-lock denture, in which a lock retainer is used on the left side and a telescope crown is used on the right side.

Fig. 2   Suginaka bolt dentures, which can be combined with the different retainers.

It is very difficult to insert/remove Suginaka bolt lock dentures with first molar and second molar or second molar missing (distal extension missing) because of inability to have a hand only on the lingual arm leading to the minor connector.

Therefore, if a temporary base plate is provided for stabilizing the lock denture in place and facilitating handling of the lock retainer, probably allowing easy denture insertion/removal.

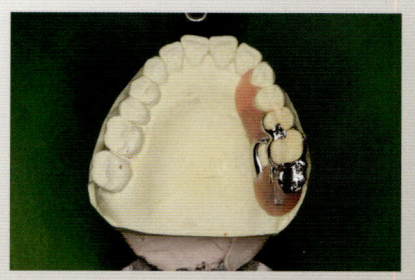

Fig. 3 A temporary base is provided in the lingual mesial region of the maxillary distal extension denture base with #27 missing.

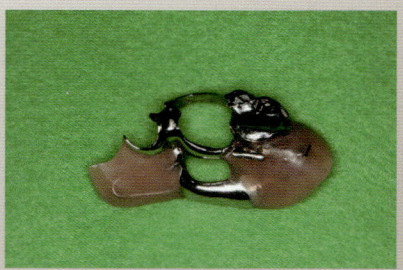

Fig. 4 The temporary base is cut as becoming accustomed to insertion/removal.

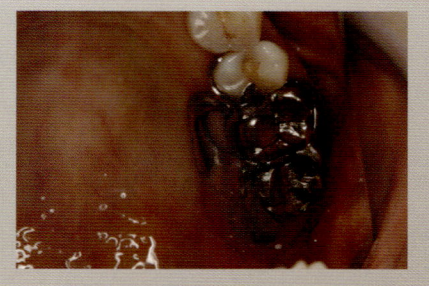

Fig. 5 Suginaka bolt lock denture inserted on missing tooth #27 region after the interim base was removed.

Bolt hook opening tool

A hook of the Suginaka bolt can be placed on either buccal or lingual side. However, when the Suginaka bolt is connected to a projection provided on the mesial surface of the abutment tooth, the hook is directed to the distal, thus it is difficult to operate the hook. In addition, when providing a projection on the distal surface, as the hook is directed to the mesial, it seems easy to pull out the lever with a fingernail, but some patients cannot do it. In such situation, you should teach them to use an instrument for operating a hook till they become accustomed to open the hook with their fingernail (**Fig. 6**).

However, early insertion of Suginaka bolt dentures, even with an instrument for operating a hook, they will become possible to pull out the lever with their fingernail as the time goes on. When the hook is directed labially or buccally, it is better than lingually-directed design in patients with difficulty to operate the hook with a finger nail especially in elderly patients although a poor esthetic result is shown.

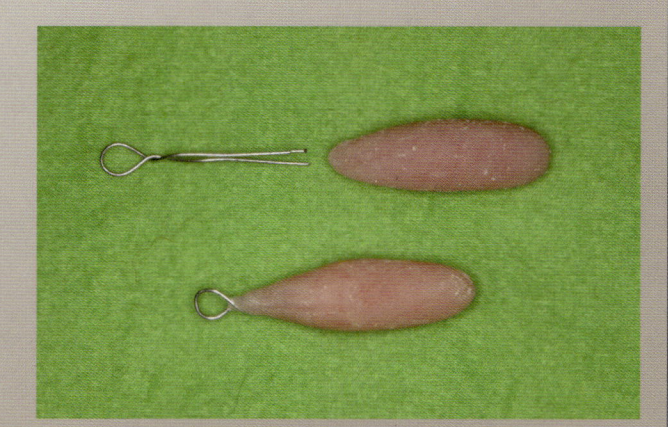

Fig. 6 How to make an instrument for operating a bolt hook
A loop is formed with a straight wire of 0.5 mm in diameter, then the residual wire ends are twisted, after that, dough of self-curing resin is wrapped around the twisted wires for fabricating an operating grip.

Chapter 7

Clinical cases with Suginaka Bolt (Riegel)

The Suginaka bolt can be indicated especially to the loss of teeth more than two in number. But, in both cases of attachment or lock dentures, even in a case of single tooth missing, with a sufficient denture base span, one can utilize the Suginaka bolt even in distal extension case of a single missing second molar.

In Suginaka bolt attachment dentures, a retentive projection can be designed from the distal surface of the lateral incisor to the mesial surface of the second molar (Fig. 1). However, if the maxillary lateral incisor is used as an abutment tooth, since the hook is located at the position of the maxillary canine, the maxillomandibular relationship must always be considered to maintain for its space.

This chapter will present clinical cases of Suginaka bolt dentures, focusing distal extension RPD's.

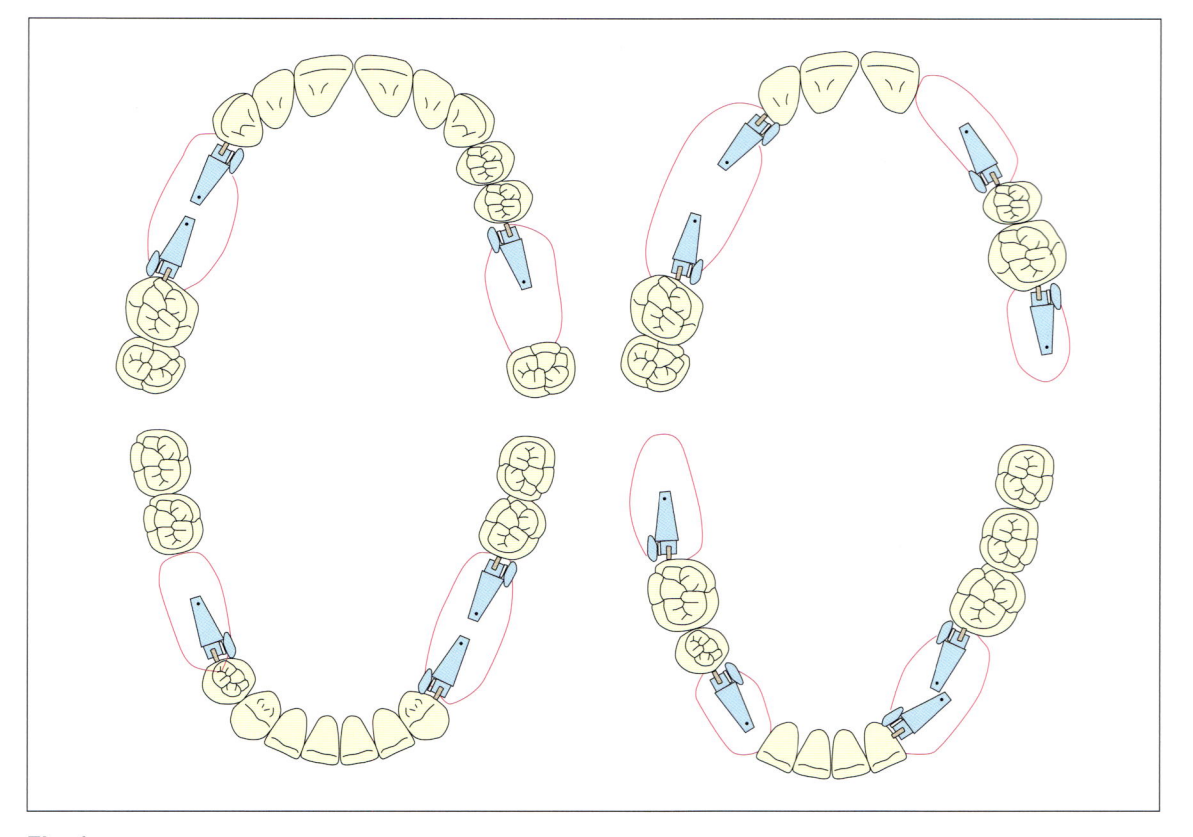

Fig. 1
Sites where a retentive projection can be placed in Suginaka bolt dentures.

COLUMN

How to lute the double crowns

When inserting 4/5 outer crown-type and Cone-crown-type double crowns, it is essential to always insert the integrated denture with the inner crown fitted into the outer crown. If the inner crown is inserted first, a slight discrepancy between the inner and outer crowns might occur, leading to possible inadaptation of denture and abnormal load on the abutment tooth (**Fig. 2**).

Fig. 2 Method for setting the double crown

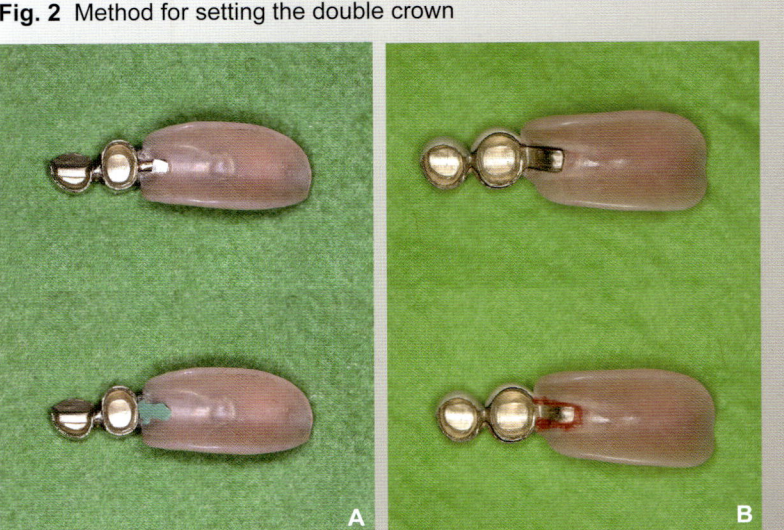

A: Cone-crown-type double crown with a rod projection

Above: Cocoa butter is applied to the inner surface of the outer crown, into which the inner crown is fitted, and the Suginaka bolt is closed.

Below: An agar impression material is packed into the dead space located below the retentive section of the Suginaka bolt and the rod projection seen from the denture basal surface. After luting, the excessive agar is cut with a carving knife just after the mucosal surface. It is ready to fabricate the denture !

B: Cone-crown-type double crown with plate projection

Above: Cocoa butter is applied to the inner surface of the outer crown, into which the inner crown is fitted, and the Suginaka bolt is closed.

Below: Utility wax or bees wax is packed into the space between the plate projection and the denture basal surface observed from the denture basal surface. It is ready to fabricate the denture !

COLUMN

Should dentures be removed by night ?

It is written in many textbook of removable prosthodontics that the dentures should be removed by night promoting the denture-bearing mucosa to rest and recovery of the denture bearing tissues . However, the author believes that as for removable partial dentures, they should be inserted during sleeping. This is because while night sleeping with dentures removed even one night, the mucosa under the denture base released from pressure to its former state, the opposing tooth at the missing site is extruded, and the abutment tooth is only slightly displaced. Consequently, next morning, there is a feeling that the occlusion is elevated when inserting dentures.

After a while, it goes away. This suggests that the opposing tooth may be affected with occlusal trauma. Therefore, if the period of removal of dentures is to be prolonged, the opposing tooth may be significantly extruded and the abutment tooth may also be displaced to much. Under these circumstances, limited insertion of the denture in use results in the increased risk of the abutment tooth affected with occlusal trauma.

Thus, the author considers that partial dentures should be always worn except during the oral hygiene.

1. Suginaka bolt attachment dentures

1) Suginaka bolt clasp dentures

①Unilateral distal extension missing case: Missing tooth #37; Patient: 70-year-old man
Tooth #36: Full metal crown with a rod projection
Teeth #35, #36: Extended-arm clasp

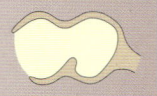

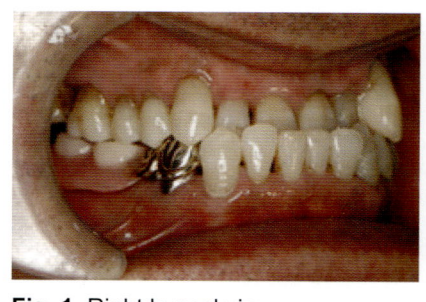

Fig. 1 Right buccal view.

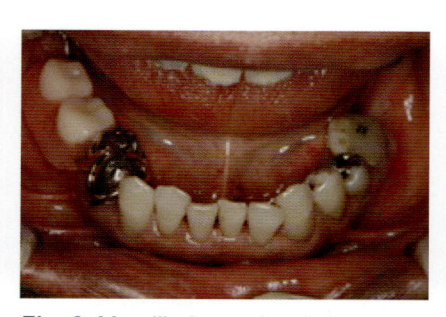

Fig. 2 Mandibular occlusal view.

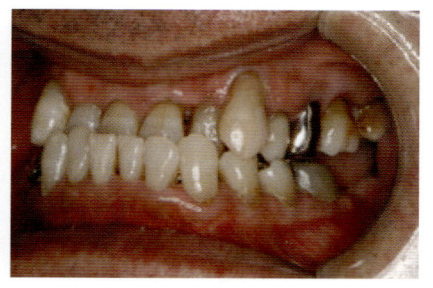

Fig. 3 Missing tooth #37 Left buccal view.

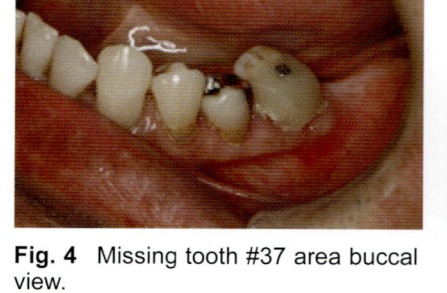

Fig. 4 Missing tooth #37 area buccal view.

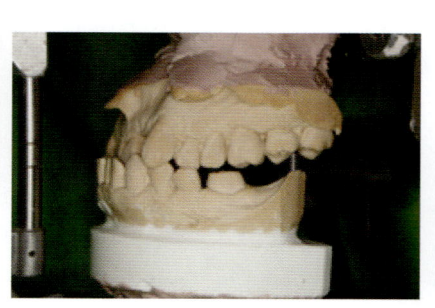

Fig. 5 Buccal view of the working model for abutment tooth #36.

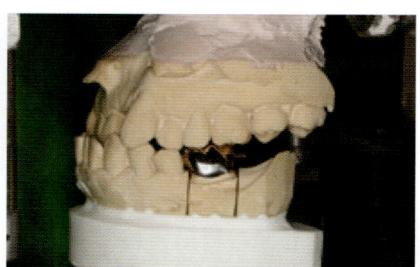

Fig. 6 Buccal view of the full metal crown with a rod projection inserted on tooth #36.

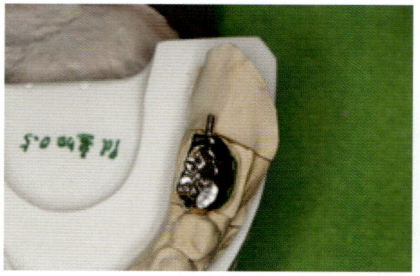

Fig. 7 Occlusal view of the full metal crown with a rod projection and the mesial rest inserted on tooth #36.

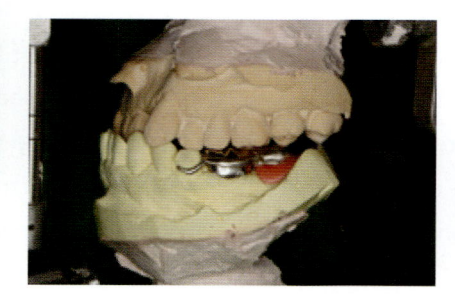

Fig. 8 Buccal view of the clasp denture with an extended-arm clasp placed on #35, #36, with a metal tooth replacing the missing tooth #37.

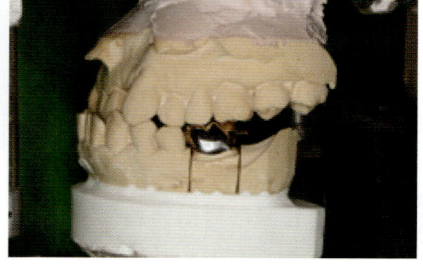

Fig. 9 Occlusal view of the clasp denture with an extended-arm clasp on #35, #36, a metal tooth replacing the missing tooth #37. A hook is directed buccally.

48

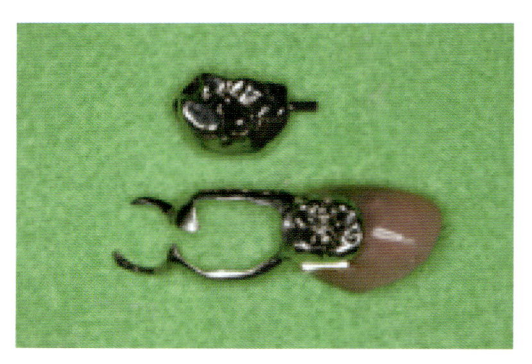

Fig. 10 Completed full metal crown with a rod projection for tooth #36 and the clasp denture with an extended-arm clasp for missing tooth #37.

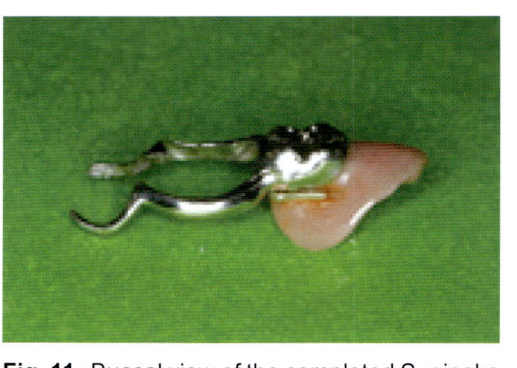

Fig. 11 Buccal view of the completed Suginaka bolt clasp denture for missing tooth #37.

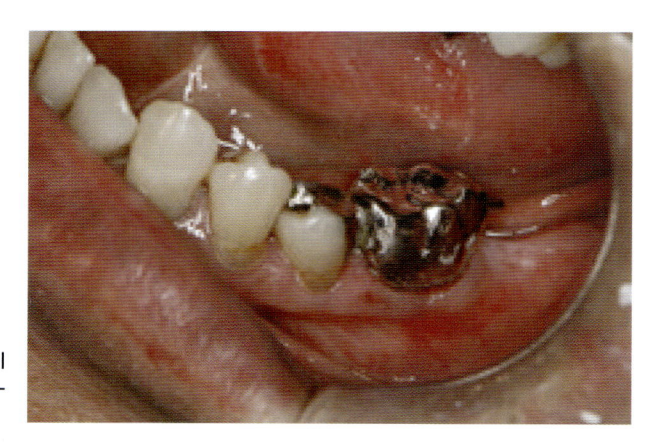

Fig. 12 Buccal view of the full metal crown with a rod projection on tooth #36.

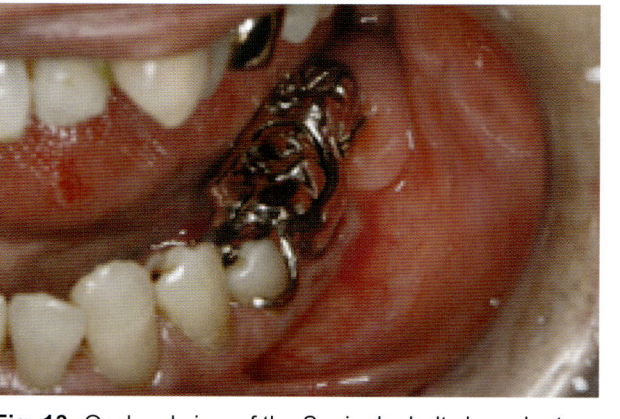

Fig. 13 Occlusal view of the Suginaka bolt clasp denture for the missing tooth #37 region.

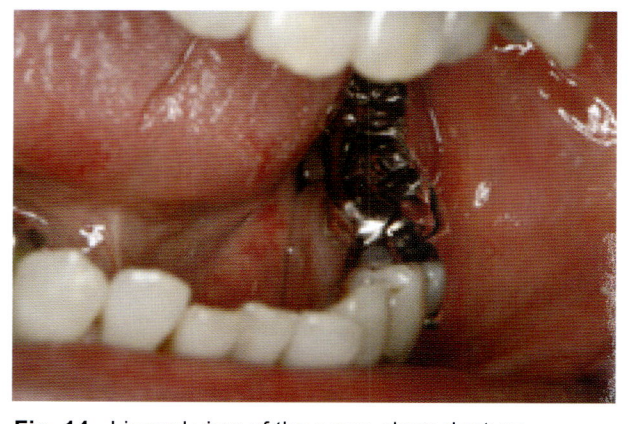

Fig. 14 Lingual view of the same clasp denture.

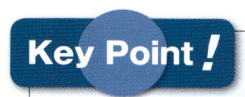

Key Point !

When restoring a single missing tooth in a distal extension denture using an extended-arm clasp, the connecting rigidity is decreased to allow sinking of denture base, since a rest is prepared on the mesial occlusal surface of the abutment tooth adjacent to the missing area. An extended-arm clasp is designed on the survey line and its clasp tip must not be placed within the undercut area. A removal hook should be directed buccally for ease to handling.

1. Suginaka bolt attachment dentures

1) Suginaka bolt clasp dentures

②Unilateral distal extension missing case: Missing tooth #47; Patient: 77-year-old man
Tooth #46: Class 2 inlay with a rod projection
Teeth #45, #46: Extended-arm clasp

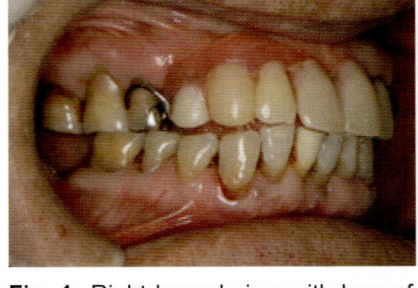

Fig. 1 Right buccal view with loss of tooth #47.

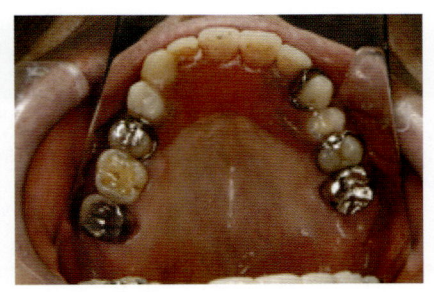

Fig. 2 Maxillary occlusal view.

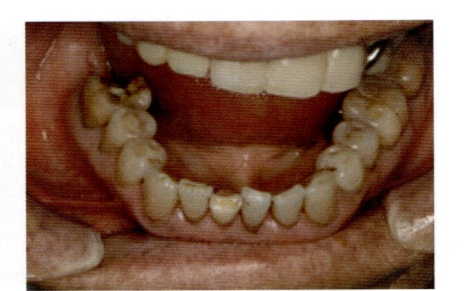

Fig. 3 Mandibular occlusal view.

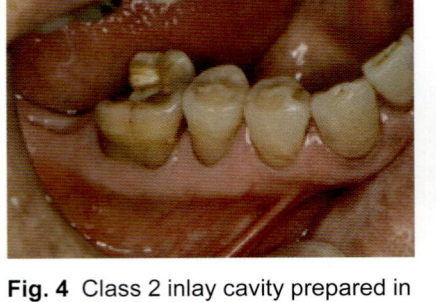

Fig. 4 Class 2 inlay cavity prepared in tooth #46 (pulpless tooth).

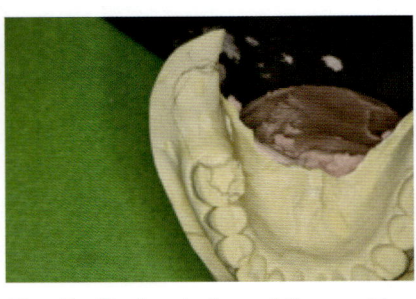

Fig. 5 Occlusal view of the working model fabricated after taking an impression. Tooth #46 is an abutment tooth.

Fig. 6 Occlusal view of Class 2 inlay with a rod projection into tooth #46. A mesial rest seat is prepared on tooth #46.

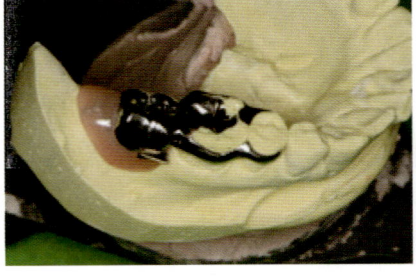

Fig. 7 Buccal view of the clasp denture with an extended-arm clasp on teeth #45, #46, a metal tooth replacing the missing tooth #47. A hook is directed to the buccal.

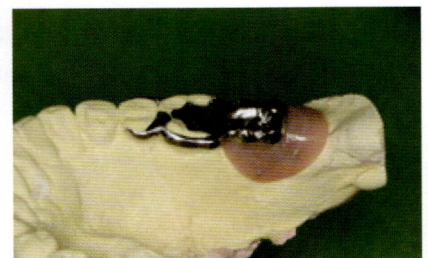

Fig. 8 Lingual view of the clasp denture with a metal tooth replacing the missing tooth #47. The mesial rest from the lingual arm is provided.

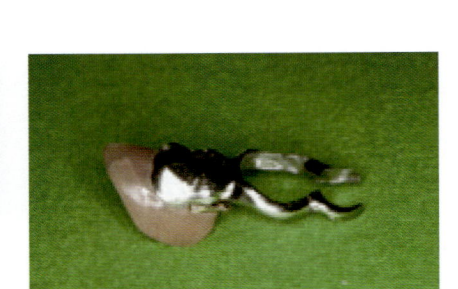

Fig. 9 Buccal view of the Suginaka bolt clasp denture for missing tooth #47, to that an extended-arm clasp for teeth #45 and #46 is attached.

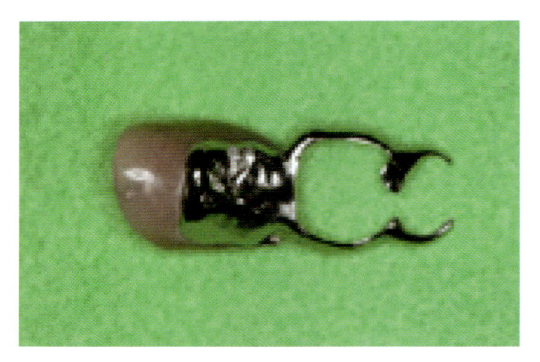

Fig. 10 Occlusal view of the same clasp denture.

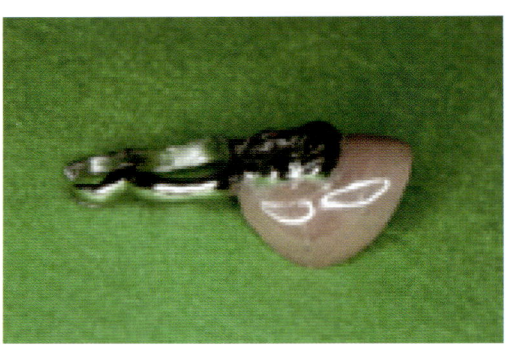

Fig. 11 Lingual view of the same clasp denture.

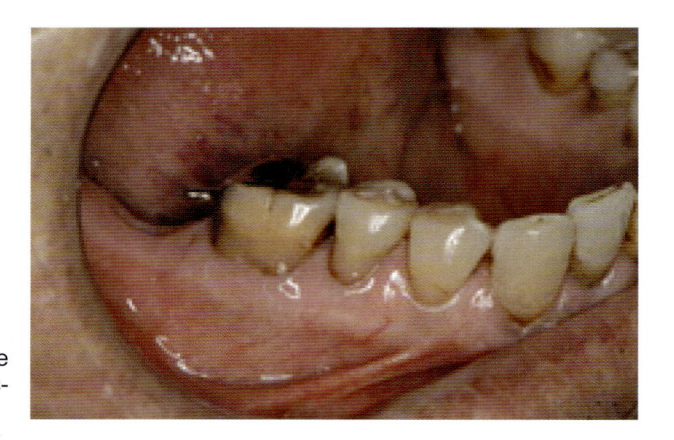

Fig. 12 Buccal view of the Class 2 inlay with a rod projection on tooth #46.

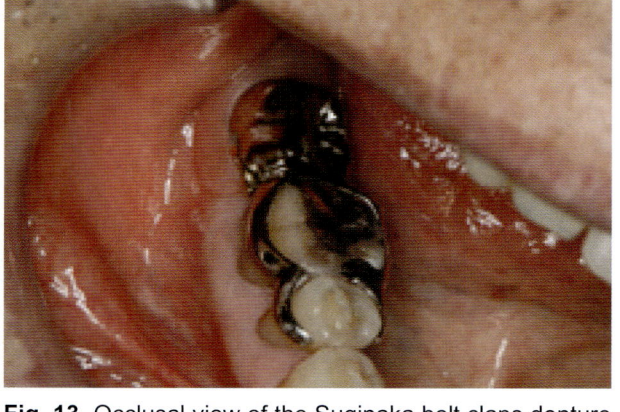

Fig. 13 Occlusal view of the Suginaka bolt claps denture replacing the missing tooth #47.

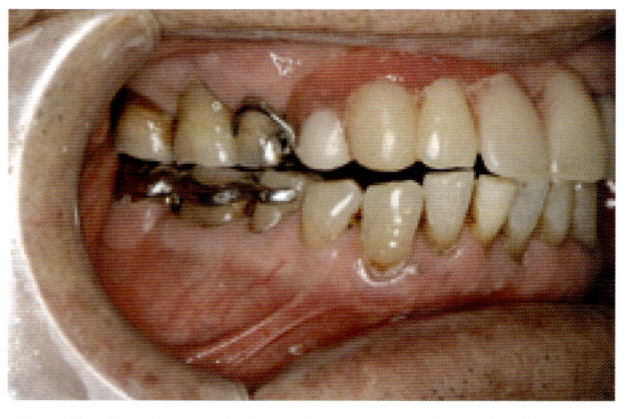

Fig. 14 Right buccal view of the same clasp denture.

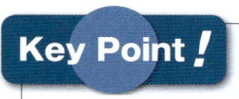

Key Point ! When an abutment tooth is a pulpless tooth with a deep cavity, inlays for any cavity preparation forms as well as Class 2 inlays are available with sufficient retention,. However, when an abutment tooth is vital, Class 2 inlays might fall out because of the shallow cavity. Therefore, it may be necessary to prepare retentive pinholes into the cavity floor. A hook should be directed to the buccal for easy handling.

1. Suginaka bolt attachment dentures

1) Suginaka bolt clasp dentures

③Unilateral distal extension missing case: Missing teeth #47-#48; Patient: 62-year-old man
Tooth #46: Full metal crown with a rod projection
Teeth #45, #46: Extended-arm ring clasp

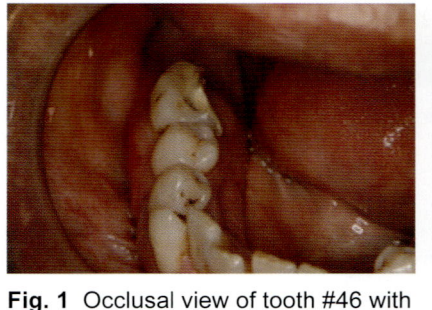

Fig. 1 Occlusal view of tooth #46 with a fractured crown.

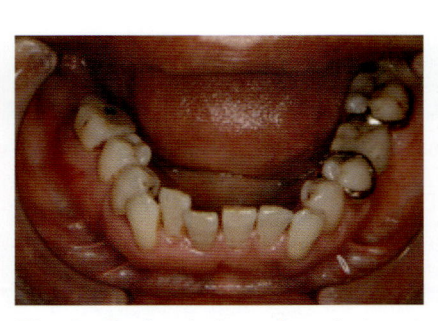

Fig. 2 Occlusal view after abutment build-up on tooth #46.

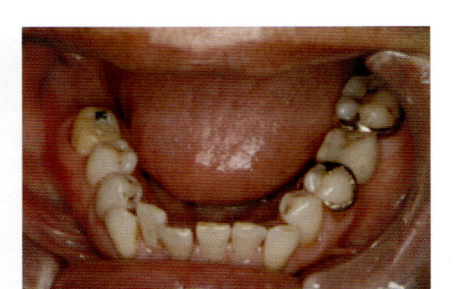

Fig. 3 Occlusal view of the finished abutment preparation for full metal crown of tooth #46.

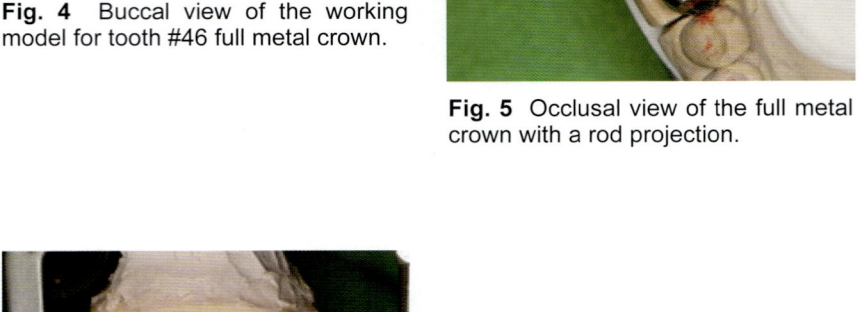

Fig. 4 Buccal view of the working model for tooth #46 full metal crown.

Fig. 5 Occlusal view of the full metal crown with a rod projection.

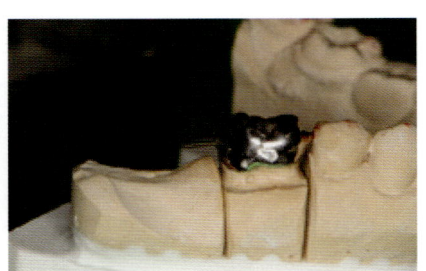

Fig. 6 Buccal view of the same crown. At this point, a groove for an extended-arm ring clasp is prepared.

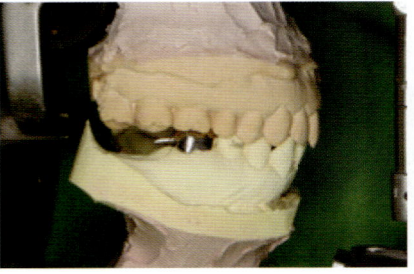

Fig. 7 Buccal view of the working model for fabricating an extended-arm ring clasp placed on teeth #45, #46, and a Suginaka bolt clasp denture replacing the missing teeth #47-#48.

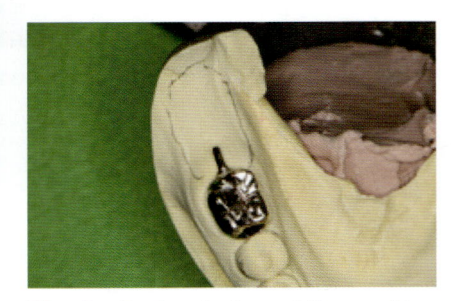

Fig. 8 Occlusal view of the working model for fabricating a Suginaka bolt clasp denture replacing the missing teeth #47-#48 region.

Fig. 9 Buccal view of the finished artificial teeth set-up for the Suginaka bolt clasp denture replacing the missing teeth #47-#48.

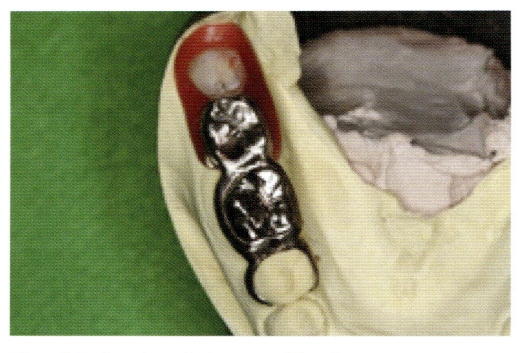

Fig. 10 Occlusal view as Fig. 9.

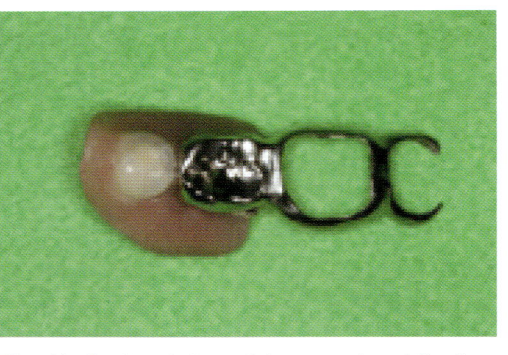

Fig. 11 Occlusal view of the completed Suginaka bolt clasp denture for missing teeth #47-#48.

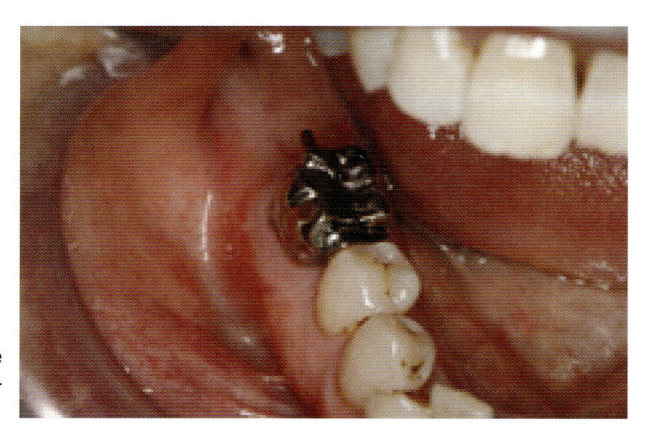

Fig. 12 Occlusal view of the full metal crown with a rod projection replacing the tooth #46.

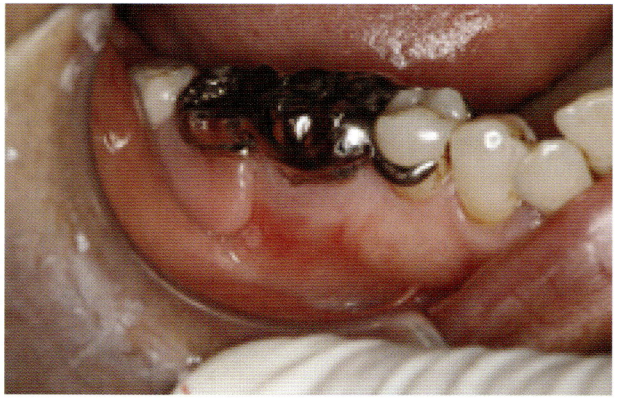

Fig. 13 Buccal view of the Suginaka bolt clasp denture replacing the missing teeth #47-#48.

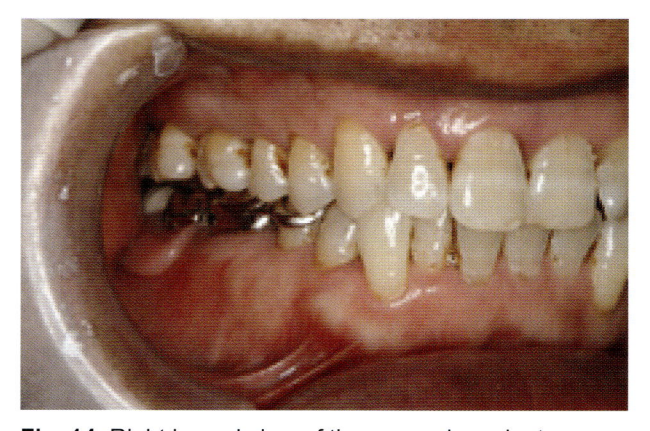

Fig. 14 Right buccal view of the same clasp denture.

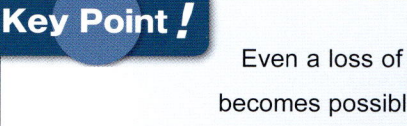

Key Point !

Even a loss of wisdom tooth, artificial teeth set-up including a wisdom tooth becomes possible if with a sufficient occlusal vertical dimension. When an extended-arm ring clasp is combined with a full cast crown with a projection, the ring clasp can be placed on the mesial marginal ridge of the restoration. In this case, no distal rest is placed for facilitating denture sinking and rotating. Of course, the clasp arms should be placed on the survey line.

1. Suginaka bolt attachment dentures

1) Suginaka bolt clasp dentures

④Unilateral distal extension missing case: Missing teeth #26-#27; Patient: 62-year-old woman
Tooth #25: Class 2 inlay with a rod projection
Teeth #24, #25: Extended-arm clasp

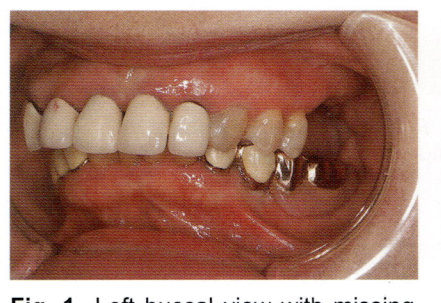

Fig. 1 Left buccal view with missing teeth #26-#27.

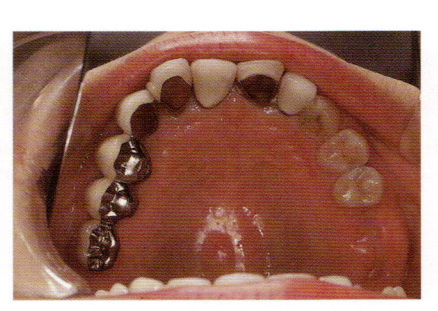

Fig. 2 Maxillary occlusal view with missing teeth #26-#27.

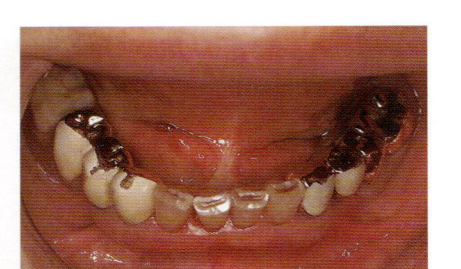

Fig. 3 Mandibular occlusal view.

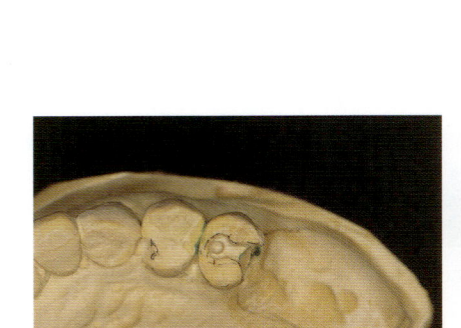

Fig. 4 Class 2 inlay cavity, in which a pinhole was prepared into the mesial cavity floor of tooth #25.

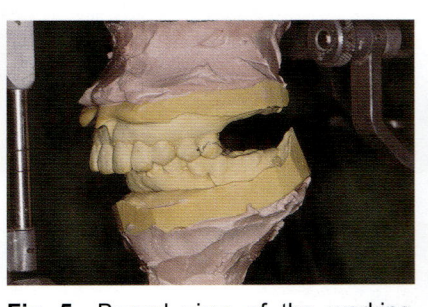

Fig. 5 Buccal view of the working model fabricated after taking an impression. In this case ,the teeth #26, #27 are lost and the teeth #24, #25 are abutment teeth.

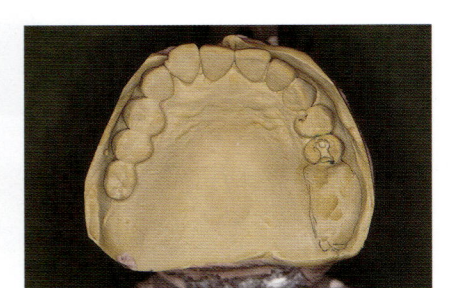

Fig. 6 Occlusal view of working model.

Fig. 7 Occlusal view of tooth #25, with a pinhole preparation for increasing retention of the inlay.

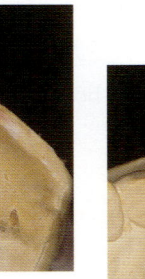

Fig. 8 Occlusal view of Class 2 inlay with a rod projection inserted in tooth #25. A rest seat prepared on the distal marginal ridge.

Fig. 9 An extended-arm clasp placed on teeth #24, #25. Artificial teeth set on the missing teeth #26-#27 (A metal tooth was made on the missing tooth #26 area). The buccal arm is shortened slightly, taking aesthetics into consideration.

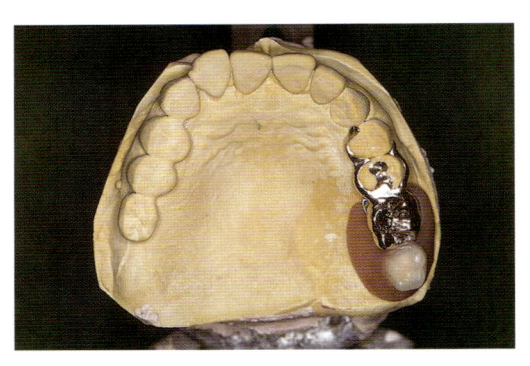

Fig. 10 Occlusal view of the completed Suginaka bolt clasp denture replacing the missing teeth #26-#27.

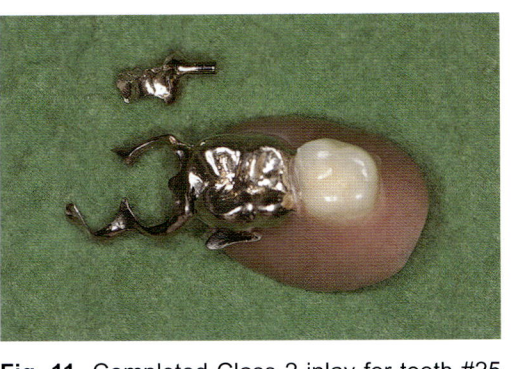

Fig. 11 Completed Class 2 inlay for tooth #25 and Suginaka bolt clasp denture for missing teeth #26-#27.

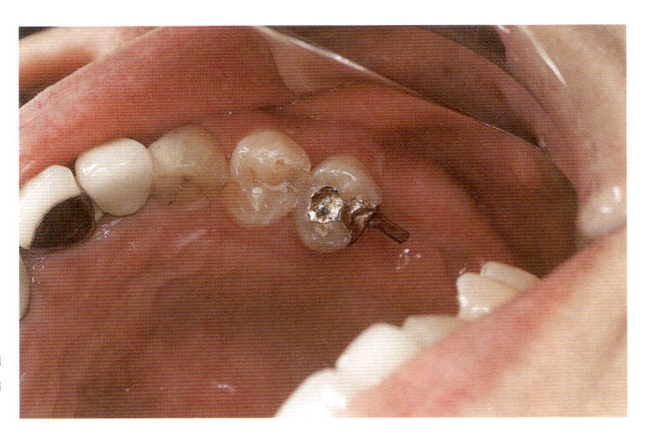

Fig. 12 Class 2 inlay with a rod projection inserted on tooth #25.

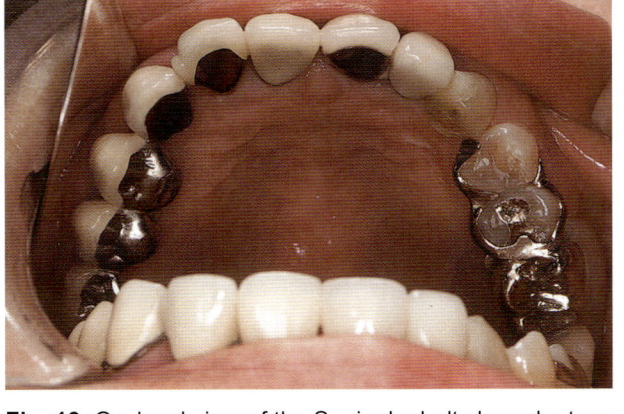

Fig. 13 Occlusal view of the Suginaka bolt clasp denture on the missing teeth #26-#27 region.

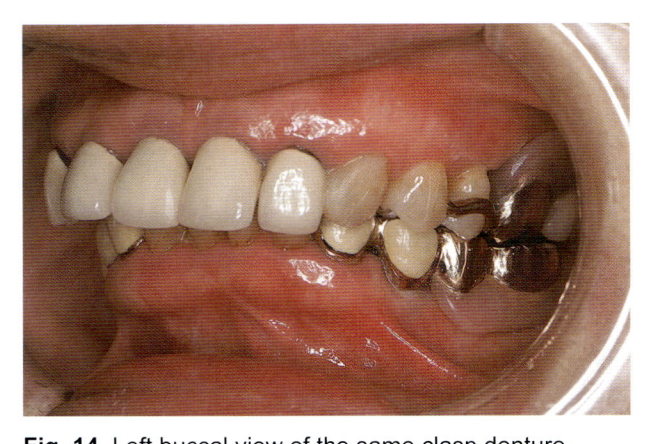

Fig. 14 Left buccal view of the same clasp denture.

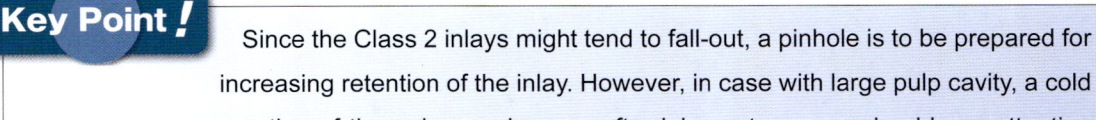

Key Point !

  Since the Class 2 inlays might tend to fall-out, a pinhole is to be prepared for increasing retention of the inlay. However, in case with large pulp cavity, a cold reaction of the pulp may happen after inlay set on, one should pay attention to it.

  If there happened something like that , a lock retainer should be used. Although the extended-arm clasp is designed on the survey line like this case, the tip of the buccal clasp arm can be stopped in the interproximal area.

1. Suginaka bolt attachment dentures

1) Suginaka bolt clasp dentures

⑤Unilateral distal extension missing case: Missing teeth #36-#37; Patient: 67-year-old woman
Tooth #35: Class 2 inlay with a rod projection
Teeth #34, #35: Extended-arm clasp

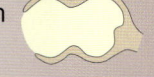

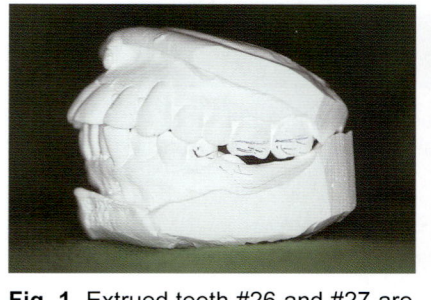

Fig. 1 Extrued teeth #26 and #27 are corrected to restore missing teeth #36-#37.

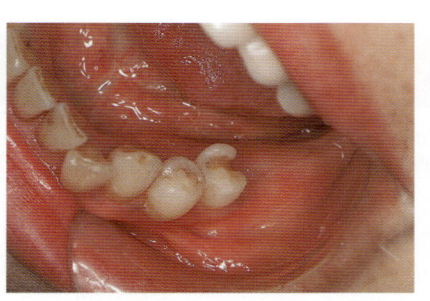

Fig. 2 Occlusal view of the same case. Class 2 cavity preparation of toorh #35.

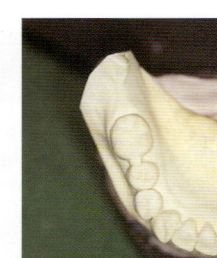

Fig. 3 Occlusal view of the mandibular working cast for fabricating a removable distal extension denture restoring missing teeth #36-# 37 , an inlay for #35.

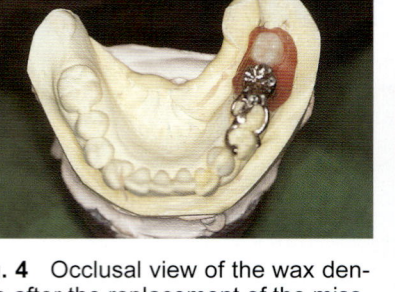

Fig. 4 Occlusal view of the wax denture after the replacement of the missing teeth #36-#37 with the artificial teeth. The class 2 inlay was placed on #35 and the extended-arm clasp was placed on #34 and #35. The extended-arm clasp with both mesial and distal rests were placed on #35 and the interproximal hook was placed between #33 and #34.

Fig. 5 Buccal view of the same case. The missing tooth#36 was replaced with the metal tooth.

Fig. 6 Completed class 2 inlay and Suginaka bolt clasp denture for missing teeth #36-#37.

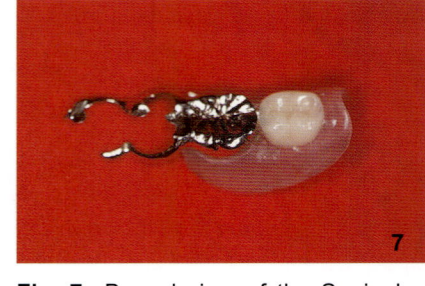

Fig. 7 Buccal view of the Suginaka bolt clasp denture for missing teeth #36-#37.

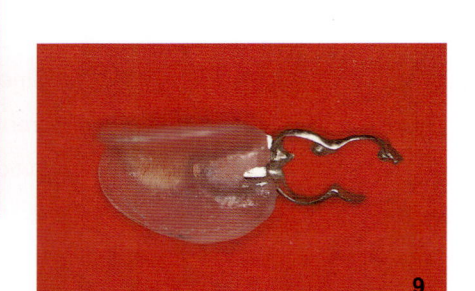

Fig. 8 Lingual view of the same case.

Fig. 9 Mucosal view of the same case.

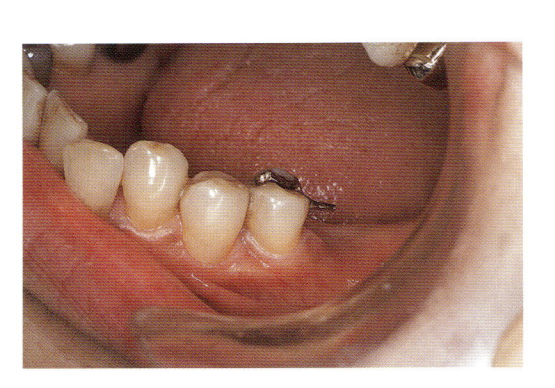

Fig. 10 Buccal view of the class 2 inlay with a rod projection placed on tooth #35.

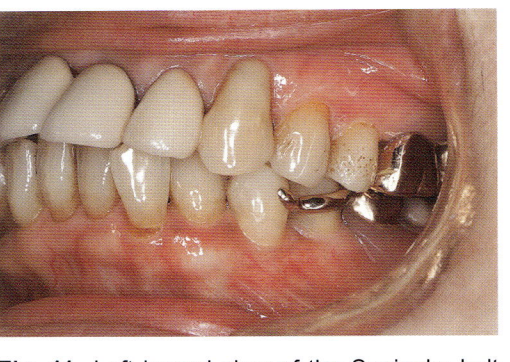

Fig. 11 Left buccal view of the Suginaka bolt clasp denture placed on the missing teeth #36-#37 region.

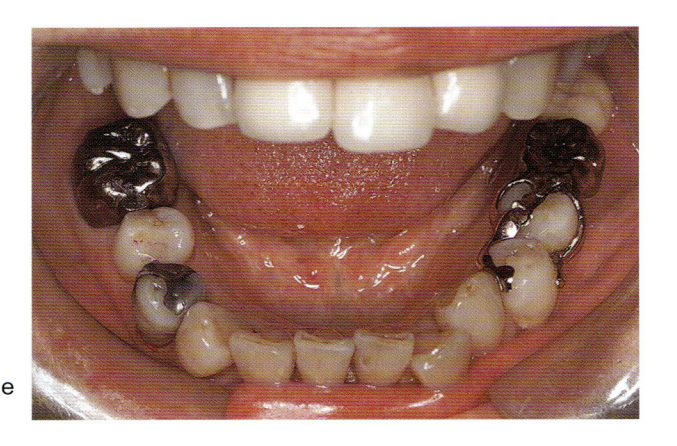

Fig. 12 Occlusal view of the same case.

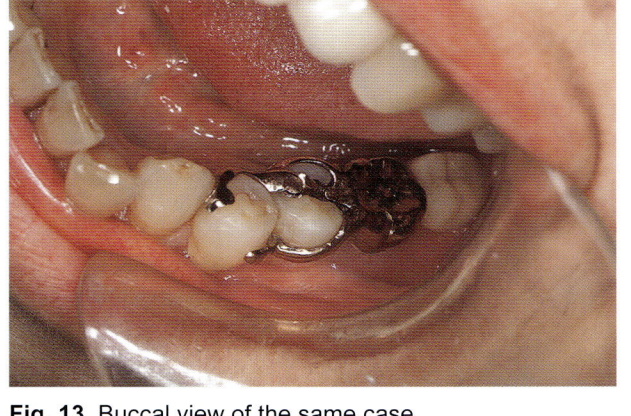

Fig. 13 Buccal view of the same case.

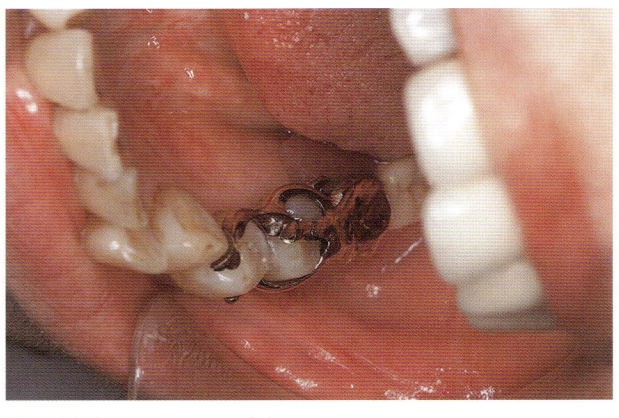

Fig. 14 Lingual view of the same case.

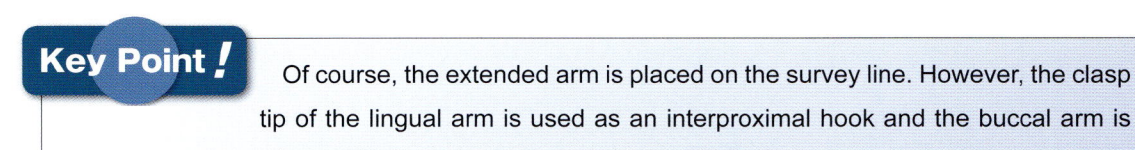

Key Point !   Of course, the extended arm is placed on the survey line. However, the clasp tip of the lingual arm is used as an interproximal hook and the buccal arm is stopped just short to the center of the crown on the mesial abutment tooth in this case.

1. Suginaka bolt attachment dentures

1) Suginaka bolt clasp dentures

⑥Unilateral distal extension missing case: Missing teeth #26-#27; Patient: 67-year-old woman
Tooth #25: Full metal crown with a plate projection
Teeth #24, #25: Extended-arm ring clasp

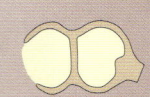

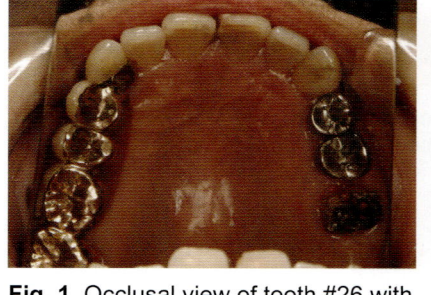

Fig. 1 Occlusal view of tooth #26 with root facture in maxilla.

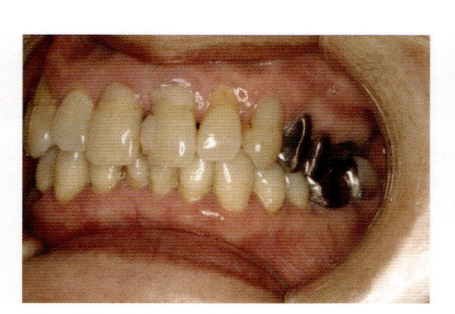

Fig. 2 Left buccal view.

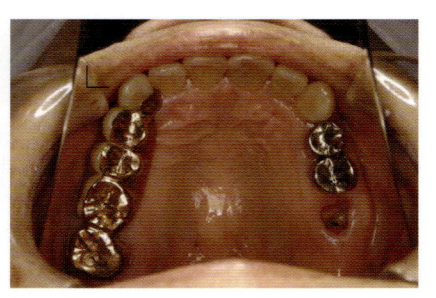

Fig. 3 Occlusal view one month after removal of #26.

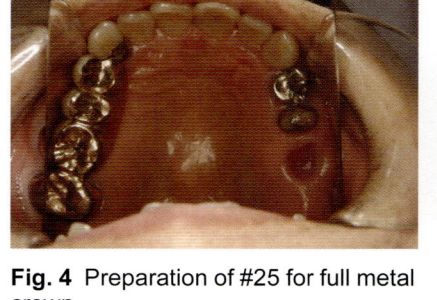

Fig. 4 Preparation of #25 for full metal crown.

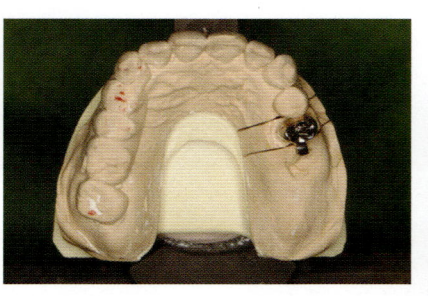

Fig. 5 Occlusal view of the full metal crown with a plate projection placed on #25. Rest seat preparation on distal marginal ridge.

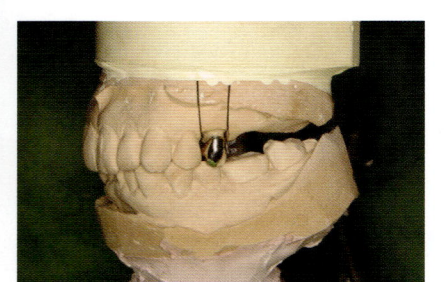

Fig. 6 Buccal view of #25. The mesial marginal ridge is formed so that an extended-arm ring clasp can be placed on it.

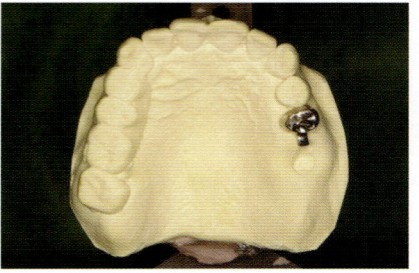

Fig. 7 A working cast is fabricated with a full metal crown placed on #25 receiving denture for missing teeth #26-#27.

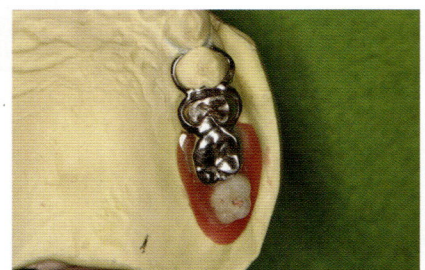

Fig. 8 Wax denture after the replacement of the missing teeth #26-#27 with the artificial teeth. The extended-arm ring clasp was placed on teeth #24, #25. The missing tooth #26 was replaced with the facing-type metal tooth involving a Suginaka bolt attachment.

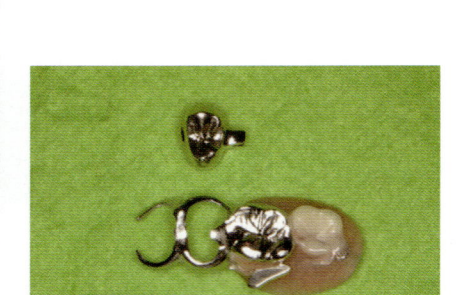

Fig. 9 Completed full metal crown with a plate projection placed on tooth #25 and Suginaka bolt clasp denture for missing teeth #26-#27, in which lever is opened.

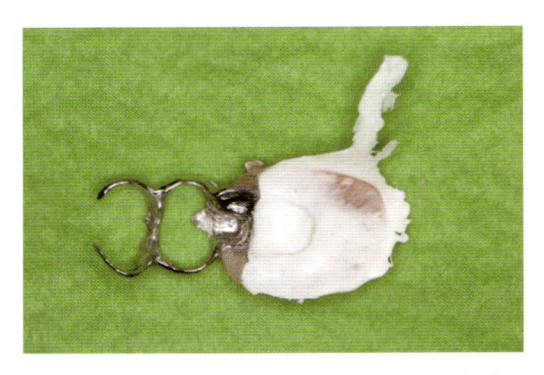

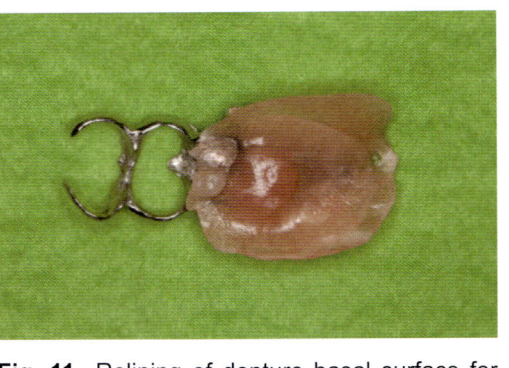

Fig. 10 Because one month has passed after removal of tooth #26, fit of denture basal surface is checked during placing Suginaka bolt clap denture.

Fig. 11 Relining of denture basal surface for missing teeth #26-#27 (before trimming).

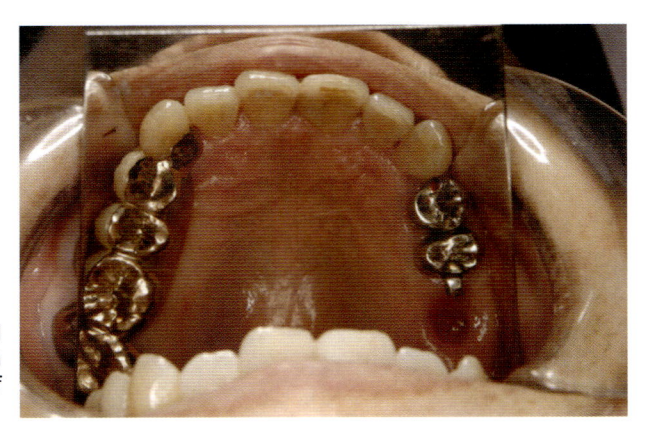

Fig. 12 Placement of full metal crown with a plate projection on tooth #25. Occlusal view of maxilla.

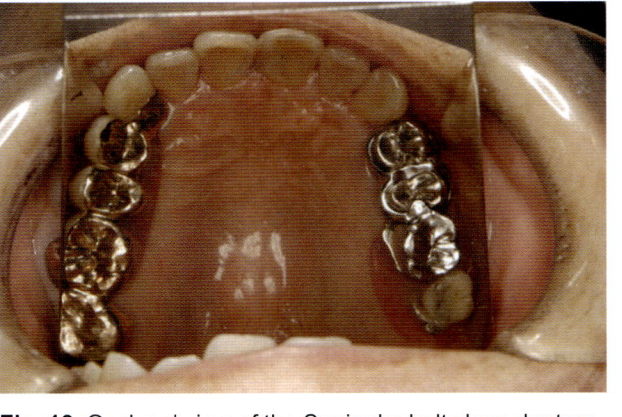

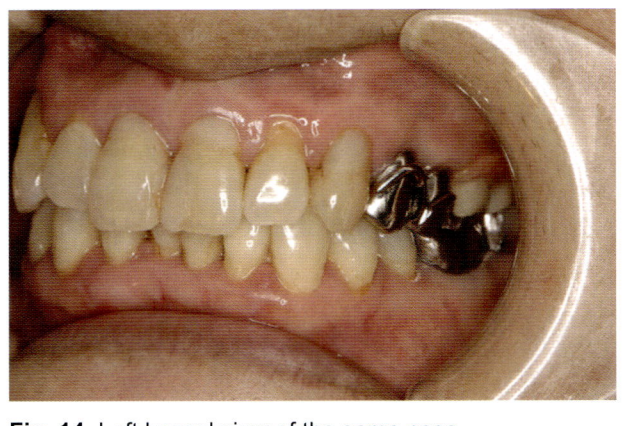

Fig. 13 Occlusal view of the Suginaka bolt clasp denture, in which an extended-arm ring clasp was placed on teeth #24, #25 in maxilla.

Fig. 14 Left buccal view of the same case.

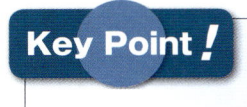
Key Point !
　　Both the clasp arm and tip of the extended-arm ring clasp have to be placed above the survey line, In case, the denture relining was required repeatedly because the denture was completed one month after removal of tooth #26. After this case, the author re-realized that healing of extraction wound is required above 3 months. In addition, because of short base, a mesial rest should have been set rather than a distal rest.

1. Suginaka bolt attachment dentures

1) Suginaka bolt clasp dentures

⑦Unilateral distal extension missing case: Missing teeth #36-#37; Patient: 59-year-old man

Tooth #34: Full metal crown
Tooth #35: Full metal crown with a rod projection
Teeth #34, #35: Extended-arm ring clasp

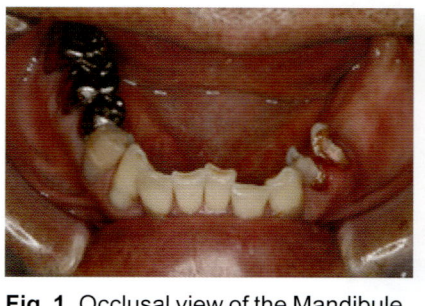

Fig. 1 Occlusal view of the Mandibule.

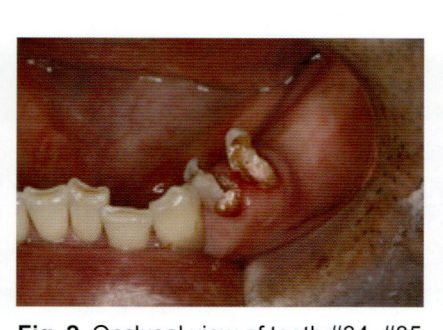

Fig. 2 Occlusal view of teeth #34, #35 with coronal fracture.

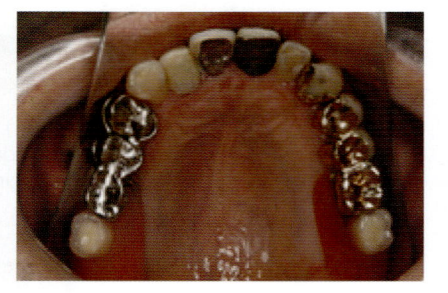

Fig. 3 Occlusal view of the Maxilla.

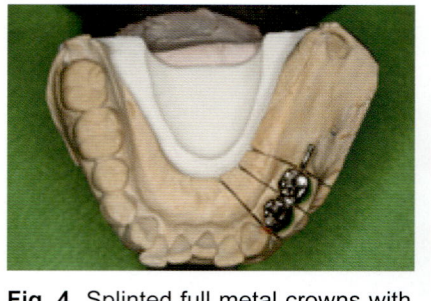

Fig. 4 Splinted full metal crowns with a rod projection on teeth #34, #35.

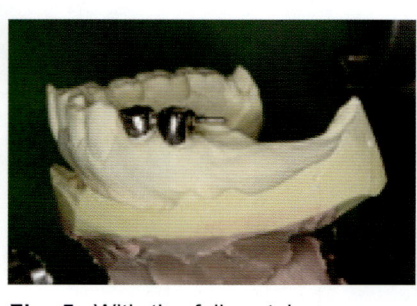

Fig. 5 With the full metal crowns on the working cast receiving the denture replacing the missing teeth #36-#37.

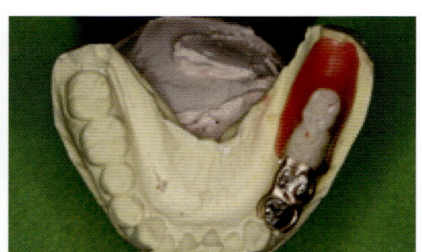

Fig. 6 Occlusal view of the wax denture for try-in after the replacement of the missing teeth #36-#37 with the artificial teeth. The extended-arm ring clasp was placed on teeth #34, #35.

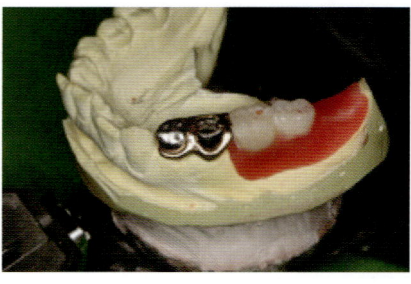

Fig. 7 Buccal view of the denture, the missing tooth #36 was replaced with a metal tooth covered fully with a hybrid resin.

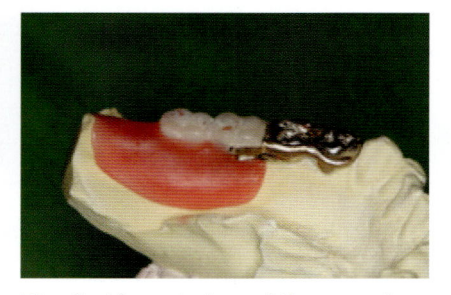

Fig. 8 Lingual view of the wax denture, a Suginaka bolt attachment was embedded into the denture base.

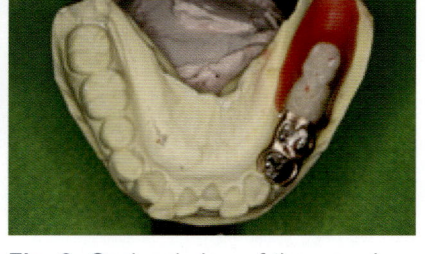

Fig. 9 Buccal view of the completed Suginaka bolt clasp denture.

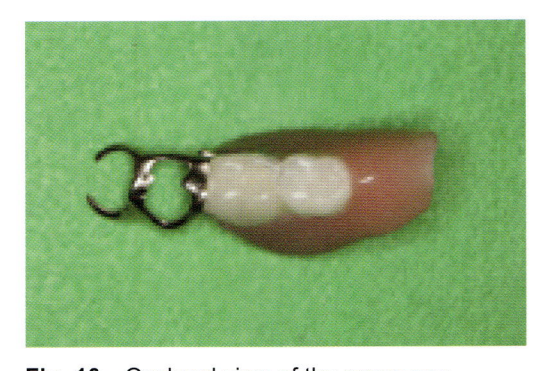

Fig. 10 Occlusal view of the same one.

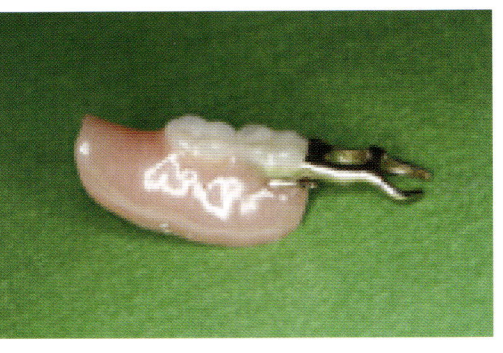

Fig. 11 Lingual view of the same one.

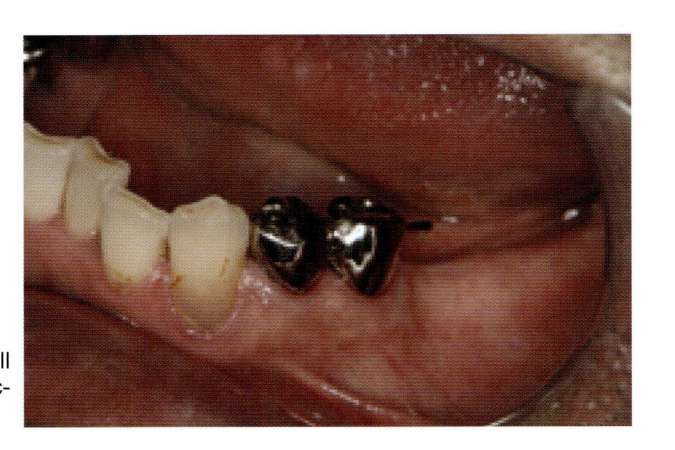

Fig. 12 Buccal view of the full metal crowns with a rod projection placed on teeth #34, #35.

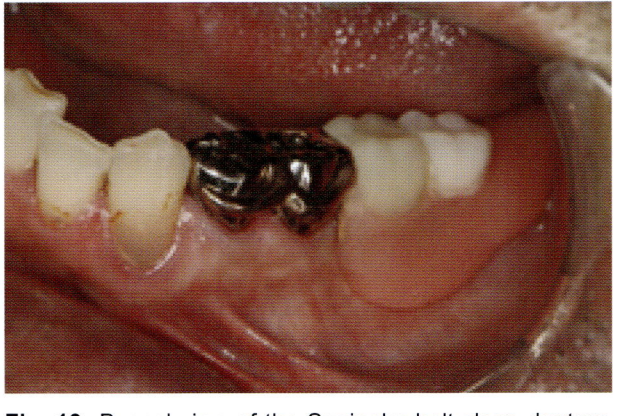

Fig. 13 Buccal view of the Suginaka bolt clasp denture placed on the missing teeth #36-#37 region, in which the extended-arm ring clasp was placed on teeth #34, #35 (both full metal crowns).

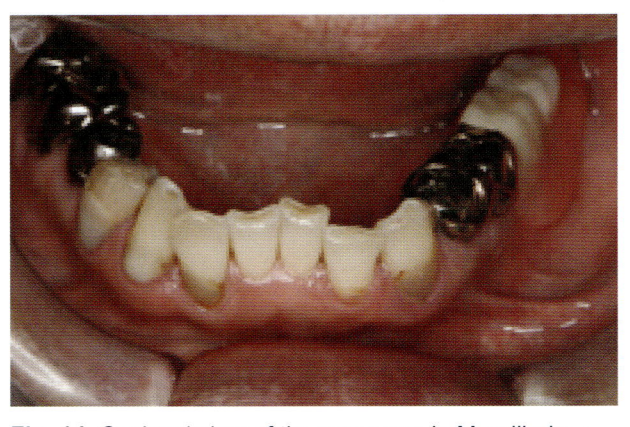

Fig. 14 Occlusal view of the same one in Mandibule.

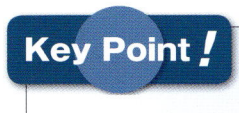

Key Point !

In case, teeth #34, #35 may be used as telescope denture abutment teeth, more tooth structure could be lost by tooth preparation due to brittle tooth substance. Therefore, the connected full metal crowns and a clasp or lock retainer should be used, avoiding telescope crowns.

1. Suginaka bolt attachment dentures

1) Suginaka bolt clasp dentures

⑧Unilateral distal extension missing case: Missing teeth #45-#47; Patient: 63-year-old man
Tooth #44: Class 2 post inlay with a plate projection
Teeth #43, #44: Extended-arm ring clasp

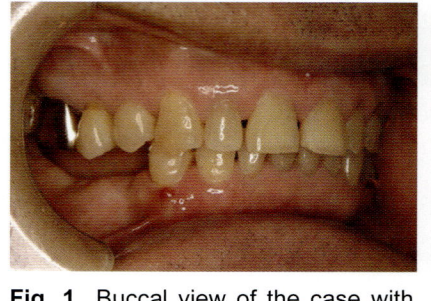

Fig. 1 Buccal view of the case with missing teeth #45-#47.

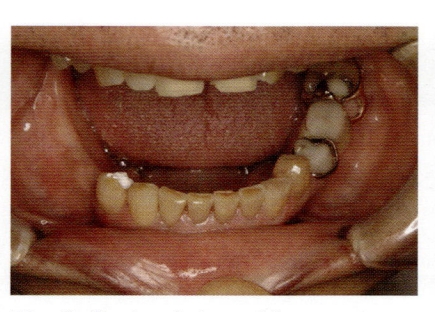

Fig. 2 Occlusal view of the same one in Mandibule Tooth #44 with infected root canal.

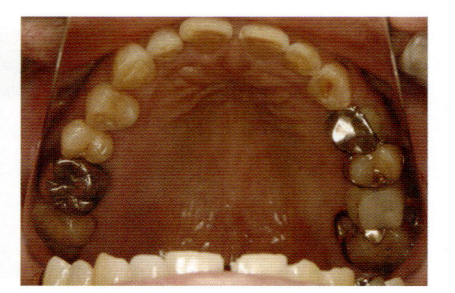

Fig. 3 Occlusal view of the Maxilla.

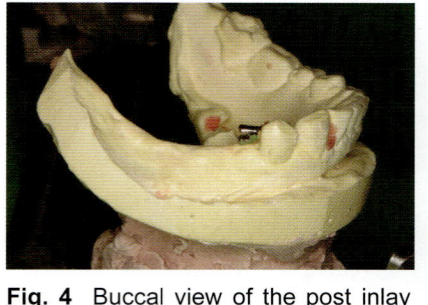

Fig. 4 Buccal view of the post inlay with a plate projection placed into tooth #44.

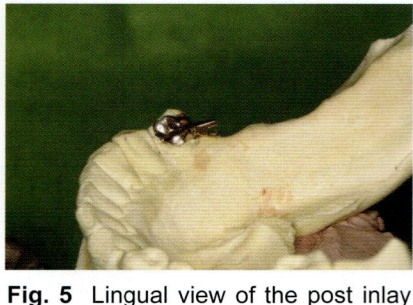

Fig. 5 Lingual view of the post inlay for tooth #44.

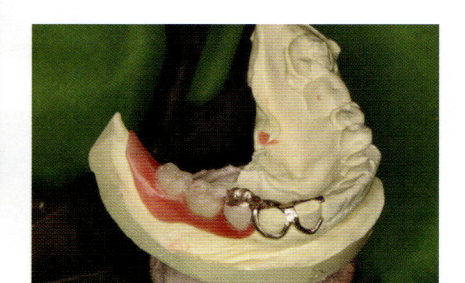

Fig. 6 Buccal view of the wax denture after the replacement of the missing teeth #46 ,#47 with the artificial teeth. The extended-arm ring clasp was on teeth #43 and #44. The missing tooth #45 was replaced with the facing metal crown involving a Suginaka bolt attachment.

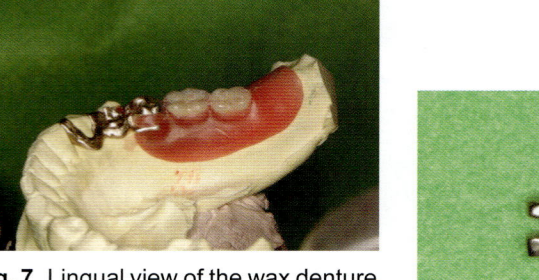

Fig. 7 Lingual view of the wax denture after the replacement of the missing teeth #45-#47 with the artificial teeth.

Fig. 8 A post inlay with a plate projection for tooth #44.

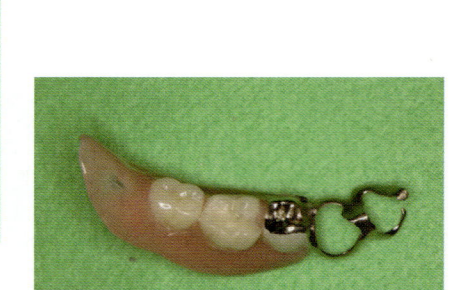

Fig. 9 Completed Suginaka bolt clasp denture for missing teeth #45-#47.

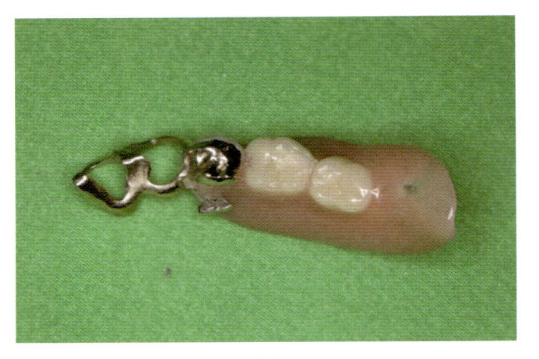

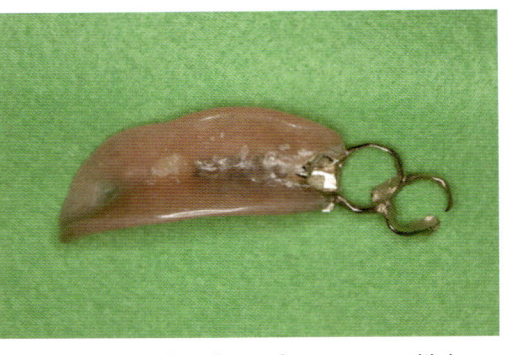

Fig. 10 Lingual view of the same one.

Fig. 11 Mucosal surface of same one with lever closed.

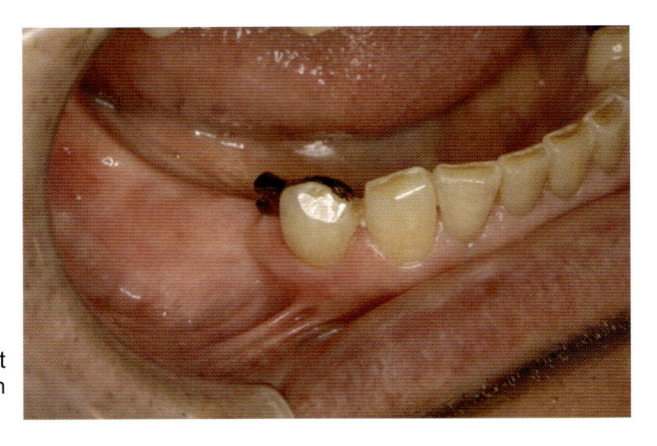

Fig. 12 Buccal view of the post inlay with a plate projection placed on teeth #44.

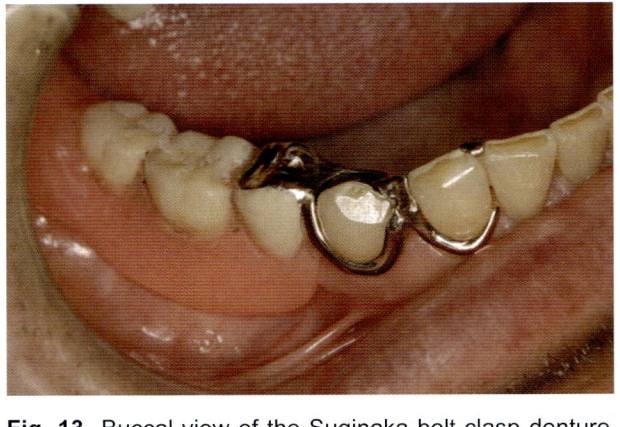

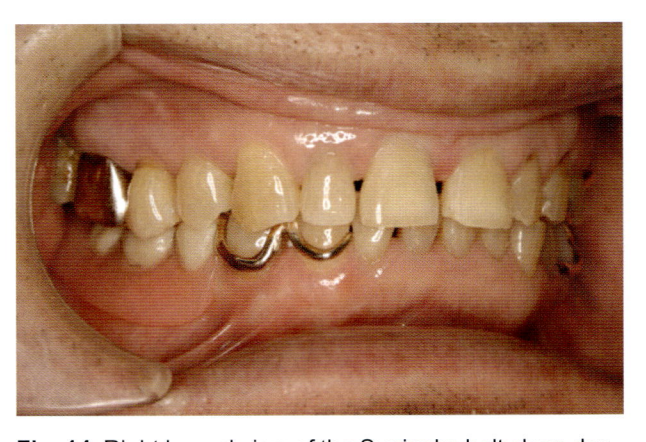

Fig. 13 Buccal view of the Suginaka bolt clasp denture with an extended-arm ring clasp (placed on teeth #43, #44) placed on missing teeth #45-#47 region.

Fig. 14 Right buccal view of the Suginaka bolt clasp denture for missing teeth #45-#47 region placed in mouth.

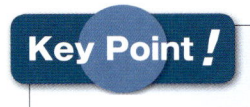 **Key Point !**

When the unilateral distal extension missing teeth #45-#47 is unilaterally restored, the hard edentulous mucosa and wide edentulous ridge allow application of an extended-arm ring arm, but in case with soft mucosa and narrow residual ridge, it is contraindicated. Similarly, in case the maxillary unilateral distal extension cases, it cannot be restored unilaterally.

1. Suginaka bolt attachment dentures

1) Suginaka bolt clasp dentures

⑨Unilateral distal extension missing case: Missing teeth #44-#47; Patient: 65-year-old man
Tooth #43: Porcelain fused to metal crown (PFM crown) with a plate projection
Teeth #43: Cingulum rest (variation of occlusal rest and lingual arm)

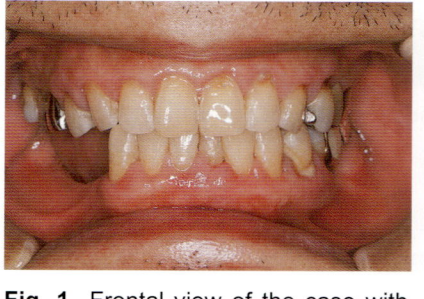

Fig. 1 Frontal view of the case with missing teeth #44-#47.

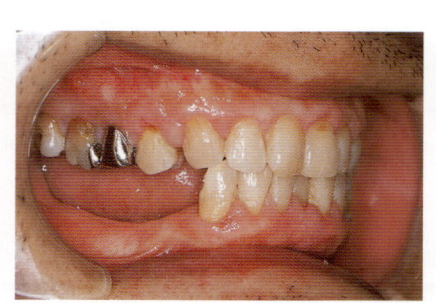

Fig. 2 Right buccal view.

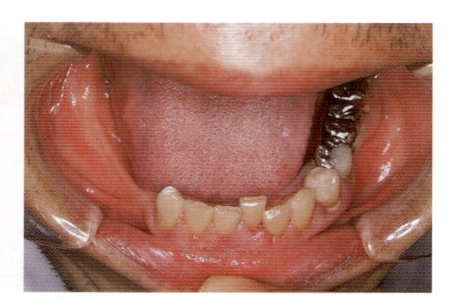

Fig. 3 Mandibular occlusal view.

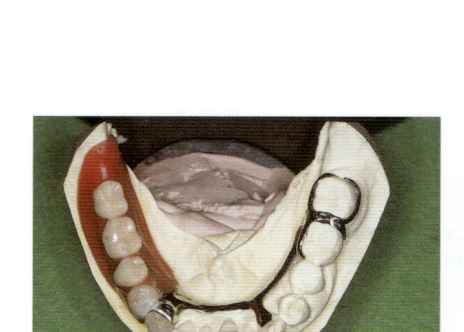

Fig. 4 Preparation of tooth #43 for PFM crown.

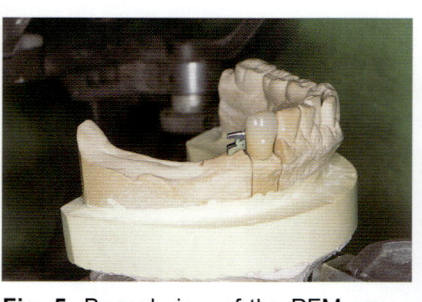

Fig. 5 Buccal view of the PFM crown with a plate projection to be placed on tooth #43.

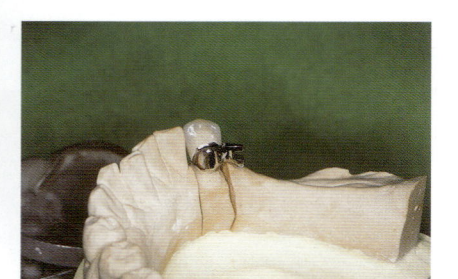

Fig. 6 Cingulum rest seat formed on lingual surface of tooth #43.

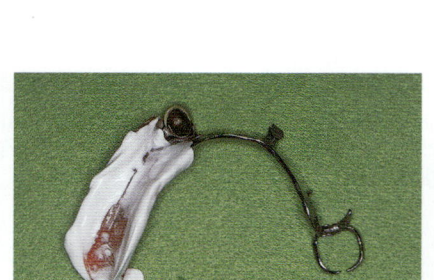

Fig. 7 Completed cast bar with a cingulum rest to be placed on tooth #43. There was an inter-arch space sufficient to involve a Suginaka bolt attachment in the missing tooth #44 region, in which the artificial tooth could be placed. Missing teeth #45-#47 were replaced with the artificial teeth.

Fig. 8 Checking denture base fit in the wax denture after the replacement of the missing teeth #44-#47 with the artificial teeth.

Fig. 9 Occlusal bite impression with the wax denture.

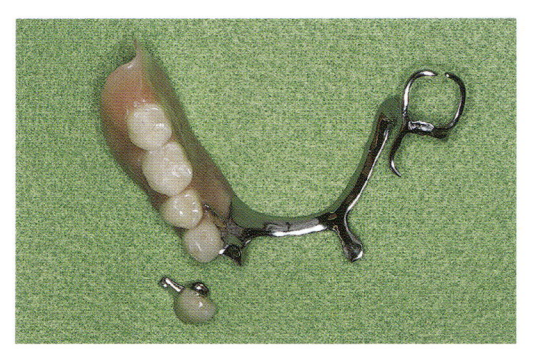

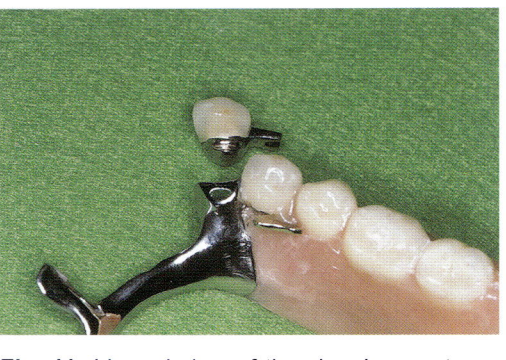

Fig. 10 A PFM crown with a plate projection to be placed on tooth #43 and completed Suginaka bolt clasp denture with missing teeth #44-#47 were replaced with the artificial teeth. Shortened buccal clasp in a double clasp for teeth #36, #37.

Fig. 11 Lingual view of the cingulum rest prepared on tooth #43. A non-metal artificial tooth was used in the missing tooth #44.

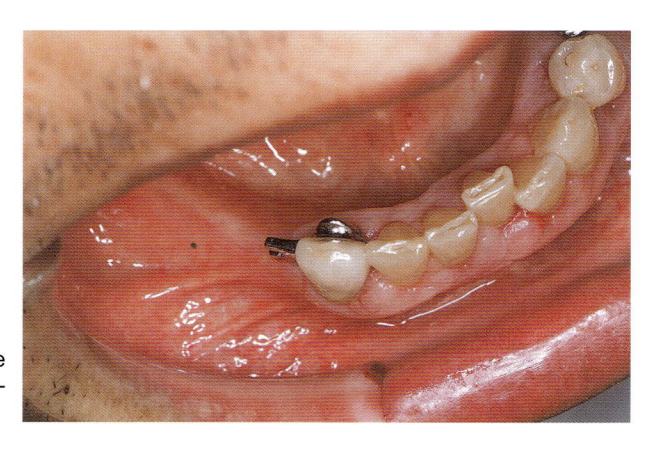

Fig. 12 Occlusal view of the PFM crown with a plate projection placed on tooth #43.

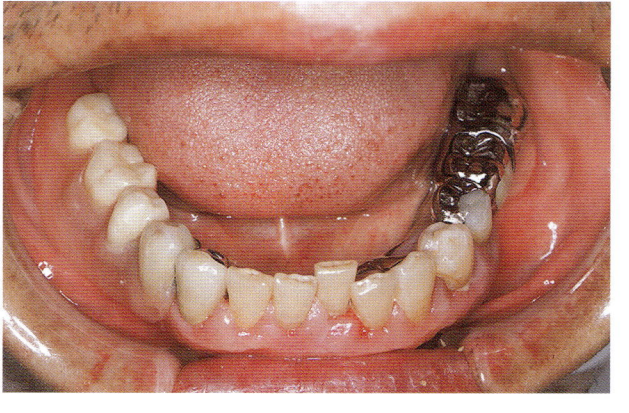

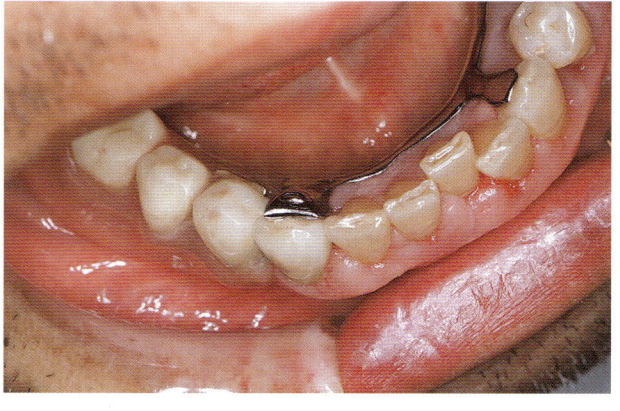

Fig. 13 Lower occlusal view of the Suginaka bolt clasp denture for missing teeth #44-#47.

Fig. 14 Lingual view of the cingulum rest placed on tooth #43.

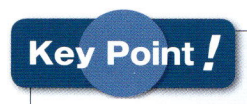
Key Point !

For crown restoration with the canine as an abutment, a cingulum rest should be provided on the lingual surface. This form is most suitable for occlusal support with the canine.

1. Suginaka bolt attachment dentures

1) Suginaka bolt clasp dentures

⑩Tooth bounded missing case: Missing teeth #36-#37; Patient: 64-year-old woman

Tooth #35: Full metal crown with a rod projection

Teeth #34, #35: Extended-arm ring clasp

Tooth #38: Akers clasp

Tooth #37: Overdenture (denture over stump)

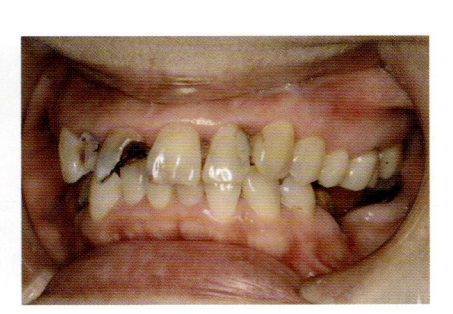

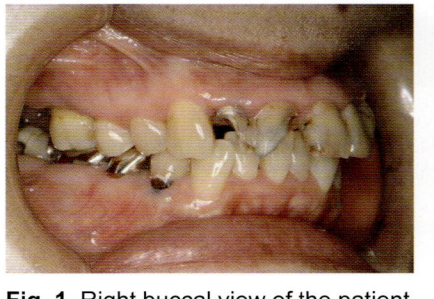

Fig. 1 Right buccal view of the patient during first visit.

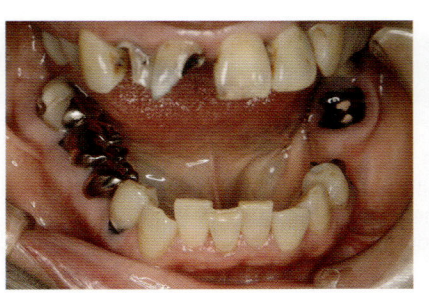

Fig. 2 Lower occlusal view at the same time.

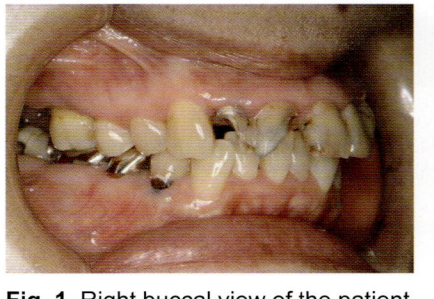

Fig. 3 Left buccal view at the same time.

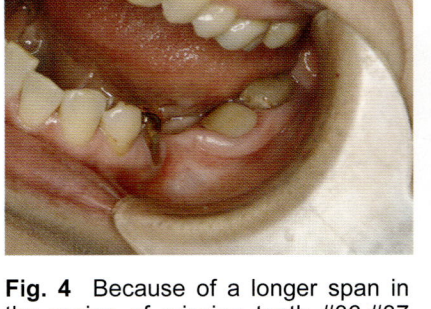

Fig. 4 Because of a longer span in the region of missing teeth #36-#37 and a shorter root of tooth #38, it was decided to fabricate a RPD rather than a bridge. An overdenture on tooth #37 inadequate as an abutment.

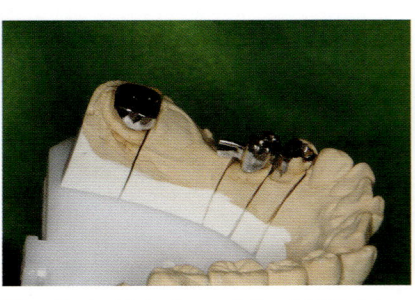

Fig. 5 Labial view of the MOD inlay placed on tooth #34, full metal crown with a rod projection placed on tooth #35, full metal crown placed on tooth #38, and guide planes parallel to each other formed on the mesial surface of tooth #38 and the distal surface of tooth #36.

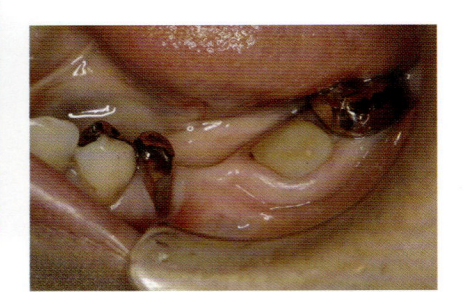

Fig. 6 Inlay placed on tooth #34 and full metal crown placed on tooth #38. An overdenture on #37.

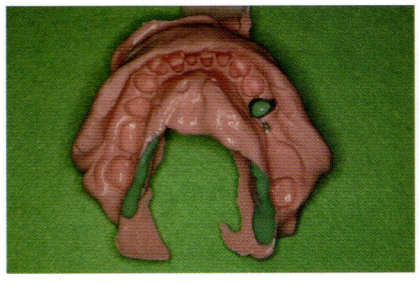

Fig. 7 Impression taking of the missing teeth #36-#37 with the full metal crown on tooth #35. Then, the crown is returned to the impression and agar impression material was packed into the crown, leaving the cervical third region of the crown, and then pouring dental stone into the impression.

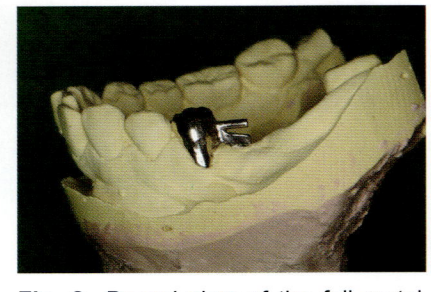

Fig. 8 Buccal view of the full metal crown with a rod projection for tooth #35 returned to the working model with missing teeth #36-#37. A plate projection was provided to eliminate the dead space located below the rod projection.

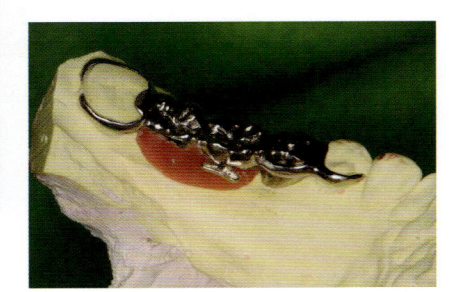

Fig. 9 Lingual view of RPD for missing teeth #36-#37 replaced with the metal teeth, in which an extended-arm ring clasp was placed on teeth #34, #35 and an Akers clasp was placed on tooth #38.

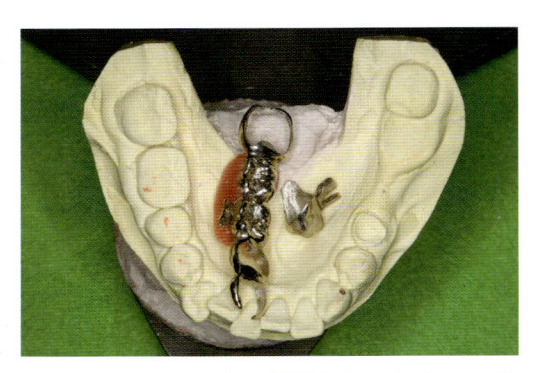

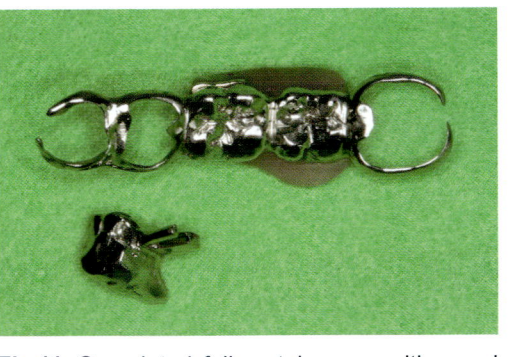

Fig. 10 During try-in of RPD for missing teeth #36-#37 replaced with the artificial teeth (metal teeth), the crown placed on #35 can be easily removed using an ultrasonic scaler.

Fig.11 Completed full metal crown with a rod projection to be placed on tooth #35 and Suginaka bolt clasp denture for missing teeth #36-#37.

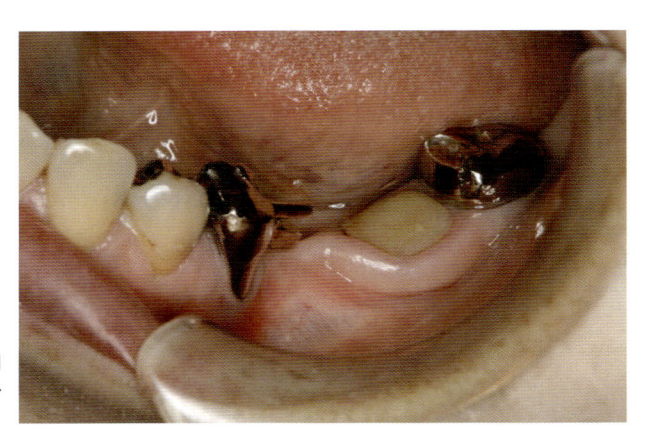

Fig. 12 Buccal view of the full metal crown with a rod projection placed on tooth #35.

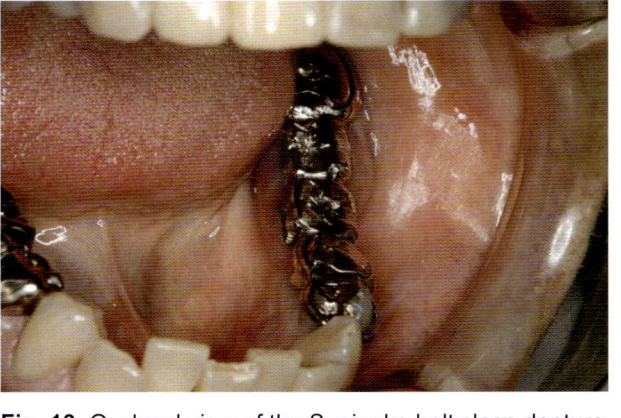

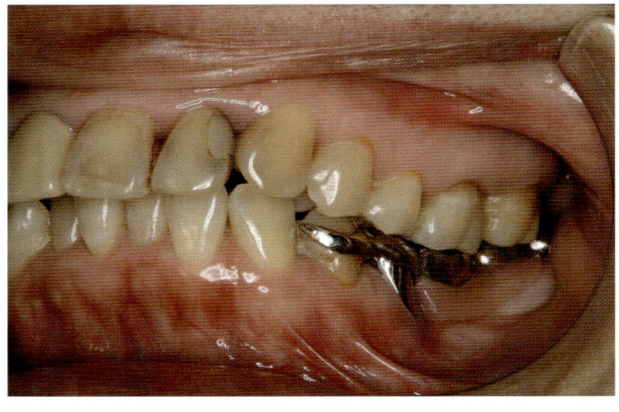

Fig. 13 Occlusal view of the Suginaka bolt clasp denture placed on the missing teeth #36-#37 region, in which the extended-arm ring clasp and the Akers clasp were used as retainers.

Fig. 14 Left buccal view of the Suginaka bolt clasp denture for an tooth bounded missing case (missing teeth #36-#37) with the extended-arm ring clasp and the Akers clasp.

 **Key Point !** The extended-arm ring clasp placed on teeth #34, #35, Akers clasp placed on tooth #38, and metal teeth for missing teeth #36-#37 are cast in once-piece. During wax-up in the mesial interproximal area of tooth #35, a space, in which an extended-arm ring clasp can pass, should be prepared. Both clasps (including the clasp tip) should be placed on the survey line.

1. Suginaka bolt attachment dentures

1) Suginaka bolt clasp dentures

⑪Bilateral distal extension missing case: Missing teeth #46-#47, #36-#37; Patient:58-year-old woman

Teeth #35, #45: MOD inlay with a rod projection

Teeth #35, #45: Lingual arm with a marginal rest

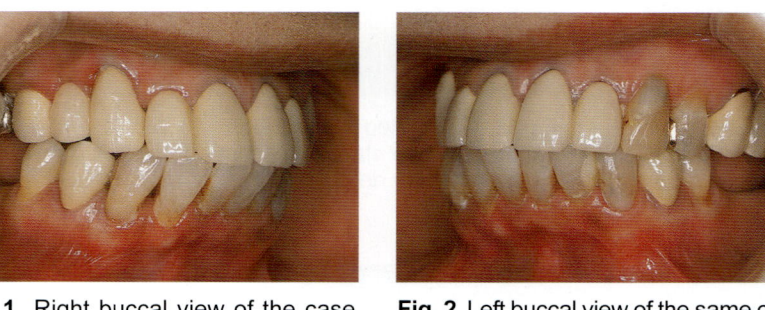

Fig. 1 Right buccal view of the case with missing teeth #46-#47, #36-#37.

Fig. 2 Left buccal view of the same one.

Fig. 3 Occlusal view of the same one.

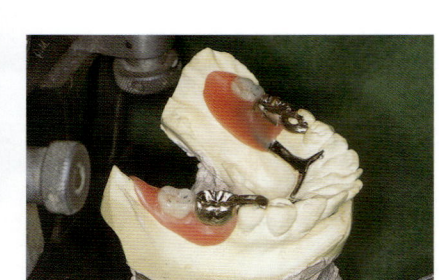

Fig. 4 Occlusal view of the MOD inlay with a rod projection placed on tooth #45.

Fig. 5 Occlusal view of the MOD inlay with a rod projection placed on tooth #35.

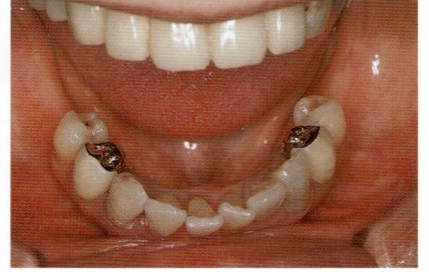

Fig. 6 Buccal view of the wax denture after the replacement of the missing tooth #46 (metal tooth) and #47 with the artificial tooth. The lingual arm with a marginal rest placed to be placed tooth #45 and the metal tooth involving a Suginaka bolt attachment were one-piece casted.

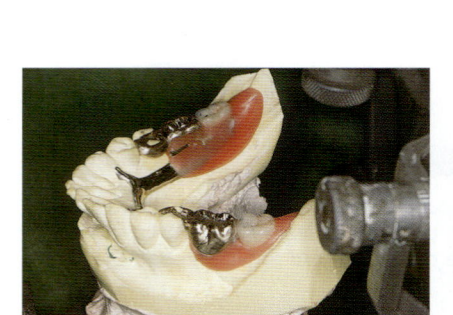

Fig. 7 Buccal view of the same one on the opposite side.

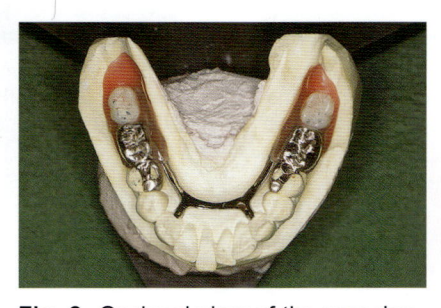

Fig. 8 Occlusal view of the wax denture after the replacement of the missing teeth #46-#47, #36-#37 with the artificial teeth. The lingual bar was placed in the denture base without soldering.

Fig. 9 Right occluso-lingual view of the completed Suginaka bolt clasp denture for missing teeth #46-#47, #36-#37.

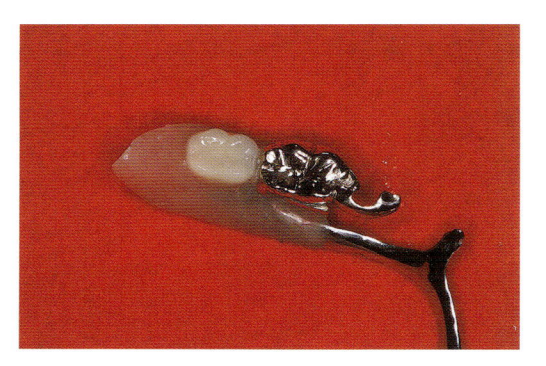

Fig. 10 Left occluso-lingual view of the same one.

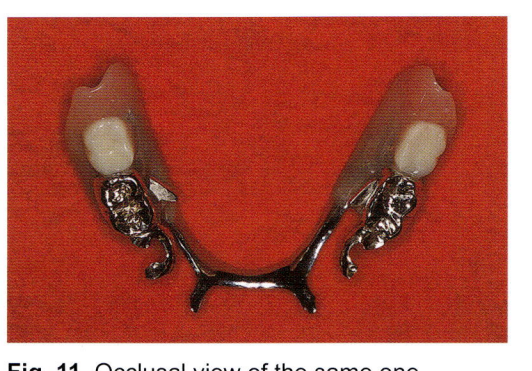

Fig. 11 Occlusal view of the same one.

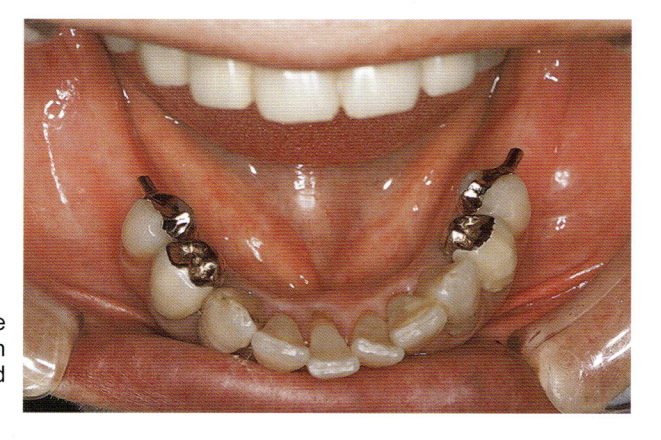

Fig. 12 Occlusal view of the MOD inlay with a rod projection placed on both teeth #35 and #45.

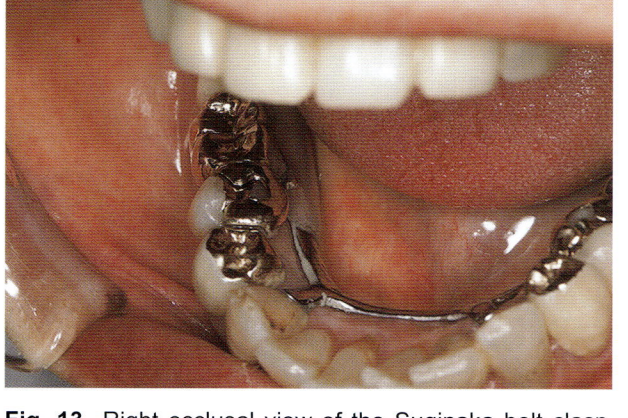

Fig. 13 Right occlusal view of the Suginaka bolt clasp denture for missing teeth #46-47, #36-#37 placed in the mouth.

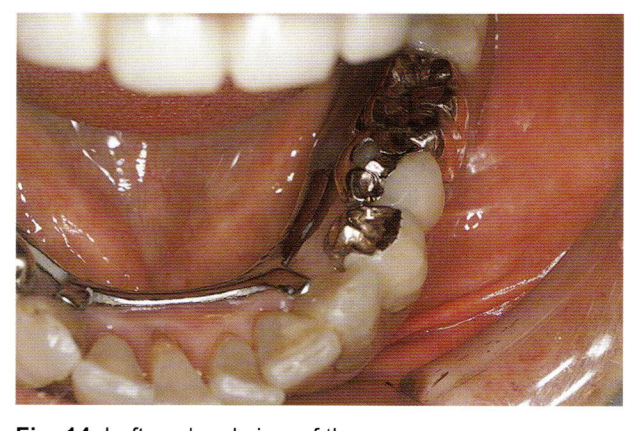

Fig. 14 Left occlusal view of the same one.

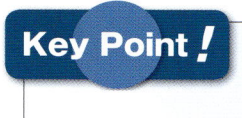

To enhance retention, the mesiodistal axial walls of the MOD inlay should be parallelly and more widely prepared.

1. Suginaka bolt attachment dentures

1) Suginaka bolt clasp dentures

⑫ Bilateral distal extension missing case: Missing teeth #45-#47, #36-#37; Patient: 58-year-old woman
Teeth #35, #44: Full metal crown with a rod projection
Teeth #35, #44: Lingual arm with a marginal rest

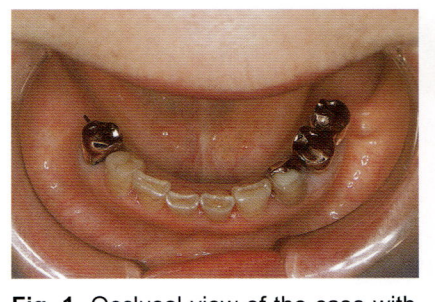

Fig. 1 Occlusal view of the case with missing teeth #45-#47, #36-#37.

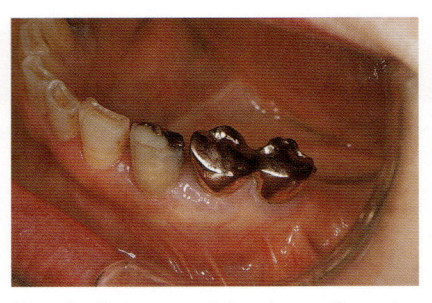

Fig. 2 Fracture of the 1mm-diameter rod projection provided on the crown placed on tooth #35.

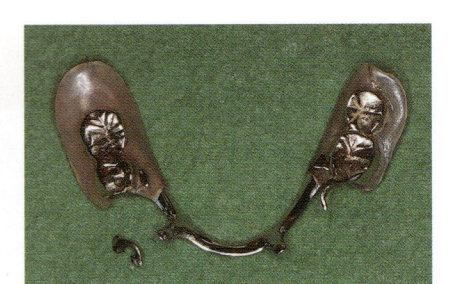

Fig. 3 Fractured lingual arm with a marginal rest placed on tooth #44 in the Suginaka bolt clasp denture for missing teeth #45-#46, #36-#37.

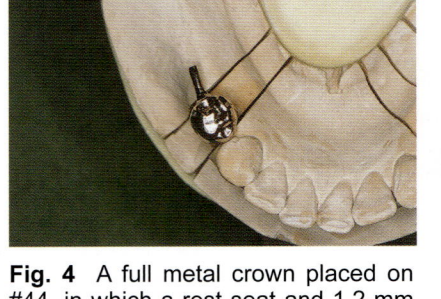

Fig. 4 A full metal crown placed on #44, in which a rest seat and 1.2-mm diameter rod projection were provided.

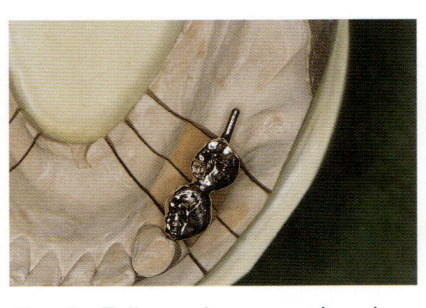

Fig. 5 Full metal crowns placed on #34 and #35, in which a rest seat and 1.2-mm diameter rod projection were provided.

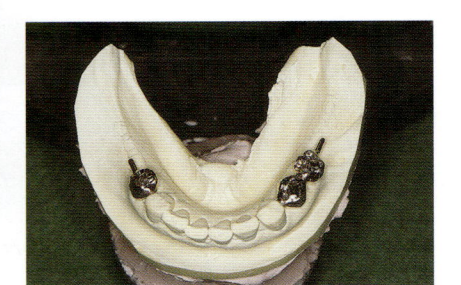

Fig. 6 Working cast for the replacement of missing teeth #45-#47, #36-#37.

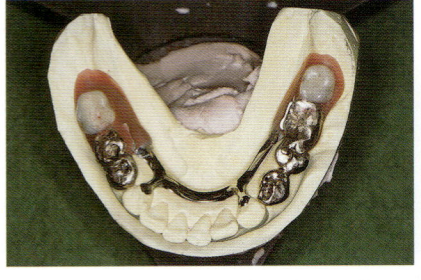

Fig. 7 Wax denture after the replacement of the missing teeth #45-#46, #36-#37 (no replacement of #47) with the artificial teeth. However, each lingual arm with a marginal rest placed on #44, #35 and each metal tooth to replace missing teeth #45 and #36 involving a Suginaka bolt attachment were cast in one-piece, respectively.

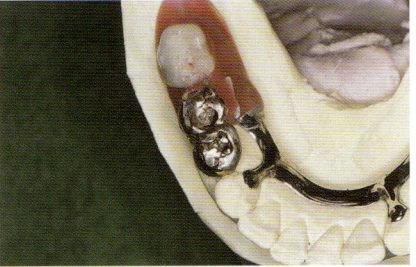

Fig. 8 Occlusal view of the lingual arm with a marginal rest placed on #44.

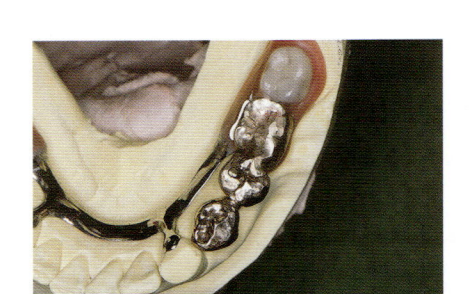

Fig. 9 Occlusal view of the lingual arm with a marginal rest placed on #35.

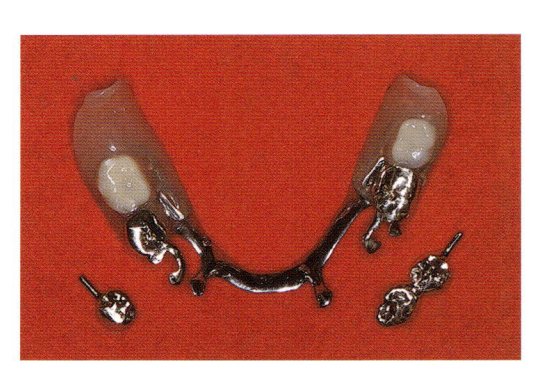

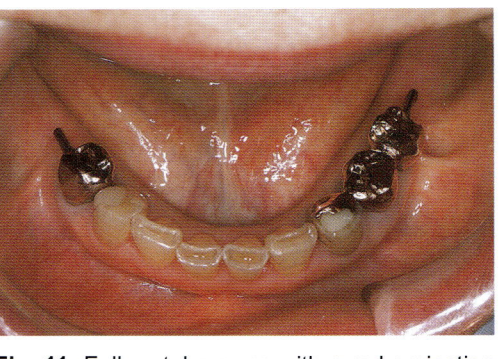

Fig. 10 Completed full metal crowns with a rod projection for #44, #34, #35 and Suginaka bolt clasp denture for missing #45-#46, #36-#37 replaced.

Fig. 11 Full metal crowns with a rod projection placed on #44, #34, and #35.

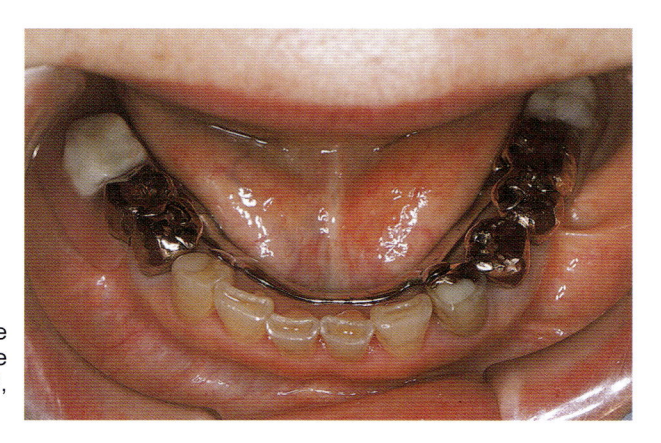

Fig. 12 Occlusal view of the Suginaka bolt clasp denture placed on the missing #45-#46, #36-#37 region.

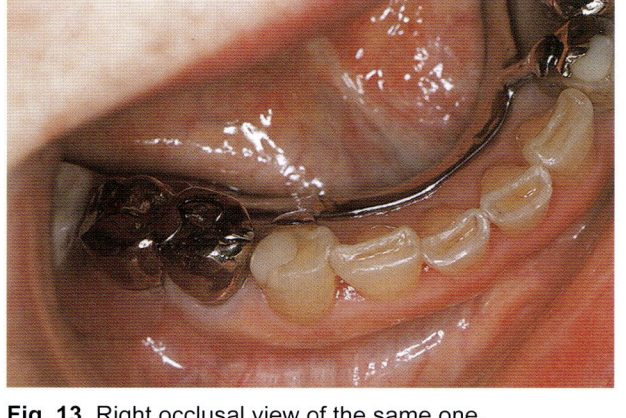

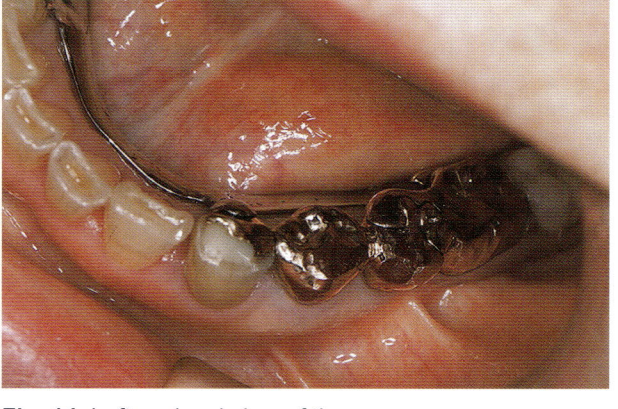

Fig. 13 Right occlusal view of the same one.

Fig. 14 Left occlusal view of the same one.

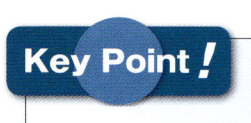 **Key Point !**

Because the use of a 1.0-mm diameter rod projection may be risky for facture, a 1.2-mm diameter one should be used. In addition, as the junction between the lingual arm and the metal tooth often causes fracture, a sufficient thickness is required for strength.

1. Suginaka bolt attachment dentures

1) Suginaka bolt clasp dentures

⑬ Bilateral distal extension missing case: Missing teeth #15-#17, #27; Patient: 52-year-old woman

Tooth #13: Porcelain fused to metal crown (PFM crown)
Tooth #14: PFM crown with a plate projection
Tooth #14: Lingual arm with an occlusal rest

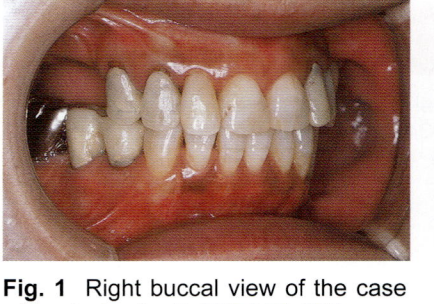

Fig. 1 Right buccal view of the case with missing teeth #15-#17, #27.

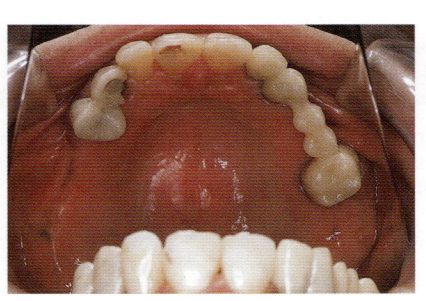

Fig. 2 Occlusal view of the same one. Temporary crowns for teeth #13, #14 and #22-26 (pontics: #24, #25).

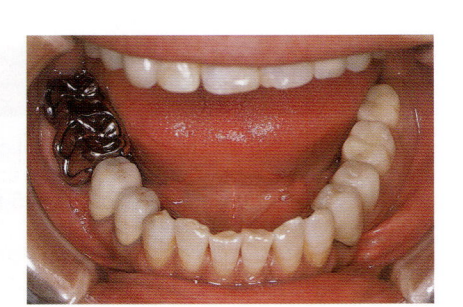

Fig. 3 Lower occlusal view.

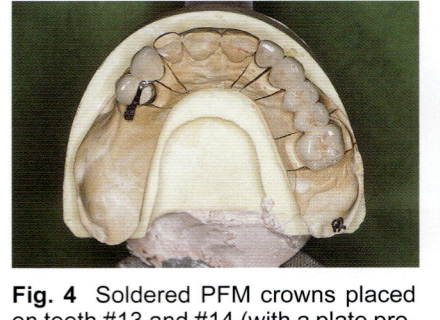

Fig. 4 Soldered PFM crowns placed on teeth #13 and #14 (with a plate projection). A fixed bridge for #22, #23, #24, #25, and #26 (pontics: #24, #25).

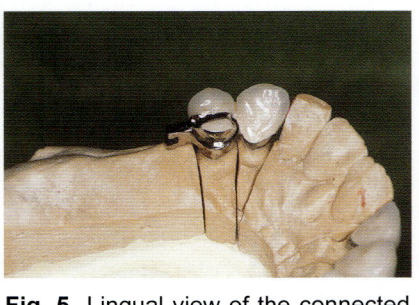

Fig. 5 Lingual view of the connected PFM crowns placed on teeth #13 and #14 (with a plate projection).

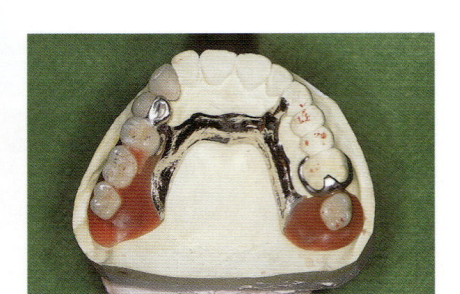

Fig. 6 Wax denture after the replacement of the missing #15-#17 with the artificial teeth (tooth #15 involves a Suginaka bolt attachment). The lingual arm with an occlusal rest, spur, and Akers clasp were placed on teeth #14, #23, and #26, respectively.

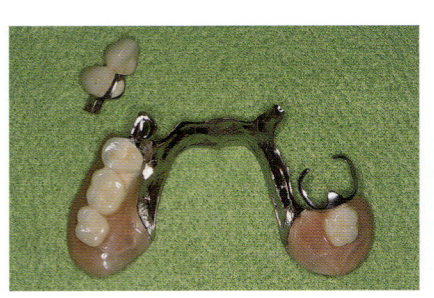

Fig. 7 Completed PFM crowns connected for teeth #13, #14 (with a plate projection) and Suginaka bolt clasp denture for teeth #15-#17, #27 replaced with the artificial teeth.

Fig. 8 Lingual view of the same one.

Fig. 9 Mucosal view of the same one.

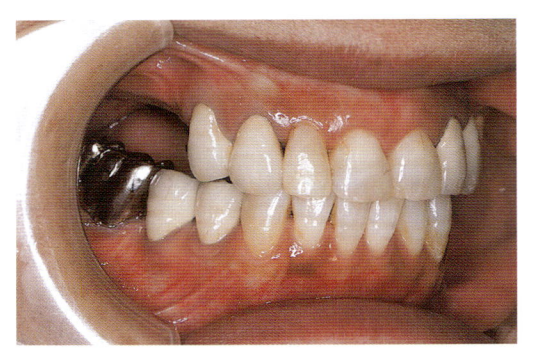

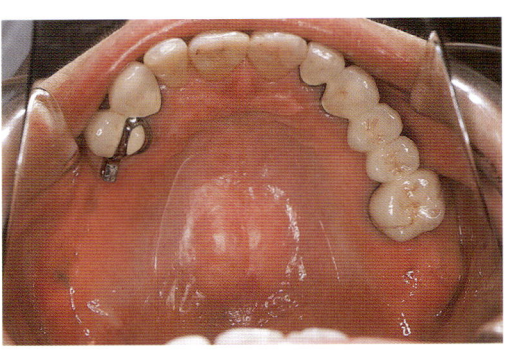

Fig. 10 Right buccal view of the connected PFM crowns with a plate projection placed on teeth #13, #14.

Fig. 11 Occlusal view of the same one.

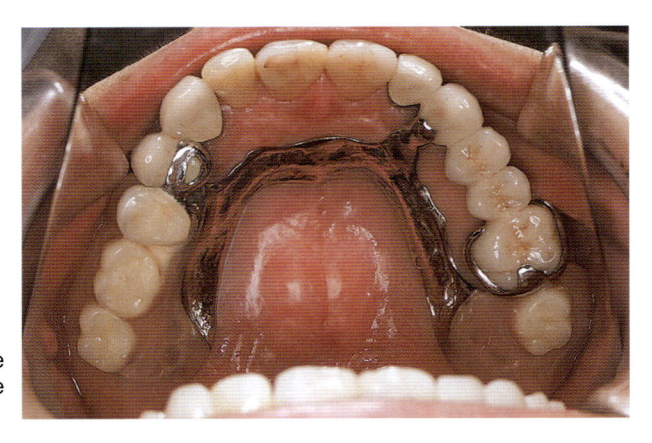

Fig. 12 Occlusal view of the Suginaka bolt clasp denture placed in the mouth.

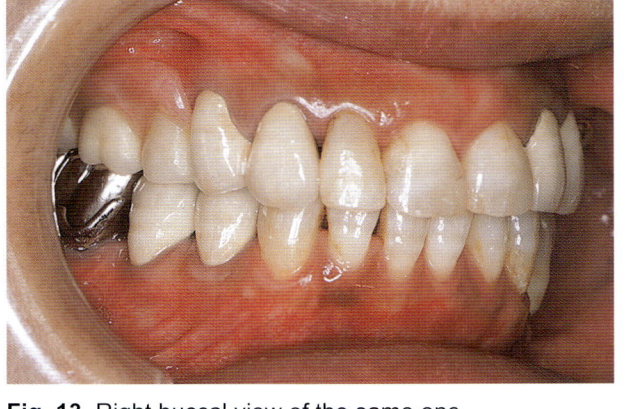

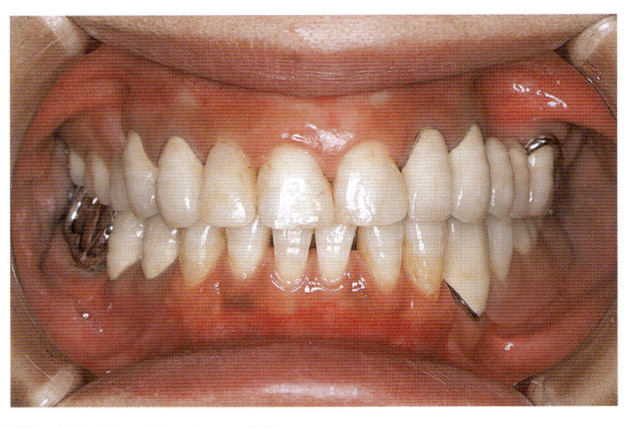

Fig. 13 Right buccal view of the same one.

Fig. 14 Frontal view of the same one.

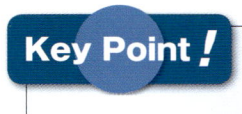 **Key Point !**

If a lingual arm with an occlusal rest to be used on the premolar is used the canine, it is a cingulum rest. The case described in 1-1) ⑨ applies to this.

1. Suginaka bolt attachment dentures

1) Suginaka bolt clasp dentures

⑭ Bilateral distal extension missing case including tooth bounded missing: Missing teeth #11-#13, #16-#17 and #21-#23, #26-#27; Patient: 52-year-old woman

Teeth #14, #24-#25: Porcelain fused to metal crown (PFM crown), lingual arm with amarginal rest

Tooth #15: 4/5 crown, lingual arm with an occlusal rest

Teeth #15, #25: Plate projection

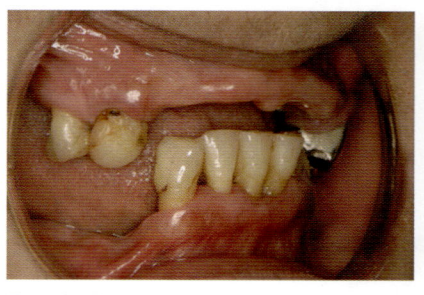

Fig. 1 Right buccal view of the case with missing teeth #11-#13, #16-#17 and #21-#23, #26-#27.

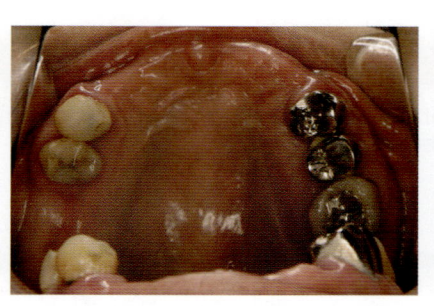

Fig. 2 Occlusal view of the same one (prior to extraction of tooth #26).

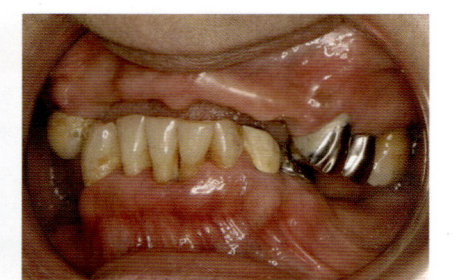

Fig. 3 Lest buccal view of the same one (prior to extraction of tooth #26).

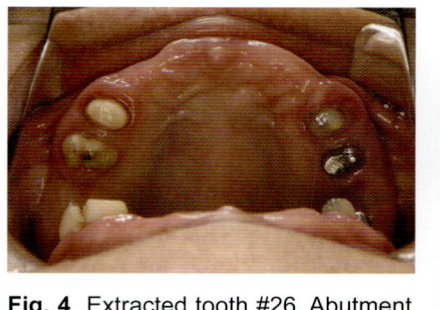

Fig. 4 Extracted tooth #26. Abutment tooth preparation of teeth #14, #15, #24, #25.

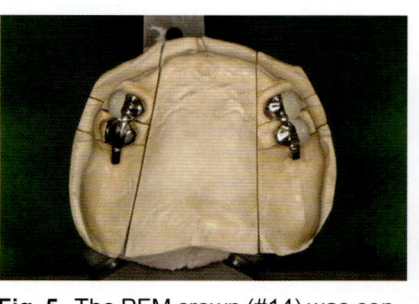

Fig. 5 The PFM crown (#14) was connected to the 4/5 inner crown with a plate projection (#15). Occlusal view of the connected PFM crowns with a plate projection placed on teeth #24, #25.

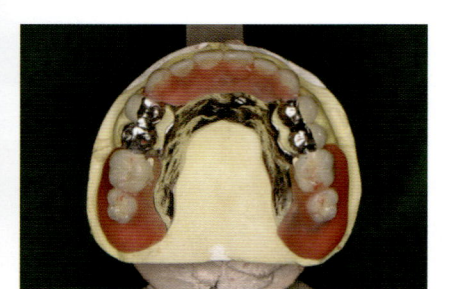

Fig. 6 Lingual arm with a marginal rest placed on teeth #14, #24, #25. The lingual arm with an occlusal rest was placed on tooth #15. The missing teeth #16, #26 were replaced with the artificial teeth involving a Suginaka riegel attachment.

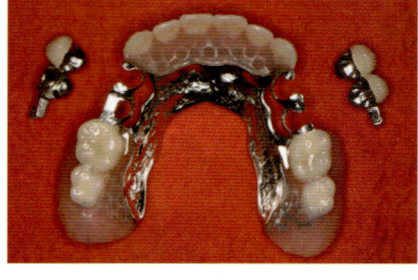

Fig. 7 Completed Suginaka bolt clasp denture consisting of the connected PFM crowns with a plate projection (teeth #14-#15, #24-#25), lingual arms with an occlusal rest (#15) and with a marginal rest (#14, #24-#25).

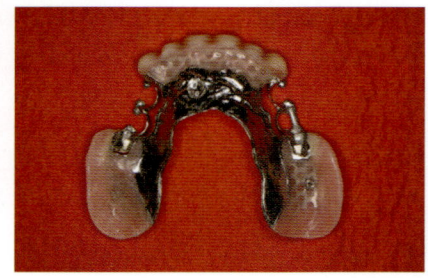

Fig. 8 Mucosal view of the completed Suginaka bolt clasp denture.

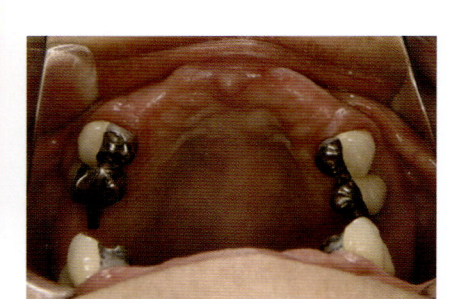

Fig. 9 Occlusal view of the PFM crown (#14) connected to the 4/5 inner crown with a plate projection (#15) and the connected PFM crowns with a plate projection (#24 and #25) placed in the mouth.

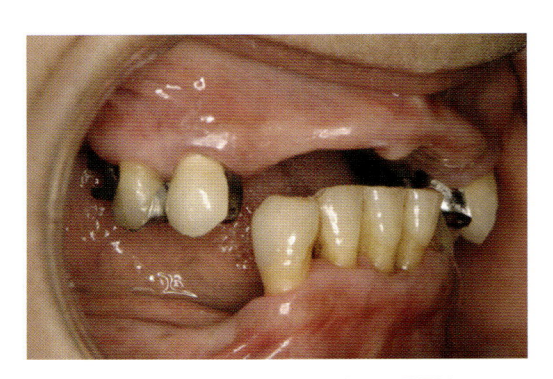

Fig. 10 Right buccal view of the PFM crown (#14) connected to the 4/5 inner crown (#15) with a plate projection placed in the mouth.

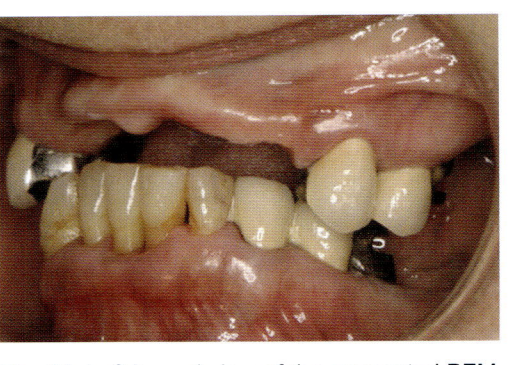

Fig. 11 Left buccal view of the connected PFM crowns with a plate projection (#24 and #25) placed in the mouth.

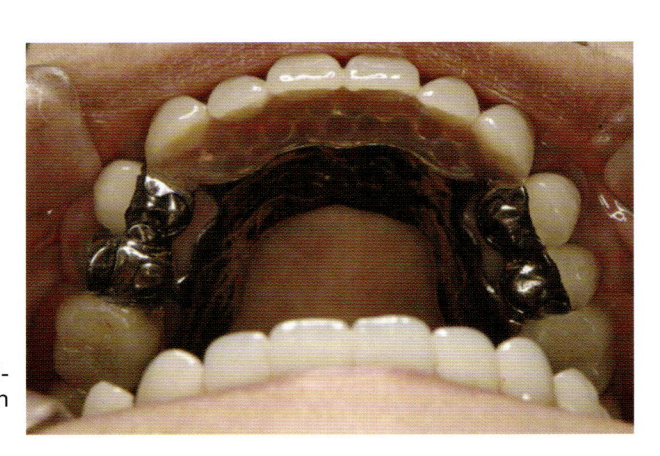

Fig. 12 Occlusal view of the Suginaka bolt clasp denture placed in the mouth.

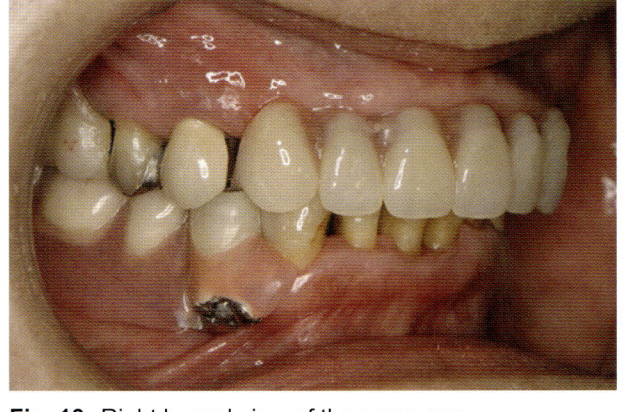

Fig. 13 Right buccal view of the same one.

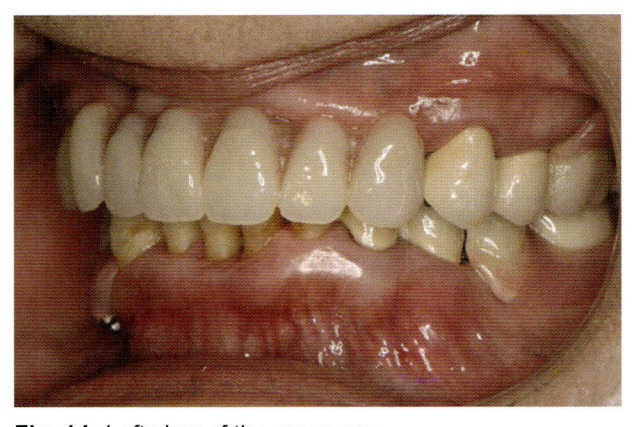

Fig. 14 Left view of the same one.

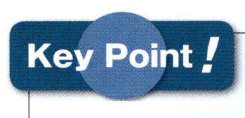

Key Point *!*

Even when the bilateral premolars are used as an abutment tooth in bilateral distal extension missing dentures, as the bilateral lingual arms are mutually-interfering, a horizontal movement can be restrained.

1. Suginaka bolt attachment dentures

2) Suginaka bolt telescope dentures

①Unilateral distal extension missing case: Missing teeth #16–#17; Patient: 58-year-old man
Tooth #14: Lingual arm with a marginal rest
Tooth #15: Cone-crown-type double crown (inner crown with a plate projection)

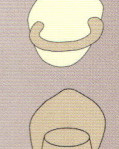

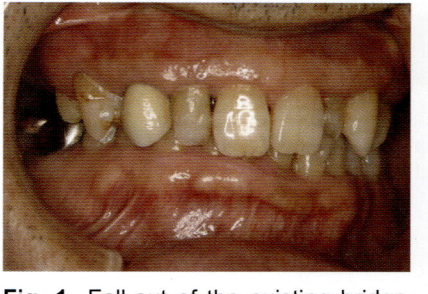

Fig. 1 Fall-out of the existing bridge (abutment teeth: #15, #17) due to root fracture of tooth #17. Right buccal view of the case.

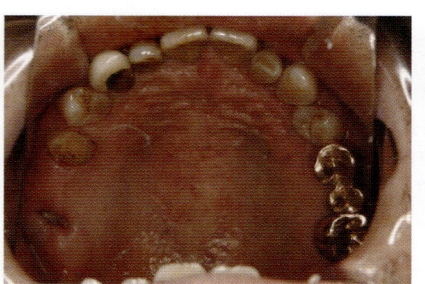

Fig. 2 Extracted tooth #17. Tooth #15 is a vital tooth. Upper occlusal view of the case.

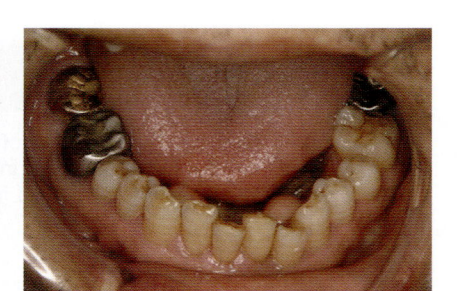

Fig. 3 Lower occlusal view of the case with the old lower denture removed.

Fig. 4 Buccal view of the abutment tooth for Cone-crown-type double crown to be placed on tooth #15.

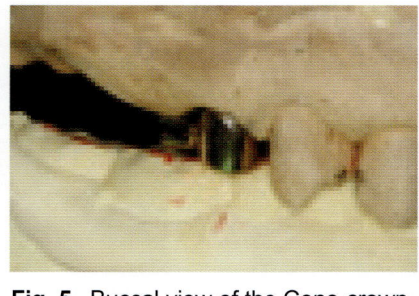

Fig. 5 Buccal view of the Cone-crown-type inner crown with a plate projection placed on tooth #15.

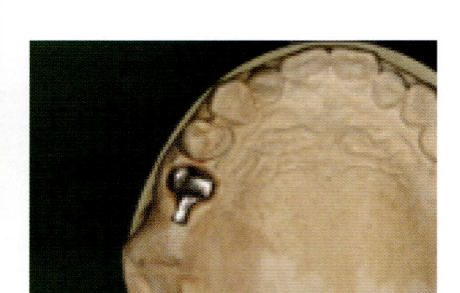

Fig. 6 Occlusal view of the same one.

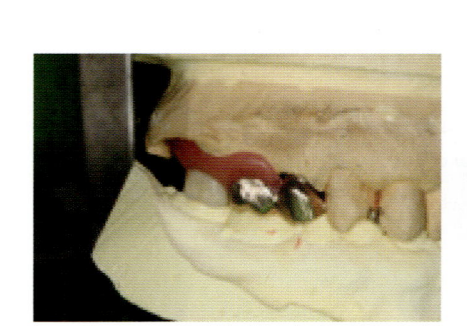

Fig. 7 Lingual arm placed on tooth #14 and Cone-crown-type outer crown placed on tooth #15. Replacement of missing teeth #16, #17 with artificial teeth (#16 replaced with a metal tooth involving the Suginaka bolt attachment).

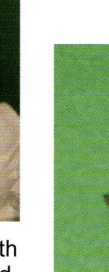

Fig. 8 No rest was placed on tooth #14 with torsion and close bite. Instead, an interproximal hook was placed between #13 and #14.

Fig. 9 Checking denture base fit of the wax denture after the replacement of the missing teeth #16–#17 with the artificial teeth.

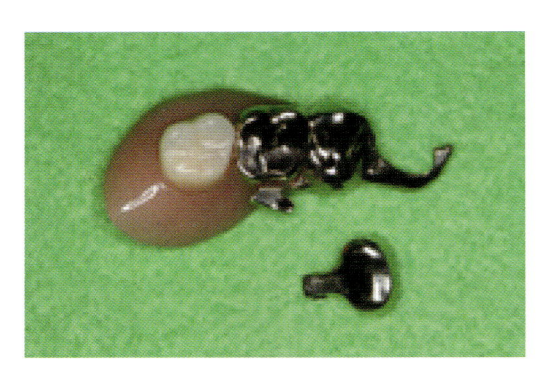

Fig. 10 Completed inner crown to be placed on tooth #15 and Suginaka bolt telescope denture for the missing teeth #16-#17 (with the lever opened).

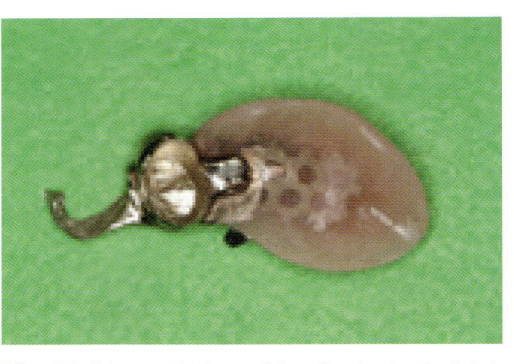

Fig. 11 Mucosal view of the Suginaka bolt telescope denture.

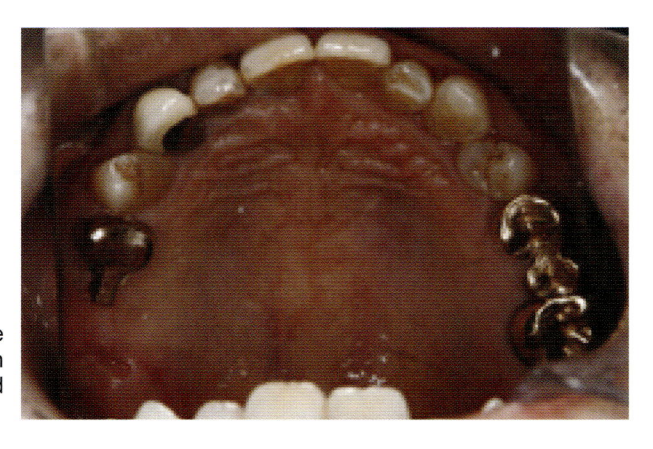

Fig. 12 Occlusal view of the Cone-crown-type inner crown with a plate projection placed on tooth #15.

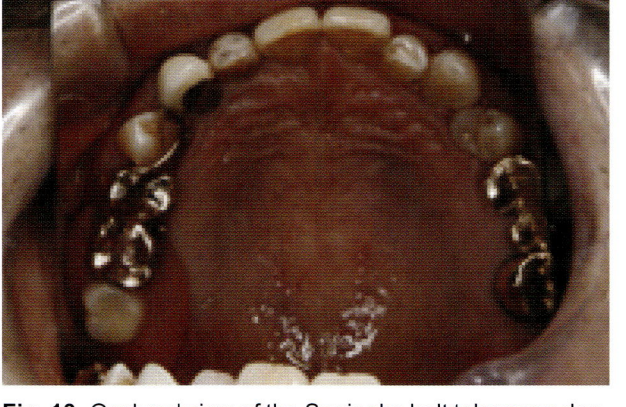

Fig. 13 Occlusal view of the Suginaka bolt telescope denture placed on the missing teeth #16-#17 region.

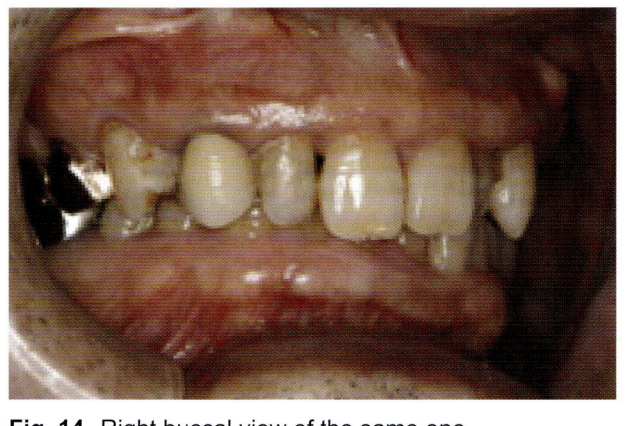

Fig. 14 Right buccal view of the same one.

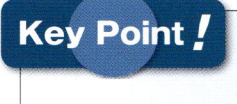

Key Point !

Because the abutment tooth is a vital tooth, no tooth fracture may be caused and also because the length of the clinical crown is short, no strong torque is applied to the abutment tooth.

When the free end missing #16-#17 is unilaterally restored using the tooth #15 that is a vital tooth and has the shorter crown length as a single abutment tooth, there is no need to connect tooth #15 with adjacent tooth.

1. Suginaka bolt attachment dentures

2) Suginaka bolt telescope dentures

②Unilateral distal extension missing case: Missing teeth #36-#37; Patient: 62-year-old woman
Tooth #34: Lingual arm with a marginal rest
Tooth #35: Cone-crown-type double crown (inner crown with a rod projection)

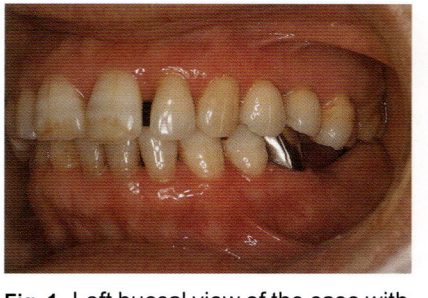

Fig. 1 Left buccal view of the case with missing teeth #36-#37.

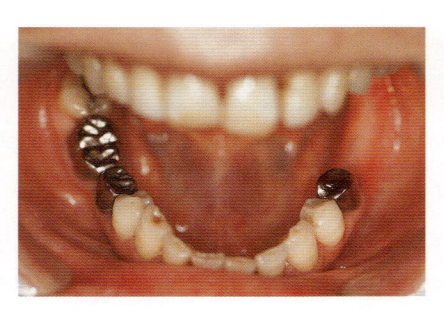

Fig. 2 Occlusal view of the same one.

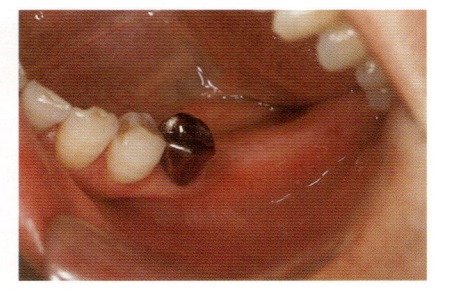

Fig. 3 Occlusal view of the case with missing teeth #36-#37.

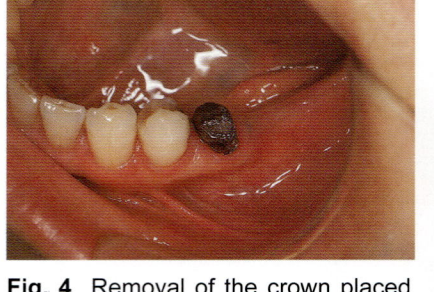

Fig. 4 Removal of the crown placed on tooth #35. Application of Silver-Fluolides following abutment preparation. Formation of a rest seat on the mesio-distal marginal ridge of tooth #44. Buccal view of the case.

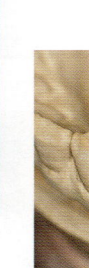

Fig. 5 Die stone model of tooth #45.

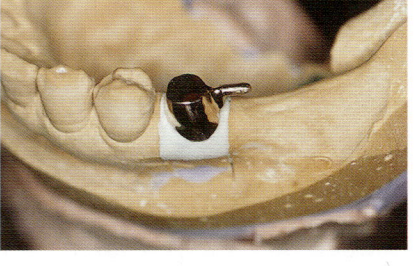

Fig. 6 Cone- crown-type inner crown with a rod projection placed on tooth #35 (a 1 mm wire in diameter was used in the case, but a 1.2 mm wire in diameter should commonly be used). Buccal view of the case.

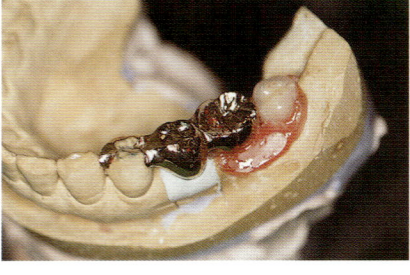

Fig. 7 The lingual arm with a marginal rest (#34), Cone-crown-type outer crown (#35), and metal tooth (for missing tooth #36) were one-piece casted. Wax denture after replacement of the missing teeth #36-37 with the metal tooth and resin tooth.

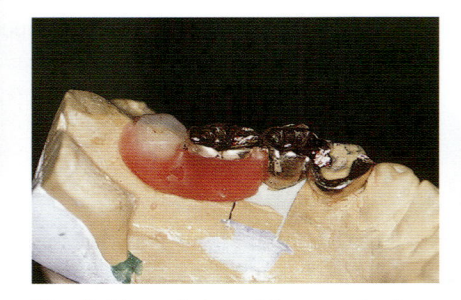

Fig. 8 Lingual view of the wax denture before a Suginaka bolt attachment is embedded in the wax base.

Fig. 9 Checking denture base fit of the wax denture.

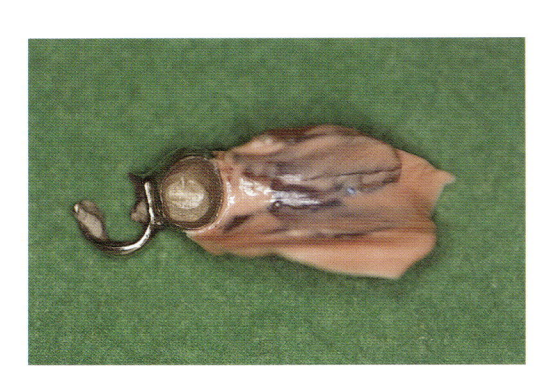

Fig.10 Impression taking of the mucosal surface of the wax denture.

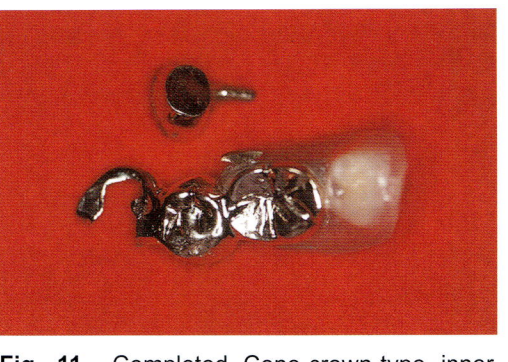

Fig. 11 Completed Cone-crown-type inner crown with a rod projection and Suginaka bolt telescope denture for missing teeth #36-#37.

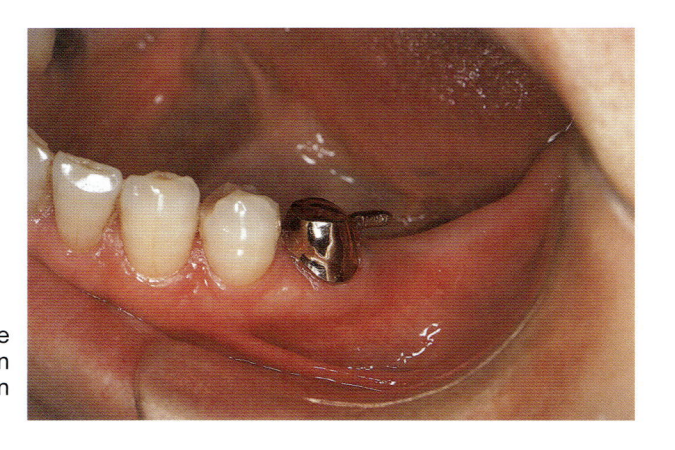

Fig. 12 Buccal view of the Cone-crown-type inner crown with a rod projection placed on tooth #35.

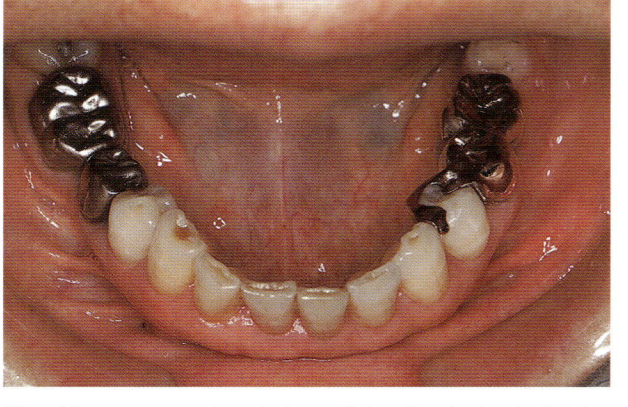

Fig. 13 Lower occlusal view of the Suginaka bolt telescope denture placed on the missing teeth #36-#37 region.

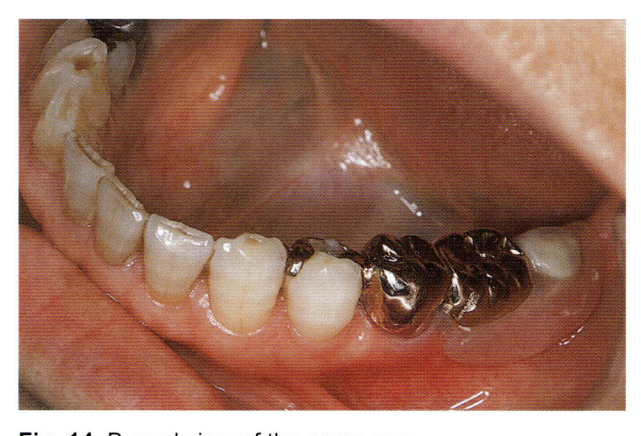

Fig. 14 Buccal view of the same one.

 **Key Point !** Because the tooth #15 is a vital tooth and has the shorter length of the clinical crown, and also the residual ridge is hard and wide, the tooth #15 can be used alone as an abutment tooth for the single telescope crown when the unilateral distal extension case is unilaterally restored.

A one mm wire in diameter was used in this case, but a 1.2 mm wire in diameter should commonly be used because there is a risk for fracture.

1. Suginaka bolt attachment dentures

2) Suginaka bolt telescope dentures

③Unilateral distal extension case: Missing teeth #26-#27; Patient: 49-year-old woman
Tooth #24: 4/5 outer crown-type double crown (4/5 type inner crown)
Tooth #25: Cone-crown-type double crown (inner crown with a rod projection)

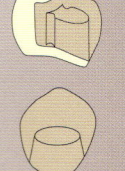

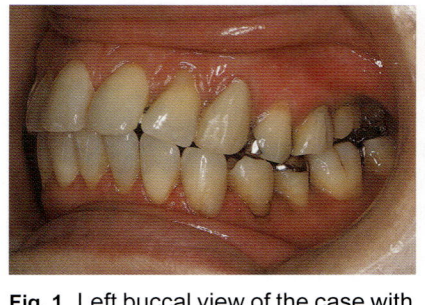

Fig. 1 Left buccal view of the case with missing teeth #26-#27 (#26 is an extension pontic).

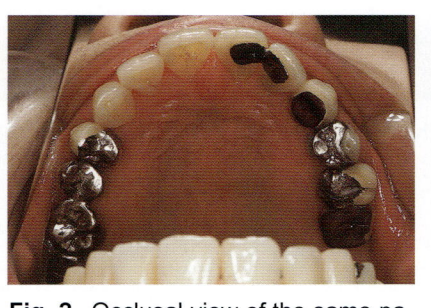

Fig. 2 Occlusal view of the same patient. The extension bridge is fractured between tooth #24 and #25.

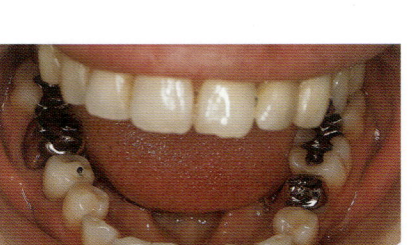

Fig. 3 Lower occlusal view of the case.

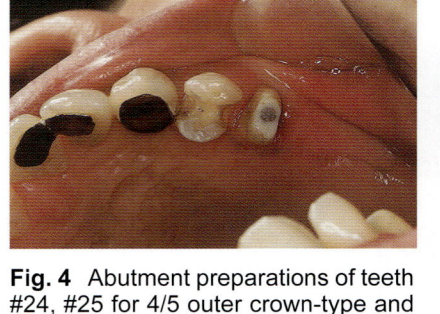

Fig. 4 Abutment preparations of teeth #24, #25 for 4/5 outer crown-type and Cone-crown-type double crowns, respectively.

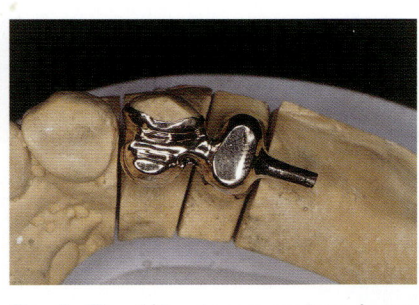

Fig. 5 The 4/5 outer crown-type inner crown for #24 was connected to the Cone-crown-type inner crown with a rod projection for #25.

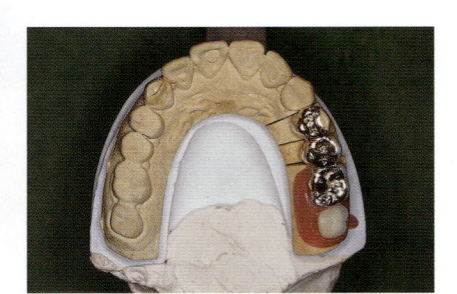

Fig. 6 The 4/5 outer crown and Cone-crown-type outer crown placed on the #24 , #25, respectively.
Wax denture after replacement of missing teeth #26-#27 with the metal tooth and resin tooth.

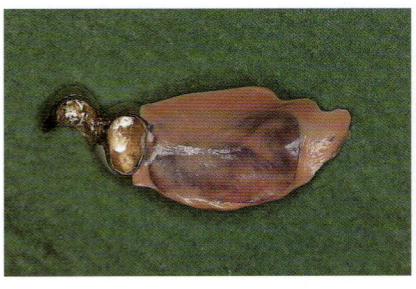

Fig. 7 Impression taking of the mucosal surface of the telescope wax denture for the missing teeth #26-#27 replaced with artificial teeth.

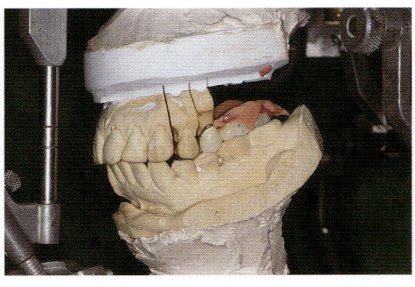

Fig. 8 The wax denture was returned to the dowel pin-type working cast model after impression taking and the impression was poured in stone. Buccal view of the working cast model.

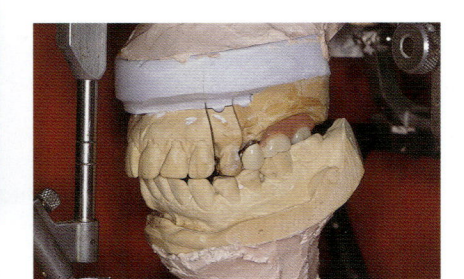

Fig. 9 The resin base for missing teeth #26-#27 was finished for completion.

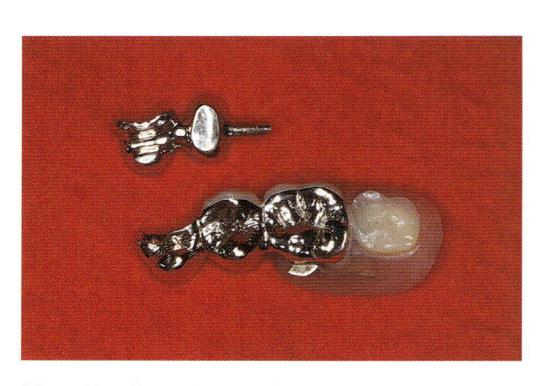

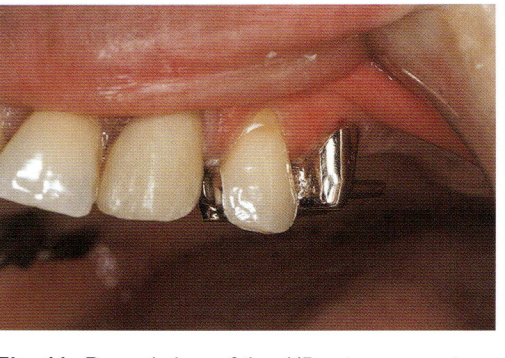

Fig. 10 Completed 4/5 outer crown-type inner crown for #24 and Cone-crown-type inner crown with a rod projection for #25 connected and Suginaka bolt telescope denture for missing teeth #26-#27.

Fig. 11 Buccal view of the 4/5 outer crown-type inner crown and Cone-crown-type inner crown with a rod projection placed on teeth #24 ,#25, respectively.

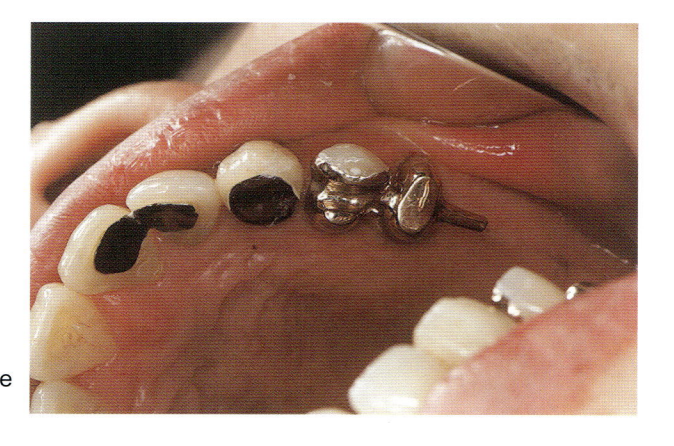

Fig. 12 Occlusal view of the same one.

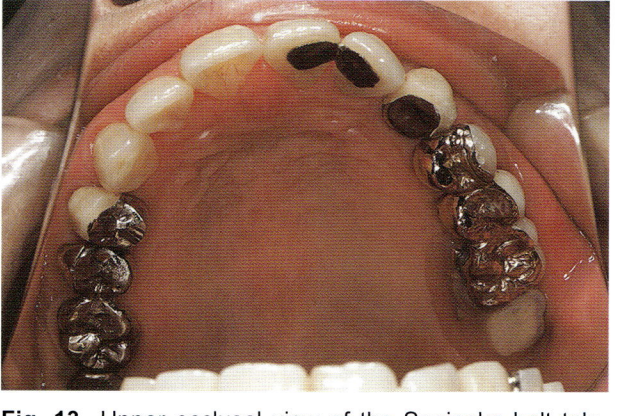

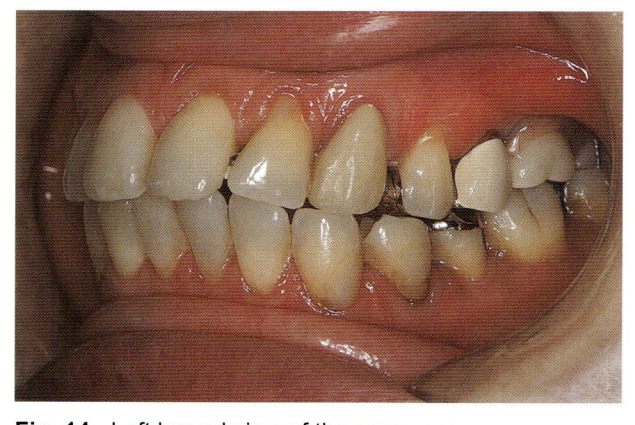

Fig. 13 Upper occlusal view of the Suginaka bolt telescope denture placed on the missing teeth #26-#27 region.

Fig. 14 Left buccal view of the same one.

 **Key Point !**   When a double crown is used as a retainer, because the connecting rigidity becomes greater, if the denture base is short, a greater torque is applied to the abutment tooth. Therefore, it is necessary to connect the inner crown with the adjacent tooth. It is, particularly, essential to connect retainers in the core construction of a pulpless tooth.

1. Suginaka bolt attachment dentures

2) Suginaka bolt telescope dentures

④ Unilateral distal extension missing case: Missing teeth #36-#37; Patient: 42-year-old woman
Tooth #34: 4/5 outer crown-type double crown (4/5-type inner crown)
Tooth #35: Cone-crown-type double crown (inner crown with a plate projection)

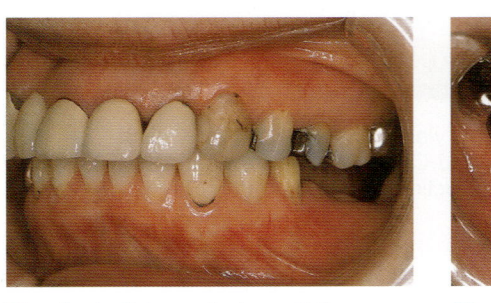

Fig. 1 Left buccal view of the case with fall-out of the bridge for teeth #35-#37 (abutment teeth: #35,#37) due to fracture of tooth #37.

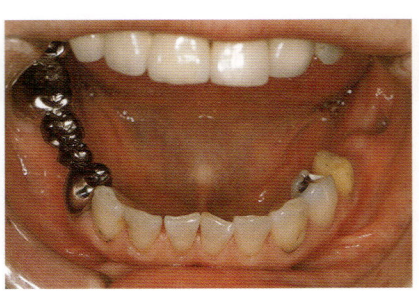

Fig. 2 Lower occlusal view of the patient after the extraction of #37.

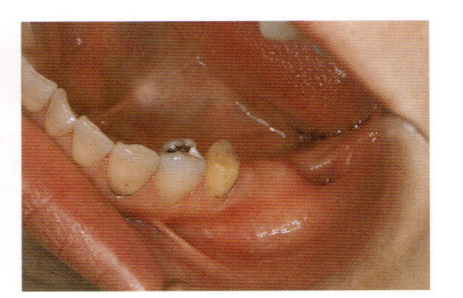

Fig. 3 Buccal view of the missing teeth #36-#37 region and tooth #35 as an abutment tooth.

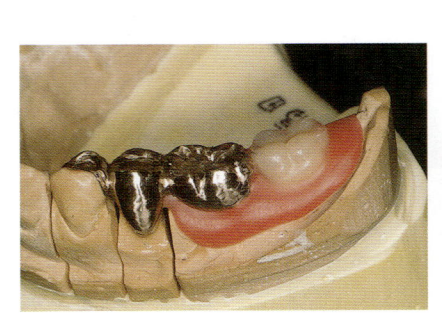

Fig. 4 Occlusal view of the abutment preparation for 4/5 crown-type (#34) and Cone-crown-type (#35) double crowns.

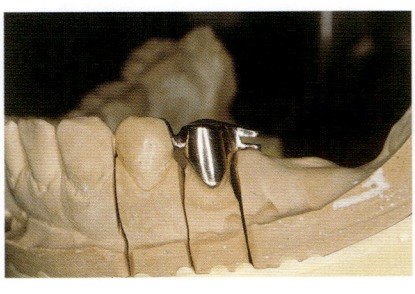

Fig. 5 Buccal view of the 4/5 crown-type inner crown for tooth #34 connected to the Cone-crown-type inner crown with a plate projection for tooth #35.

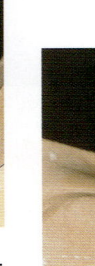

Fig. 6 Lingual view of the same one.

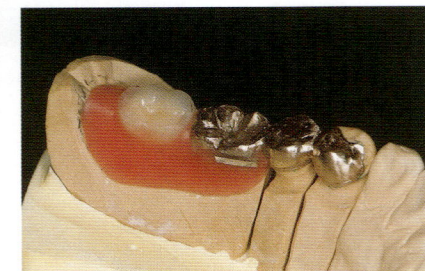

Fig. 7 The 4/5 crown-type outer crown, Cone-crown-type outer crown, and metal tooth involving a Suginaka bolt attachment were one-piece casted. Buccal view of the wax denture after replacement of the missing teeth #36 (metal tooth) and #37 with the artificial teeth.

Fig. 8 Lingual view of the wax denture, in which a Suginaka bolt attachment was embedded in the denture base placed on the missing tooth #36 region.

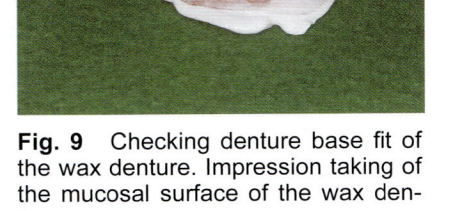

Fig. 9 Checking denture base fit of the wax denture. Impression taking of the mucosal surface of the wax denture.

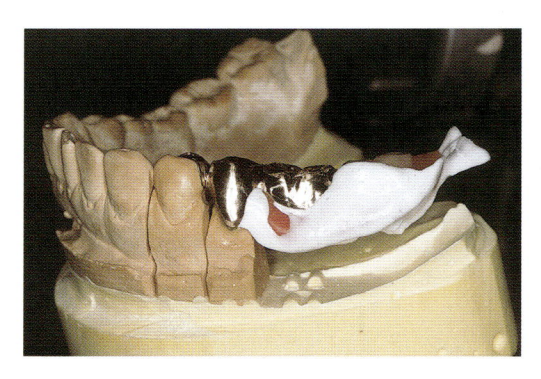

Fig. 10 The wax denture was returned to the dowel pin-type working cast model after impression taking and the impression was poured in stone.

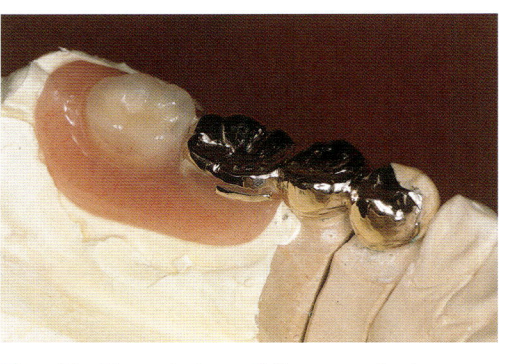

Fig. 11 Lingual view of the wax denture corrected again for finishing.

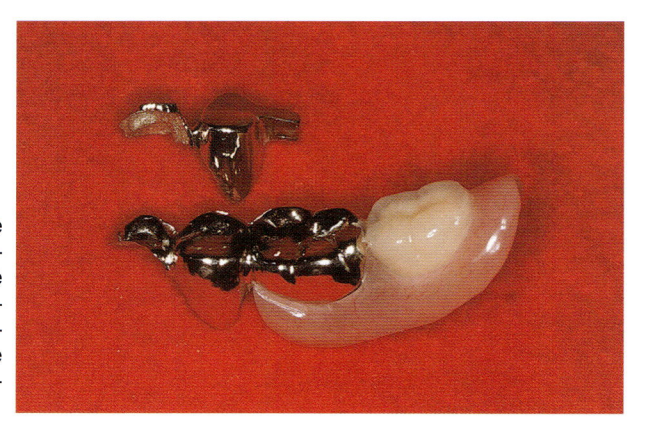

Fig. 12 The 4/5 crown-type inner crown for tooth #34 connected to the Cone-crown-type inner crown with a plate projection for tooth #35 and the completed Suginaka bolt telescope denture for missing teeth #36-#37.

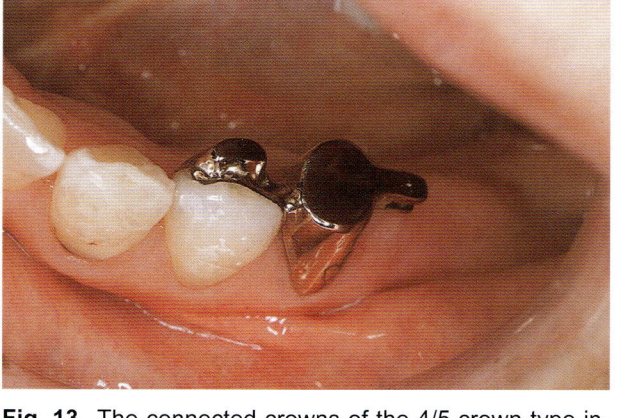

Fig. 13 The connected crowns of the 4/5 crown-type inner crown and the Cone-crown-type inner crown with a plate projection placed on teeth #34, #35, respectively.

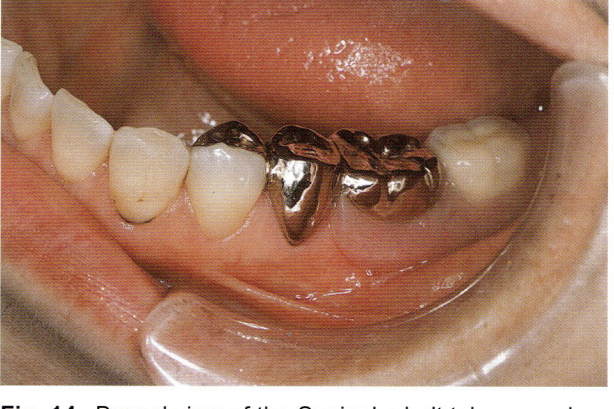

Fig. 14 Buccal view of the Suginaka bolt telescope denture place in the missing teeth #36-#37 region.

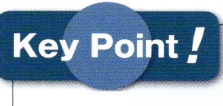 **Key Point !** In case, it passed not so long time since the tooth #37 was removed, alveolar ridge resorption would continue after the denture was delivered. Therefore, even if the tooth #35 is a vital tooth, it was not used as a single abutment for the double crown and the inner crown with a plate projection was connected to the 4/5 crown-type inner crown for the tooth #34.

1. Suginaka bolt attachment dentures

2) Suginaka bolt telescope dentures

⑤Unilateral distal extension missing case: Missing teeth #36-#37; Patient: 60-year-old woman
Tooth #34: 4/5 outer crown-type double crown (facing-type inner crown)
Tooth #35: Cone-crown-type double crown (inner crown with a plate projection)

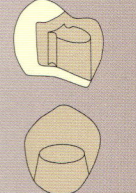

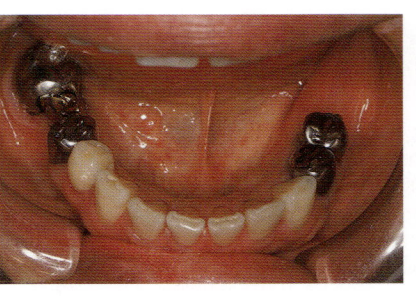

Fig. 1 Left buccal view of the case with missing teeth #36-#37.

Fig. 2 Lower occlusal view of the same one.

Fig. 3 Buccal view of the same one.

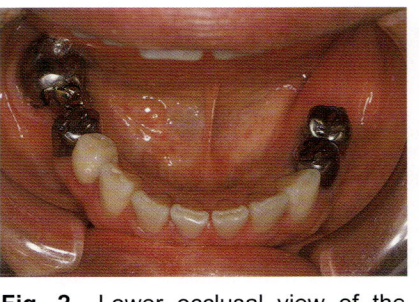

Fig. 4 Abutment preparation for double crowns to be placed on teeth #34, #35.

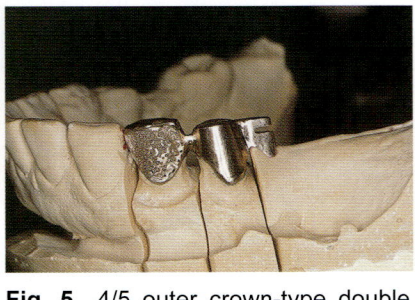

Fig. 5 4/5 outer crown-type double crown facing inner crown for #34 and Cone-crown-type double crown inner crown with a plate projection for #35. Buccal view of the connected both inner crowns.

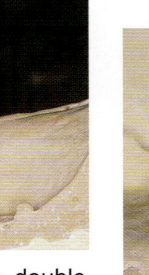

Fig. 6 Occlusal view of the same one.

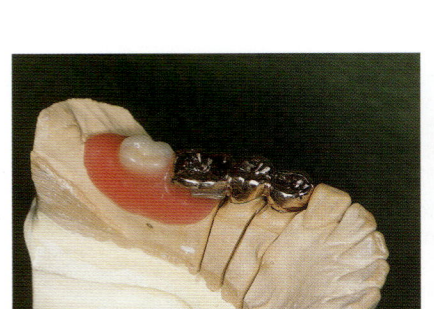

Fig. 7 The 4/5 crown-type outer crown for #34, Cone-crown-type facing outer crown for #35, and metal tooth involving a Suginaka bolt attachment for missing tooth #36 were one-piece casted. Lingual view of the wax denture after replacement of the missing teeth #36 (metal tooth) and #37 with the artificial teeth.

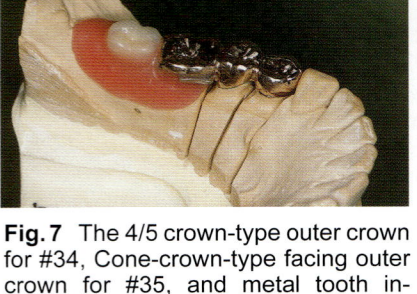

Fig. 8 Buccal view of the same one.

Fig. 9 After impression taking of the mucosal surface of the wax denture with the retainers pressed by fingers, the wax denture was returned to the dowel pin separated working cast model with the dowel pin for missing teeth #36 and #37 removed. This is not the occlusal bite impression.

84

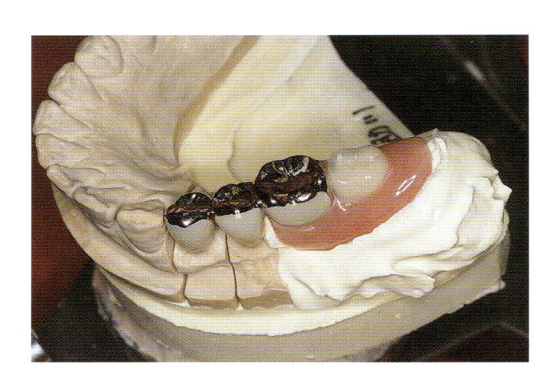

Fig. 10 The impression was poured with stone and the denture base was corrected for finishing.

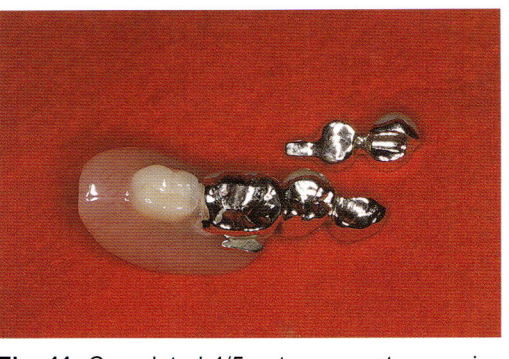

Fig. 11 Completed 4/5 outer crown-type resin-facing inner crown for #34 and Cone-crown-type inner crown with a rod projection for #35 connected. Lingual view of the completed Suginaka telescope denture for missing teeth #36-#37.

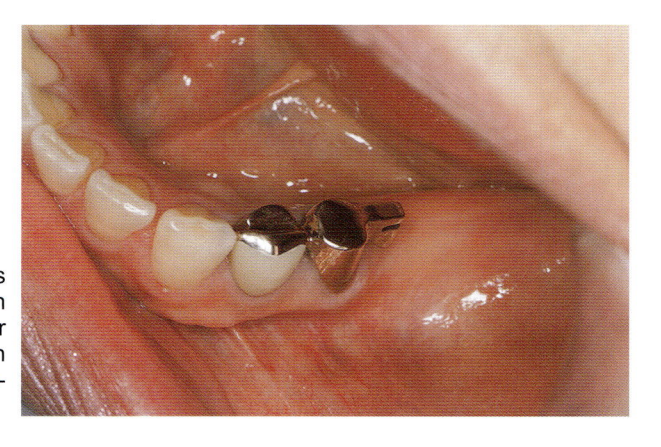

Fig. 12 The connected crowns of the resin-facing inner crown and Cone-crown-type inner crown with a plate projection placed on #34 and #35, respectively.

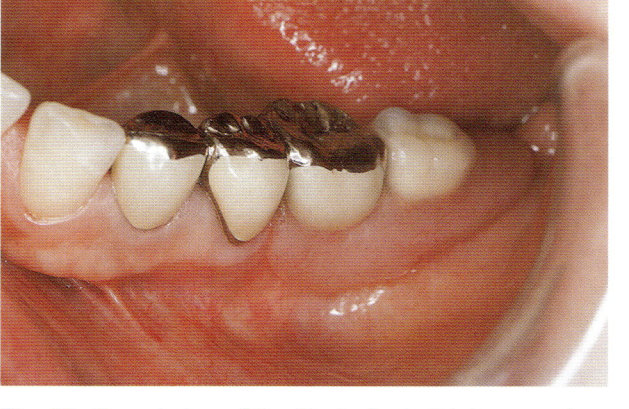

Fig. 13 Buccal view of the Suginaka bolt telescope denture in the missing teeth #36-#37 region.

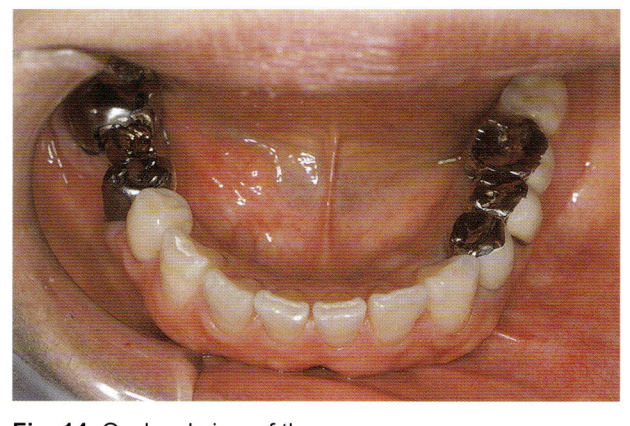

Fig. 14 Occlusal view of the same one.

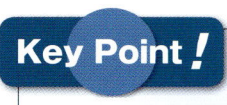

Key Point !

The process to denture set-up were performed on the dowel pin separated working cast model for fabricating the retainers and an impression of the mucosal surface of the wax denture was taken with the retainers pressed by fingers. It is essential not to take a bite-seating impression.

1. Suginaka bolt attachment dentures

2) Suginaka bolt telescope dentures

⑥Unilateral distal extension missing case: Missing teeth #46-#47; Patient: 50-year-old woman
Teeth #44, #45: Cone-crown-type double crown (inner crown with a rod projection)

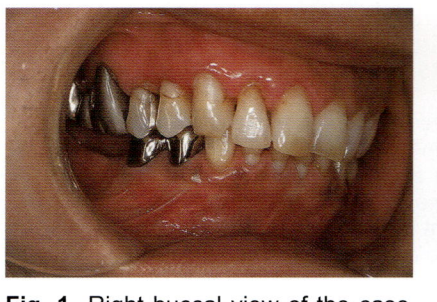

Fig. 1 Right buccal view of the case with missing teeth #46-#47.

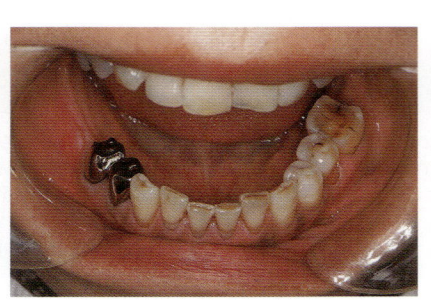

Fig. 2 Lower occlusal view of the same one.

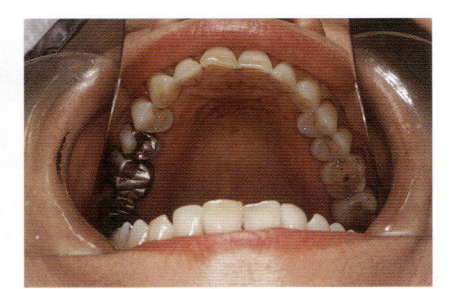

Fig. 3 Upper occlusal view of the same one.

Fig. 4 Abutment preparation following removal of restorations placed on teeth #44, #45.

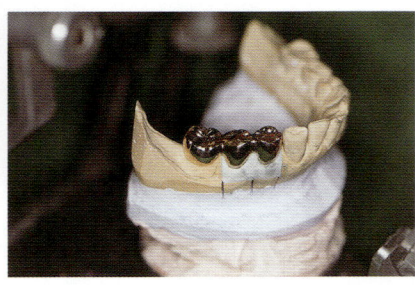

Fig. 5 The outer crowns for the connected Cone-crown-type inner crowns with a rod projection to be placed on #44 and #45 and the metal tooth involving a Suginaka bolt attachment were one-piece casted.

Fig. 6 Lingual view of the soldered outer crowns for #44, #45 and the metal tooth for #46.

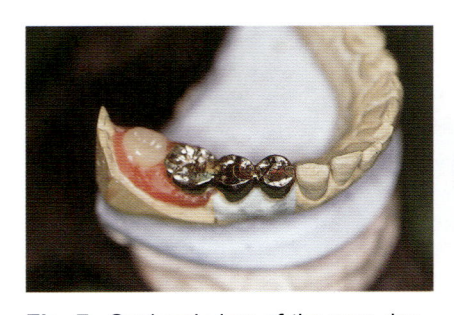

Fig. 7 Occlusal view of the wax denture after replacement of the missing teeth #46-#47 with the artificial teeth.

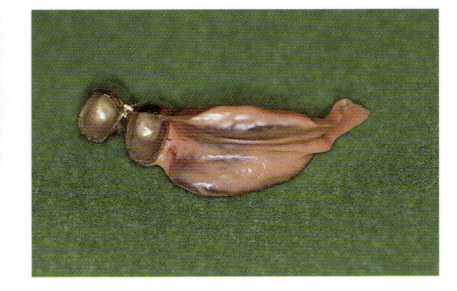

Fig. 8 Lingual view of the same one without embedding a Suginaka bolt attachment at this time.

Fig. 9 Impression taking of the mucosal surface of the wax denture.

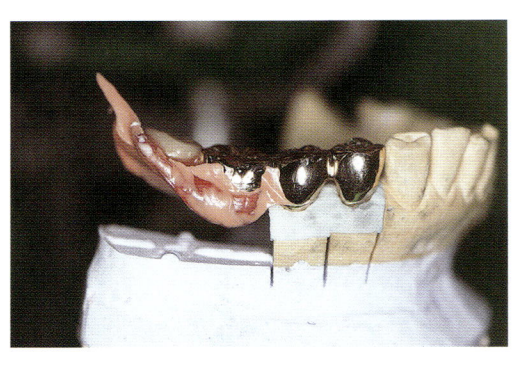

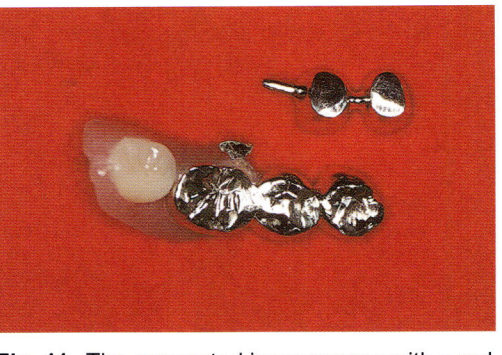

Fig. 10 The wax denture was returned to the dowel pin separated working cast model after impression taking and the impression was poured in stone, after which a Suginaka bolt attachment was embedded for finishing.

Fig. 11 The connected inner crowns with a rod projection for teeth #44, #45 and the Suginaka bolt telescope denture for missing teeth #46-#47 were completed.

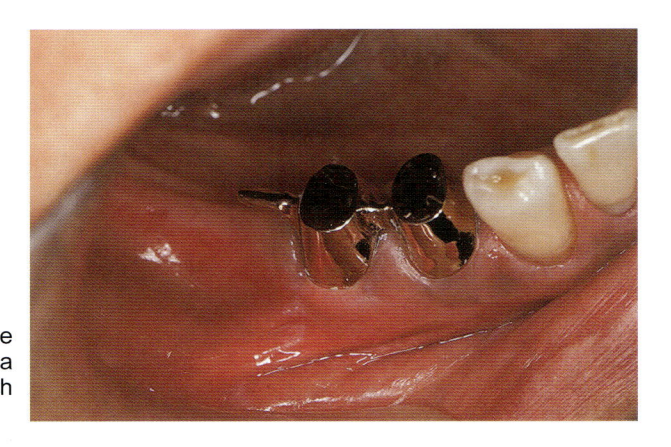

Fig. 12 Buccal view of the splinted inner crowns with a rod projection placed on teeth #44, #45.

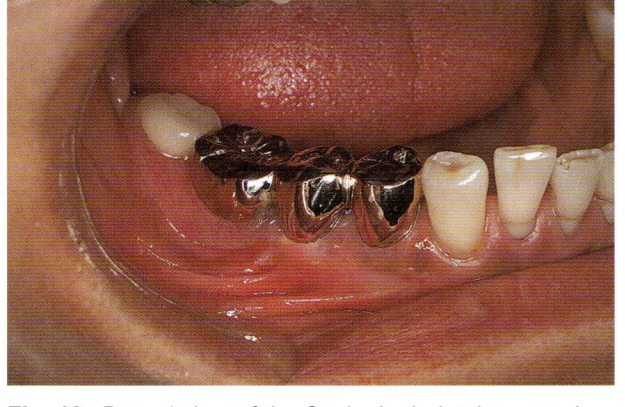

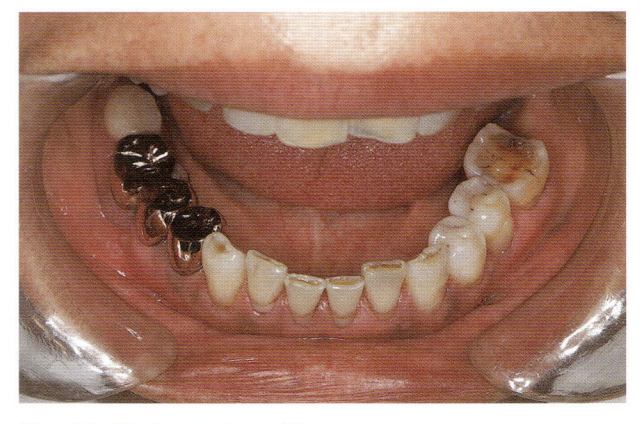

Fig. 13 Buccal view of the Suginaka bolt telescope denture in the missing teeth #46-#47 region.

Fig. 14 Occlusal view of the same one.

Key Point ! The procedure of denture set-up should be performed on the dowel pin-type working cast model for try-in and occlusal adjustment. Then, an impression of the mucosal surface of the wax denture, not a bite-seating impression, but it was taken with the retainers pressed by fingers. The wax denture was returned to the dowel pin-type working cast model without the dowel pin for missing teeth #46 and #47 removed for pouring the impression in dental stone for the altered working cast.

1. Suginaka bolt attachment dentures

2) Suginaka bolt telescope dentures

⑦Unilateral distal extension missing case: Missing teeth #46-#47; Patient: 40-year-old woman
Teeth #44, #45: Cone-crown-type double crown (inner crown with a plate projection)

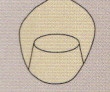

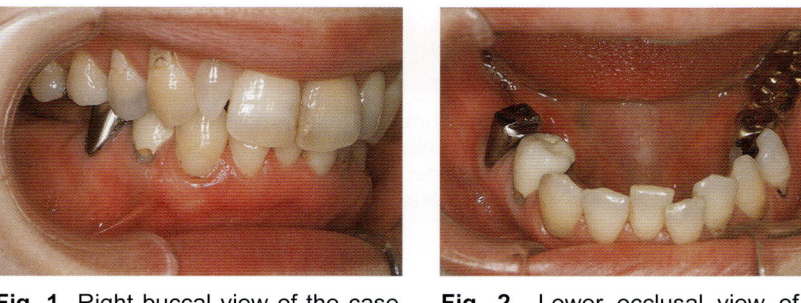

Fig. 1 Right buccal view of the case with missing teeth #46-#47.

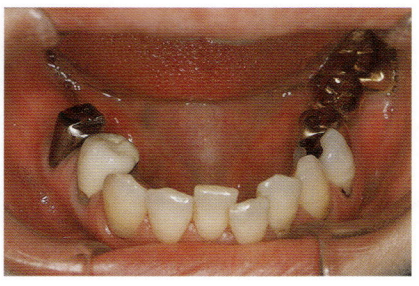

Fig. 2 Lower occlusal view of the same one.

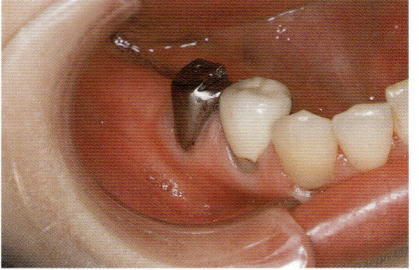

Fig. 3 Buccal view of the same one.

Fig. 4 Abutment preparation following removal of restorations on teeth #44, #45.

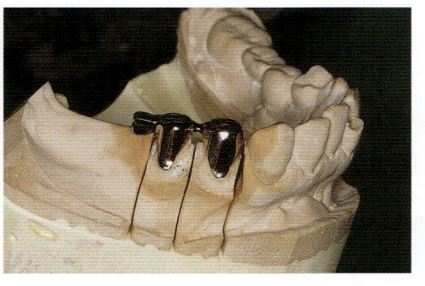

Fig. 5 Splinted Cone-crown-type inner crowns with a plate projection placed on teeth #44, #45.

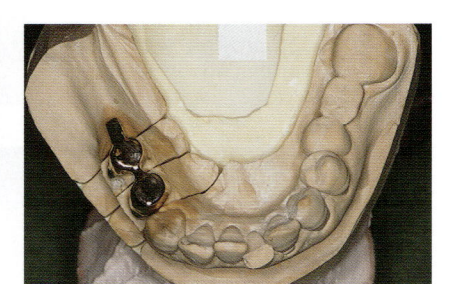

Fig. 6 Occlusal view of the same one.

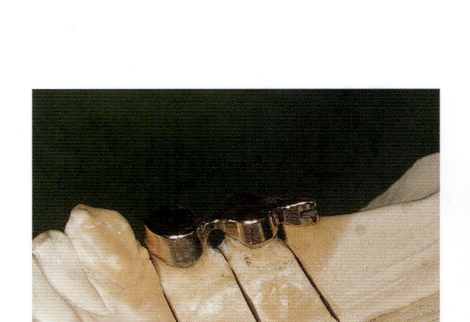

Fig. 7 Lingual view of the same one.

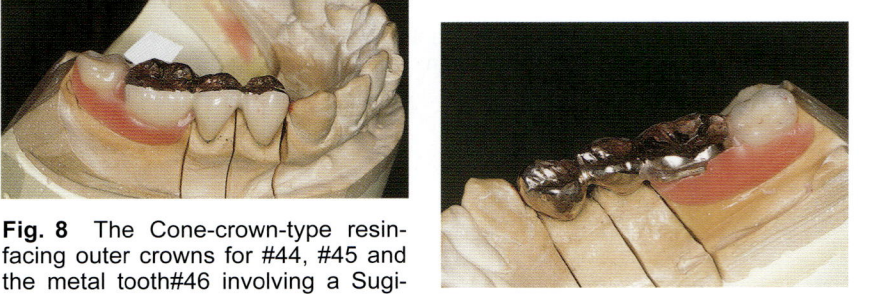

Fig. 8 The Cone-crown-type resin-facing outer crowns for #44, #45 and the metal tooth#46 involving a Suginaka bolt attachment were one-piece casted. Buccal view of the wax denture after replacement of the missing teeth #46 and #47 with artificial teeth.

Fig. 9 Lingual view of the wax denture after embedding a Suginaka bolt attachment.

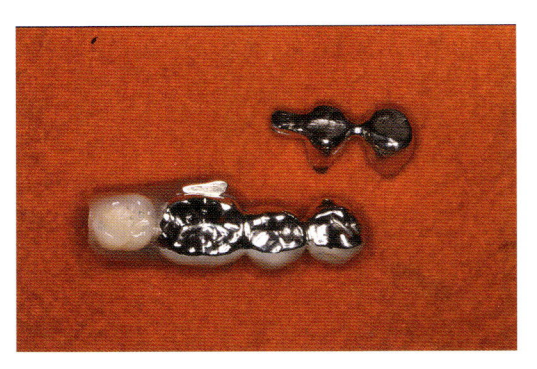

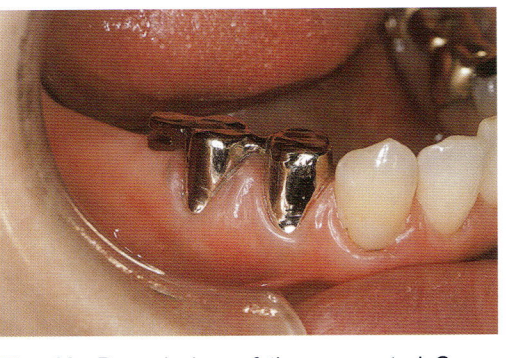

Fig. 10 The connected inner crowns with a rod projection for teeth #44, #45 and the Suginaka bolt telescope denture for missing teeth #46-#47 were completed.

Fig. 11 Buccal view of the connected Cone-crown-type inner crowns with a rod projection placed on teeth #44, #45.

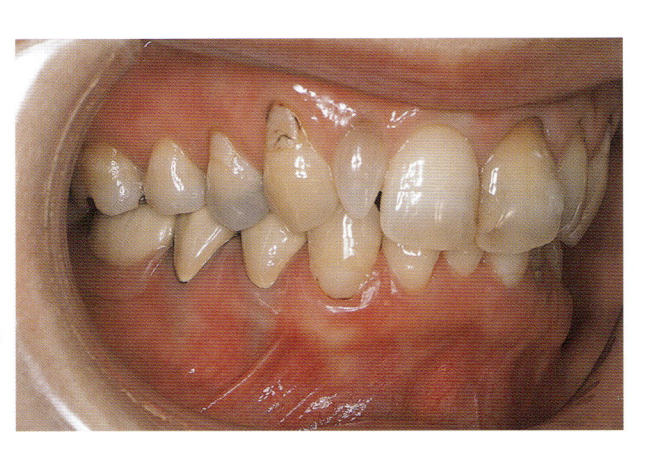

Fig. 12 Right buccal view of the Suginaka bolt telescope denture placed on the missing teeth #46-#47 region.

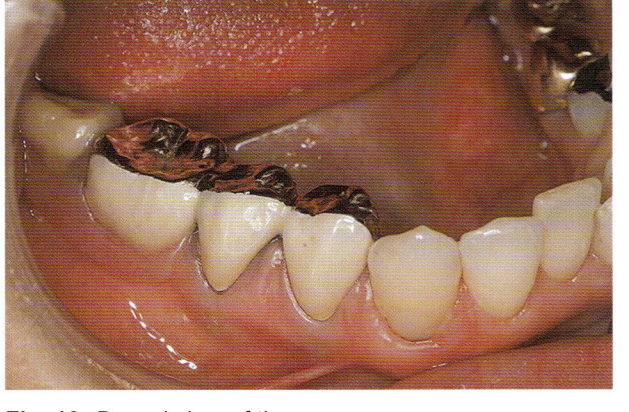

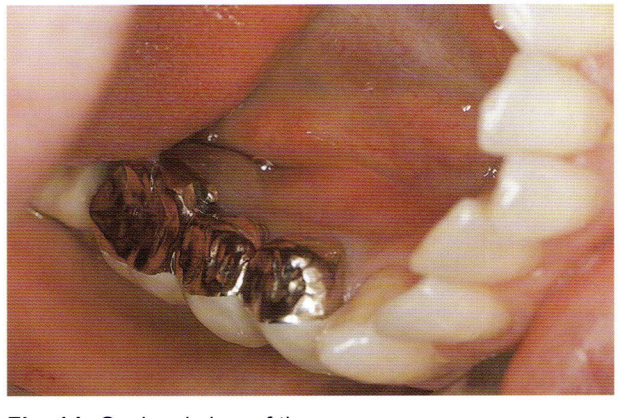

Fig. 13 Buccal view of the same one.

Fig. 14 Occlusal view of the same one.

 **Key Point !**   Procedure of denture set-up should be performed on the dowel pin-type working cast model for occlusal adjustment and an impression of the mucosal surface of the wax denture was taken with the retainers pressed by fingers. Then, the wax denture was returned to the dowel pin-type working cast model with the dowel pin for missing teeth #46 and #47 removed for pouring the impression in dental stone. The impression technique in this case was the same as that in the previous case.

1. Suginaka bolt attachment dentures

2) Suginaka bolt telescope dentures

⑧Unilateral distal extension missing case: Missing teeth #46-#47; Patient: 58-year-old man
   Tooth #43: Porcelain fused to metal crown (PFM crown)
   Teeth #44, #45: Cone-crown-type double crown (inner crown with a rod projection)

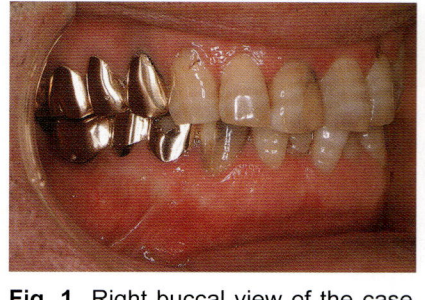

Fig. 1 Right buccal view of the case with the broken bridge for teeth #44-#46 (#46: extension pontic).

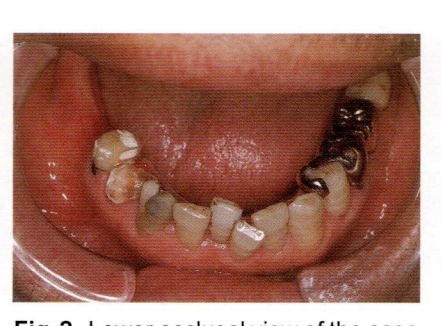

Fig. 2 Lower occlusal view of the case with the removed existing bridge and missing teeth #46-#47.

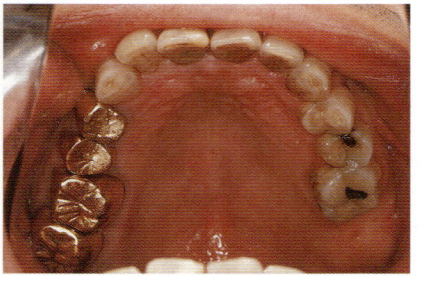

Fig. 3 Upper occlusal view.

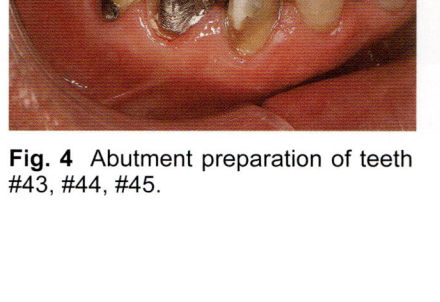

Fig. 4 Abutment preparation of teeth #43, #44, #45.

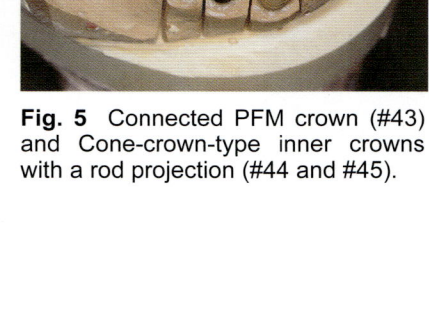

Fig. 5 Connected PFM crown (#43) and Cone-crown-type inner crowns with a rod projection (#44 and #45).

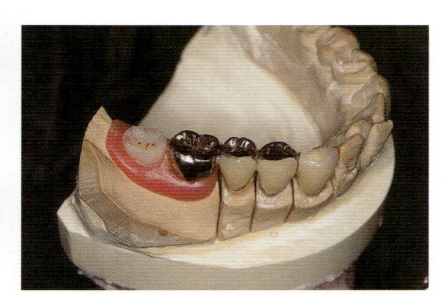

Fig. 6 The Cone-crown-type resin-facing outer crowns for #44, #45 and the metal tooth involving a Suginaka bolt attachment were one-piece casted. Buccal view of the wax denture after replacement of the missing teeth #46 (metal tooth) and #47 with artificial teeth.

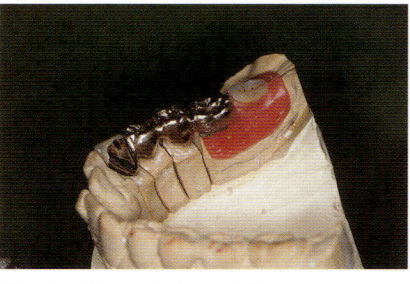

Fig. 7 Lingual view of the same one.

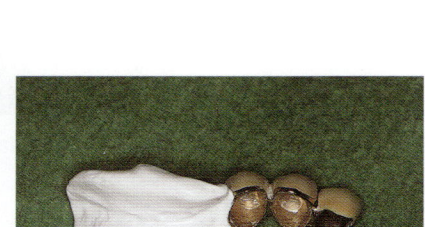

Fig. 8 Checking denture base fit of the wax denture for impression taking after its try-in and occlusal adjustment.

Fig. 9 The wax denture was returned to the dowel pin-type working cast model with the dowel pin for missing teeth #46, #47 removed for pouring the impression in dental stone.

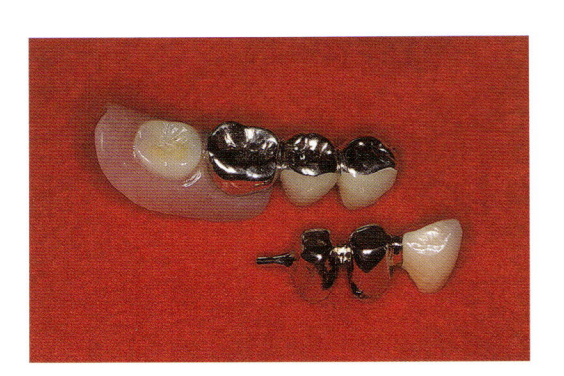

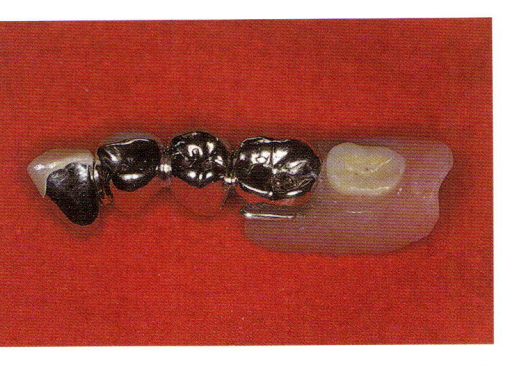

Fig. 10 The 3-unit connected PFM crown for #43 and Cone-crown-type inner crowns with a rod projection for #44, #45 and the Suginaka bolt telescope denture for missing teeth #46-#47 were completed.

Fig. 11 Lingual view of the Suginaka bolt telescope denture.

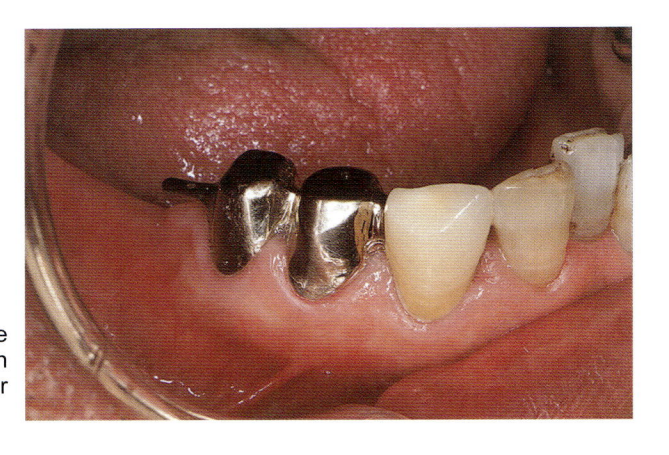

Fig. 12 Buccal view of the 3-unit connected PFM crown and Cone-crown-type inner crowns.

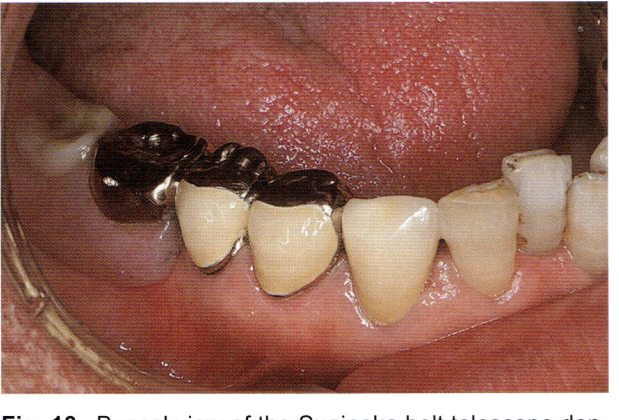

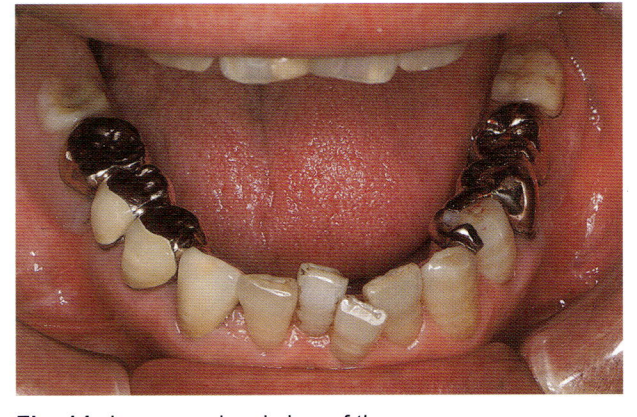

Fig. 13 Buccal view of the Suginaka bolt telescope denture placed on the missing teeth #46-#47 region.

Fig. 14 Lower occlusal view of the same one.

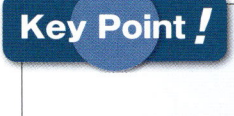 **Key Point !** The connection of the Cone-crown-type inner crown and its adjacent retainer leads to reinforcement between the retainers. Also in this case, the process to denture set-up were performed on the dowel pin-type working cast model for occlusal adjustment and an impression of the mucosal surface of the wax denture was taken with the retainers pressed by fingers.

1. Suginaka bolt attachment dentures

2) Suginaka bolt telescope dentures

⑨Unilateral distal extension missing case: Missing teeth #15-#17; Patient: 52-year-old woman
Tooth #13: Porcelain fused to metal crown (PFM crown)
Tooth #15: Implant abutment
Teeth #14, #15: Cone-crown-type double crown (inner crown with a plate projection)

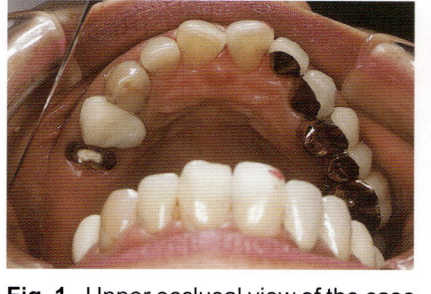

Fig. 1 Upper occlusal view of the case with the fractured tooth #15.

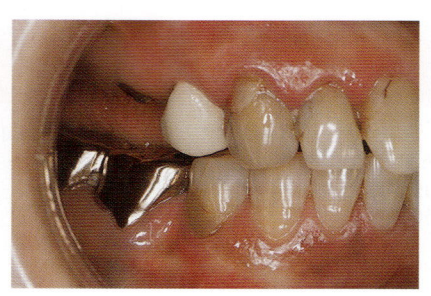

Fig. 2 Right buccal view of the same one.

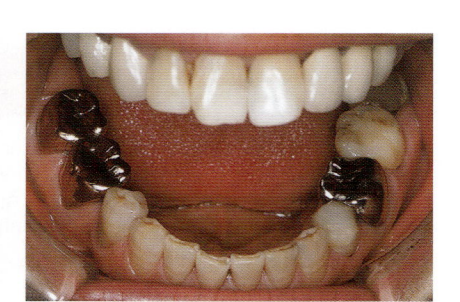

Fig. 3 Lower occlusal view.

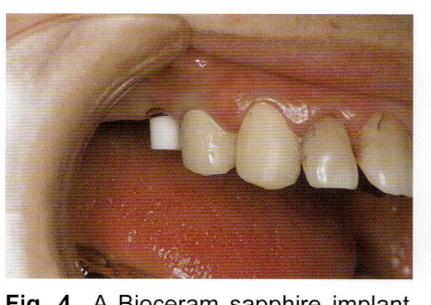

Fig. 4 A Bioceram sapphire implant was placed immediately after extraction of tooth #15.

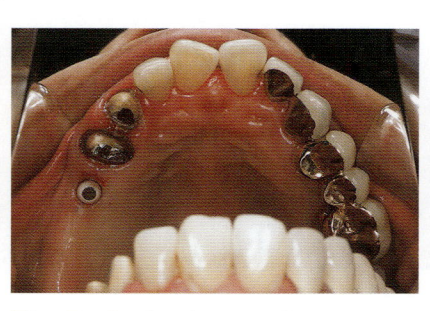

Fig. 5 Occlusal view of the patient after abutment preparations of the Bioceram sapphire implant placed in the tooth #15 region and teeth #13, #14.

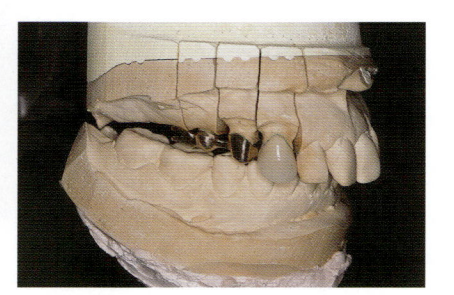

Fig. 6 Buccal view of the working cast model after the Cone-crown-type inner crown with a plate projection for tooth #15, the one for tooth #14, and the PFM crown for tooth #13 were connected.

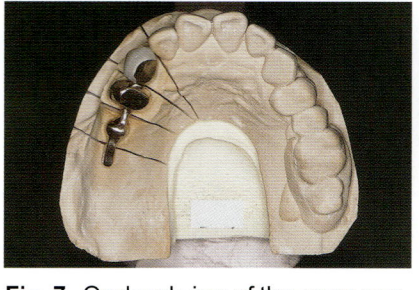

Fig. 7 Occlusal view of the same one.

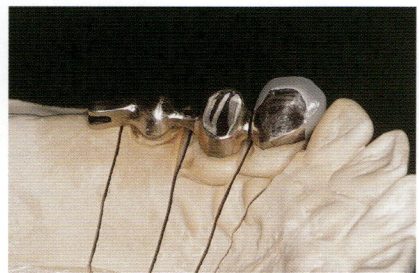

Fig. 8 Lingual view of the same one.

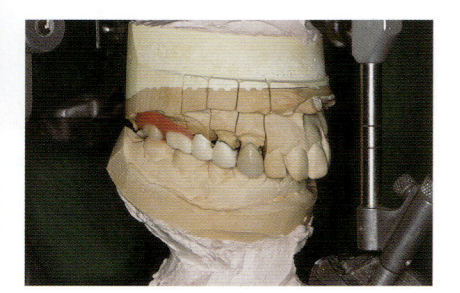

Fig. 9 Cone-crown-type resin-facing outer crowns for teeth #14, #15 and the metal tooth for missing tooth #16 involving a Suginaka bolt attachment were one-piece casted. Buccal view of the wax denture after replacement of the missing teeth #16 (metal tooth), #17 with artificial teeth.

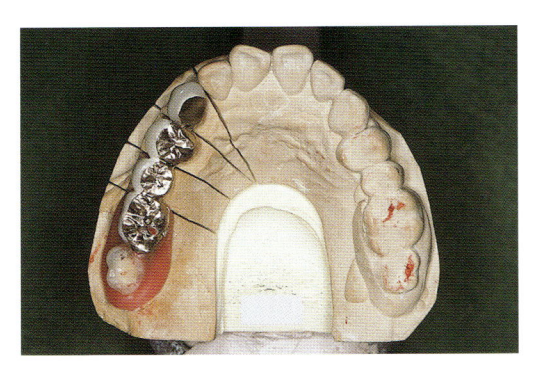

Fig. 10 Occlusal view of the same one.

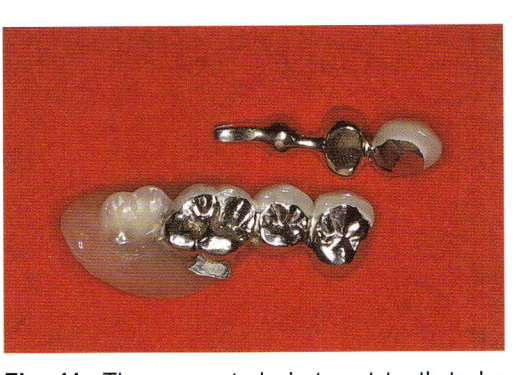

Fig. 11 The connected abutment teeth to be placed on teeth #13, #14, #15 and the Suginaka bolt telescope denture for missing teeth #16-#17 were completed.

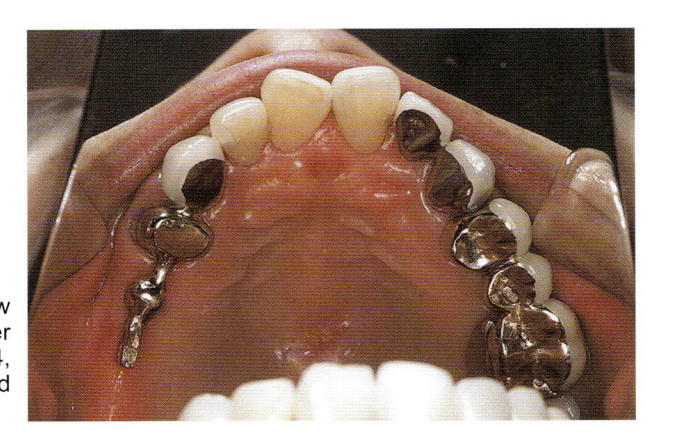

Fig. 12 Upper occlusal view of the Cone-crown-type inner crowns placed on teeth #14, #15 and the PFM crown placed on tooth #13.

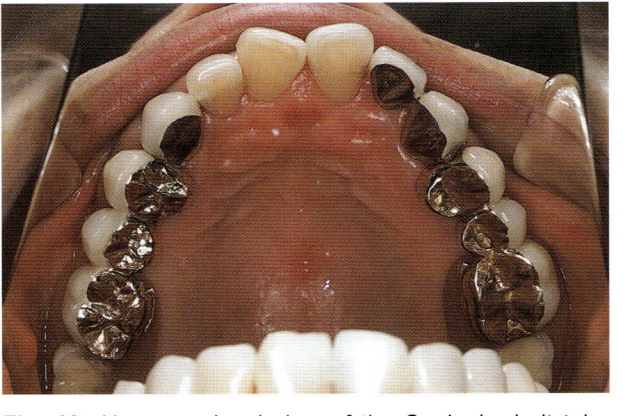

Fig. 13 Upper occlusal view of the Suginaka bolt telescope denture placed on the missing #16-#17 region.

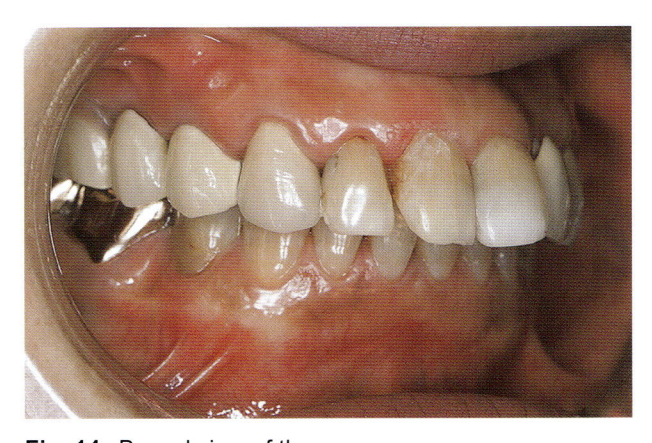

Fig. 14 Buccal view of the same one.

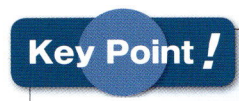

Key Point !

Although the Bioceram sapphire implant cannot be used as a single abutment tooth, placing this in the adjacent region of the abutment tooth for connection with the adjacent abutment tooth leads to an increase in strength of both abutment teeth.

1. Suginaka bolt attachment dentures

2) Suginaka bolt telescope dentures

⑩ Unilateral distal extension missing case: Missing teeth #14, #16-#17; Patient: 53-year-old woman
Tooth #13: Porcelain fused to metal crown (PFM crown)
Tooth #14: Implant abutment
Teeth #14, #15: Cone-crown-type double crown (inner crown with a rod projection)

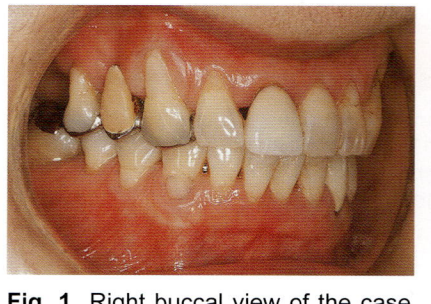

Fig. 1 Right buccal view of the case with secondary caries occurred in the existing bridge for teeth #13-#15 (#14: pontic) and missing teeth #16-#17.

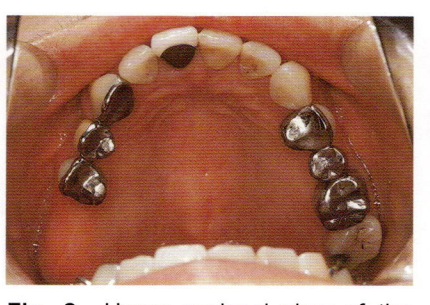

Fig. 2 Upper occlusal view of the same one.

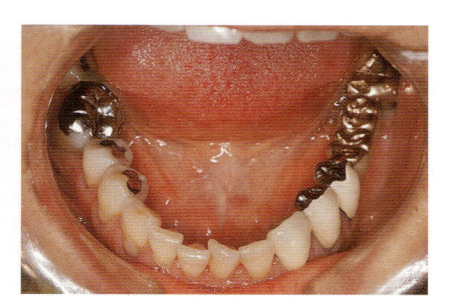

Fig. 3 Lower occlusal view of the same one.

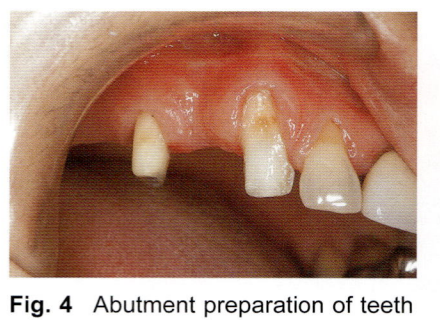

Fig. 4 Abutment preparation of teeth #13, #15 viewed buccally.

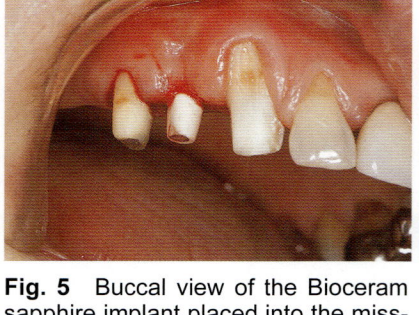

Fig. 5 Buccal view of the Bioceram sapphire implant placed into the missing #14 region for abutment preparation.

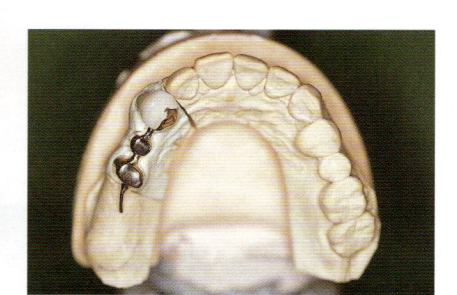

Fig. 6 Occlusal view of the connected Cone-crown-type inner crown with a rod projection for #15, Cone-crown-type inner crown for #14, and PFM crown for #13.

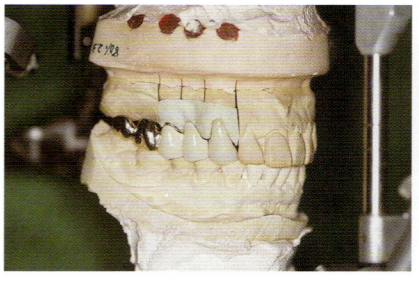

Fig. 7 Buccal view of the one-piece casted Cone-crown-type resin-facing outer crowns for #14, #15 and metal tooth replaced for missing tooth #16.

Fig. 8 Occlusal view of the same one.

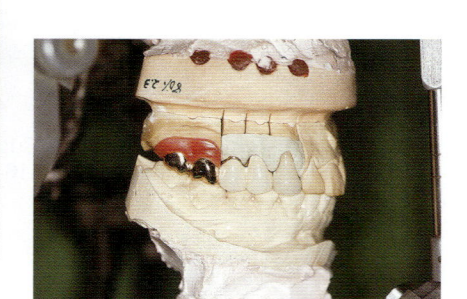

Fig. 9 Buccal view of the wax denture, in which Cone-crown-type resin-facing outer crowns with the metal tooth (for missing tooth #16) involving a Suginaka bolt attachment were placed on teeth #14, #15 and missing tooth #17 was replaced with the resin tooth.

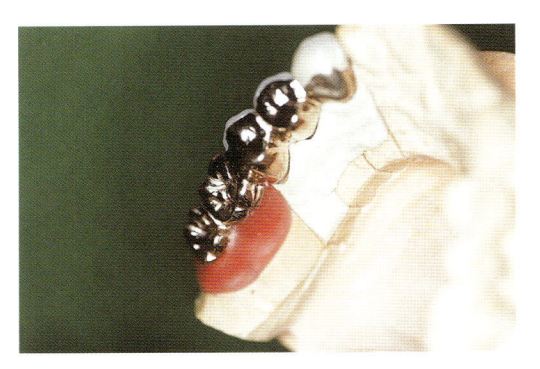

Fig. 10 Lingual view of the same one.

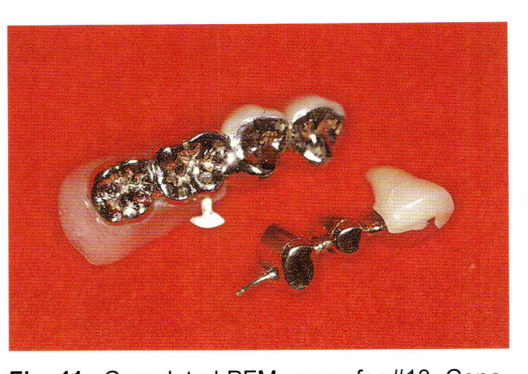

Fig. 11 Completed PFM crown for #13, Cone-crown-type inner crown with a rod projection for #14, #15 (one-piece casted), and Suginaka bolt telescope denture for missing teeth #16-#17.

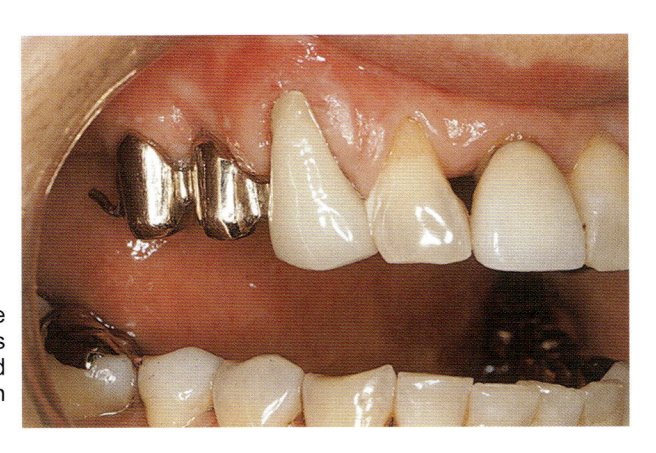

Fig. 12 Buccal view of the Cone-crown-type inner crowns placed on #14, #15 connected to the PFM crown placed on #13.

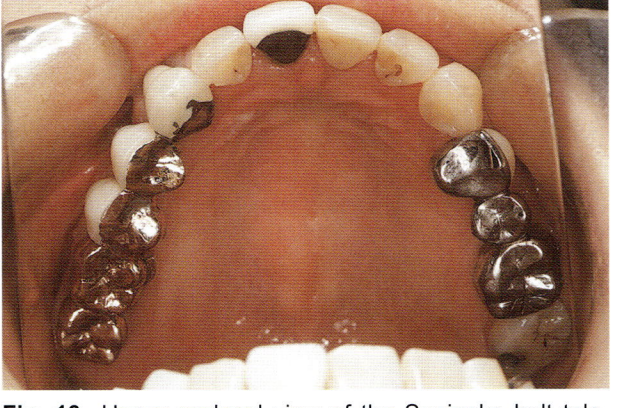

Fig. 13 Upper occlusal view of the Suginaka bolt telescope denture placed on the missing teeth #16-#17 region, in which teeth #14, #15 are used as abutment teeth.

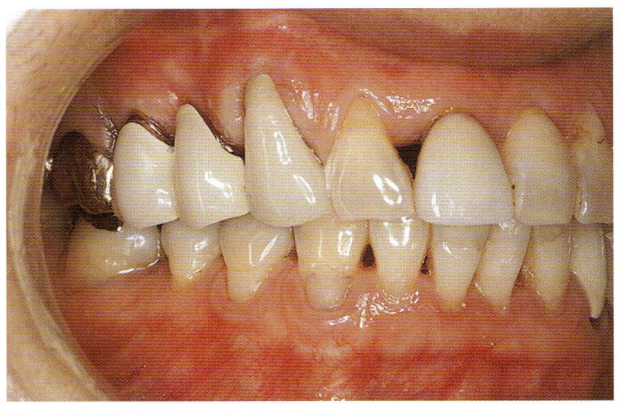

Fig. 14 Right buccal view of the same one.

Key Point !

Although the Bioceram sapphire implant cannot be used as a single abutment tooth, implant placement next to the abutment tooth for splinting of abutment teeth leads to an increase in strength of the implant itself as well as prevention of tooth mobility. As the case, placement of a Bioceram sapphire implant into the tooth #14 region results in avoidance of the solitary tooth of #15.

1. Suginaka bolt attachment dentures

2) Suginaka bolt telescope dentures

⑪Unilateral distal extension missing case: Missing teeth #35-#37; Patient: 61-year-old woman
Tooth #34: 4/5 outer crown-type double crown
Tooth #35: Implant abutment
Teeth #35: Cone-crown-type double crown (inner crown with a plate projection)

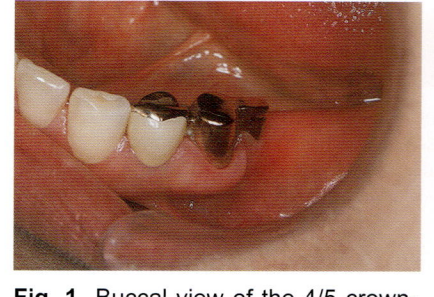

Fig. 1 Buccal view of the 4/5 crown-type inner crown for #34 and Cone-crown-type inner crown for #35, on which Suginaka bolt telescope denture for missing teeth #36-#37 was placed.

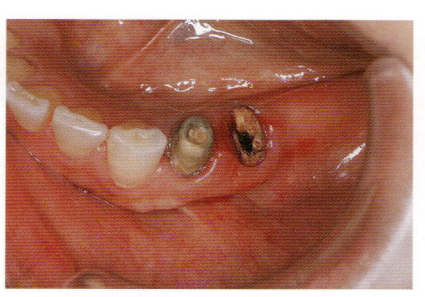

Fig. 2 Buccal view of the abutment tooth of #35 with secondary caries and root fracture.

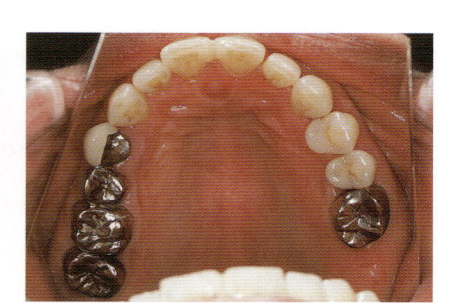

Fig. 3 Upper occlusal view.

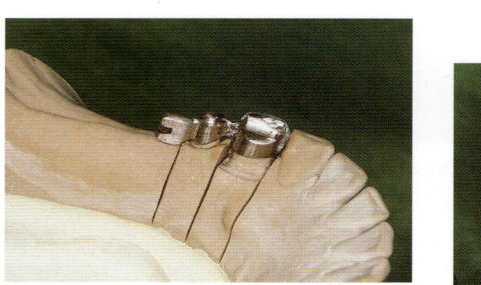

Fig. 4 A sapphire implant placed immediately after extraction of #35.

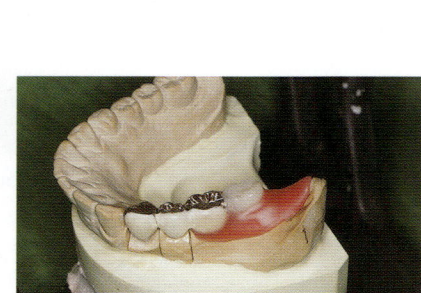

Fig. 5 Buccal view of abutment preparation of the sapphire implant placed in the missing tooth #35 region.

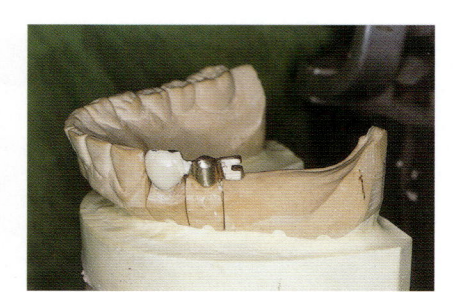

Fig. 6 The inner crown with a plate projection for missing tooth #35 (as implant abutment) was connected to the facing-type inner crown for #34.

Fig. 7 Buccal view of the same one.

Fig. 8 The 4/5 crown-type outer crown for #34, Cone-crown-type outer crown for #35, and metal tooth involving a Suginaka bolt attachment for missing tooth #36 were one-piece casted. Buccal view of the wax denture after replacement of the missing teeth #36 (metal tooth) and #37 with the artificial teeth.

Fig. 9 After try-in and occlusal adjustment of the wax denture, an impression of the mucosal surface of the wax denture was taken with the retainers pressed by fingers. Buccal view of the wax denture returned to the dowel pin working cast model.

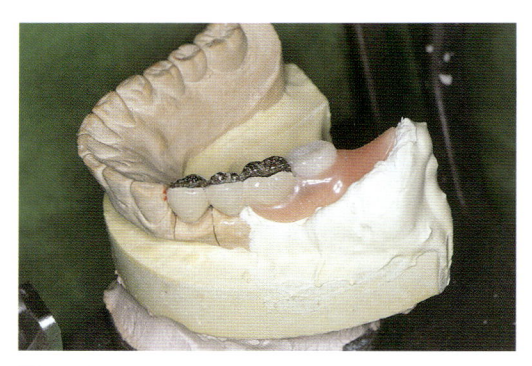

Fig. 10   Pouring dental stone into the impression followed by trimming of the denture base and polymerization.

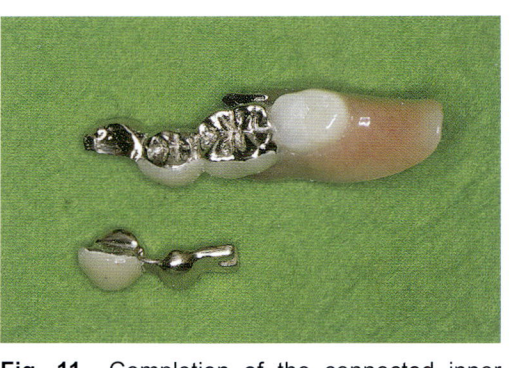

Fig. 11   Completion of the connected inner crowns for #34, #35 and Suginaka bolt telescope denture for missing teeth #36-#37.

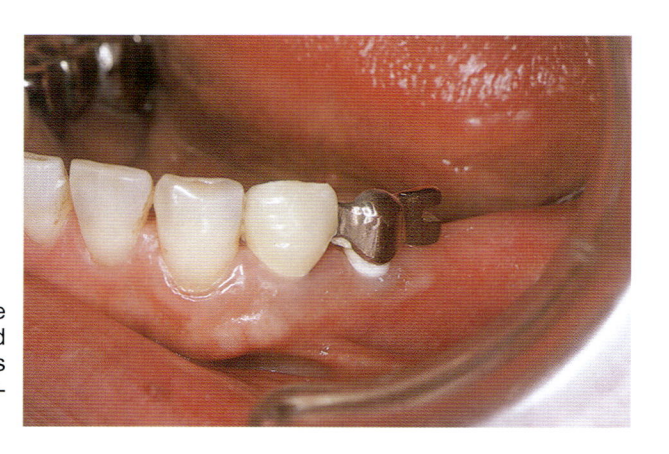

Fig. 12   Buccal view of the connected facing-type and Cone-crown-type inner crowns placed on #34, #35, respectively.

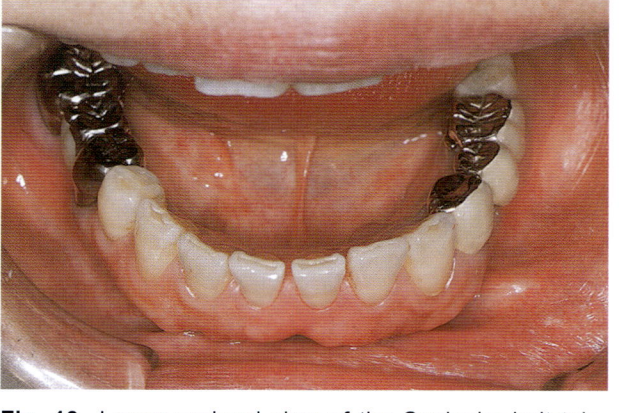

Fig. 13   Lower occlusal view of the Suginaka bolt telescope denture for missing teeth #36-#37 that used #34 and #35 as abutment teeth.

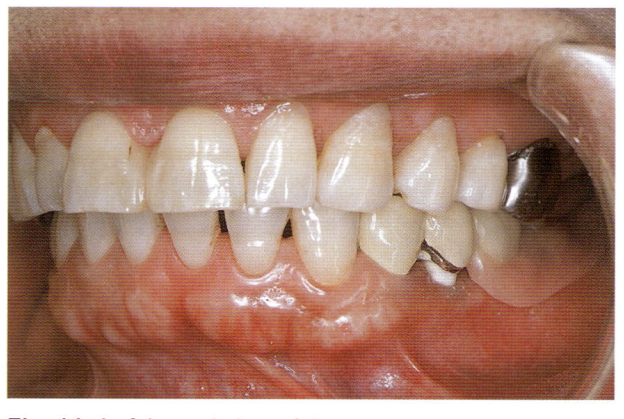

Fig. 14   Left buccal view of the same one.

Key Point !   Although the Bioceram sapphire implant cannot be used as a single abutment tooth, implant placement of the abutment tooth for splinting of adjacent abutment teeth leads to an increase in strength of the implant itself as well as prevention of tooth mobility. Use of immediate post-extraction implant placement-type ones allows initiation of prosthetic treatment before healing of the extraction socket.

1. Suginaka bolt attachment dentures

2) Suginaka bolt telescope dentures

⑫ Bilateral distal extension missing case: Missing teeth #15-#17, #26-#27; Patient: 62-year-old woman
Tooth #14: 4/5 crown-type double crown (4/5-type inner crown with a rod projection)
Tooth #23: Hard resin facing crown
Teeth #24, #25: Cone-crown-type double crown (inner crown with a rod projection)

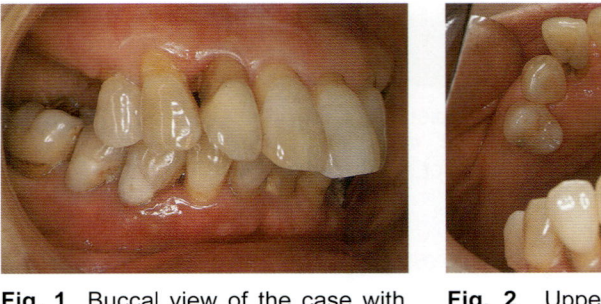

Fig. 1 Buccal view of the case with missing teeth #15-#17, #26-#27.

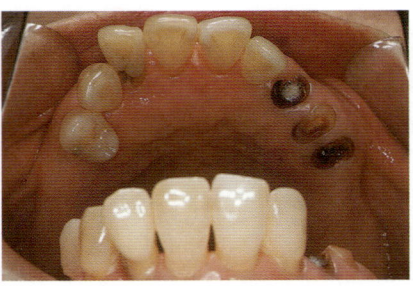

Fig. 2 Upper occlusal view of the same one.

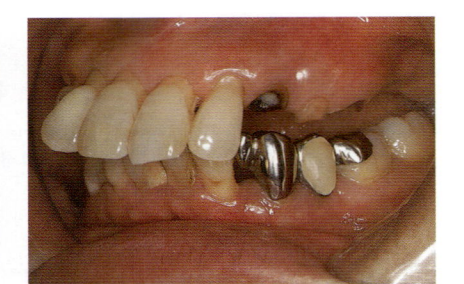

Fig. 3 Left buccal view of the same one.

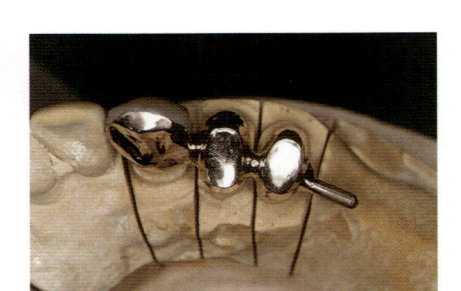

Fig. 4 Occlusal view of the abutment prepared teeth #14, #23-#25.

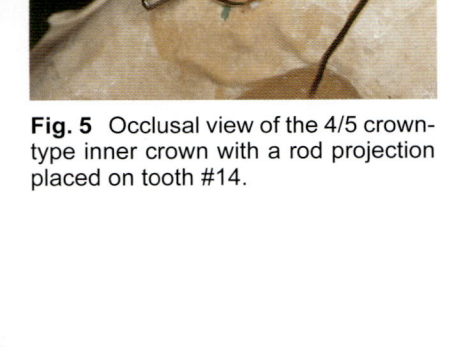

Fig. 5 Occlusal view of the 4/5 crown-type inner crown with a rod projection placed on tooth #14.

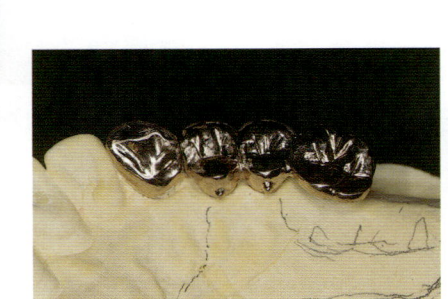

Fig. 6 Occlusal view of the resin-facing crown for #23 connected to Cone-crown-type inner crowns for # 24, #25 (with a rod projection).

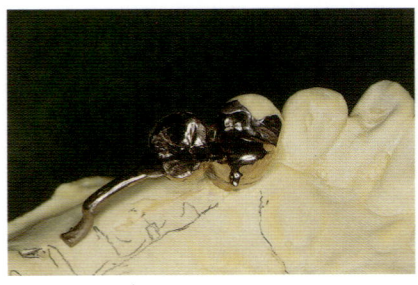

Fig. 7 The 4/5 outer crown for tooth #14 and the facing-type metal tooth for missing tooth #15 involving a Suginaka bolt attachment were one-piece casted. A lug provided for the metal tooth for missing tooth #15 acts as retention during impression taking and denture work.

Fig. 8 Lingual view of the facing-type outer crowns for teeth #24, #25 and metal tooth for missing tooth #26 involving a Suginaka bolt attachment one-piece casted.

Fig. 9 The bilateral outer crowns were soldered to the metal flame placed in the palatal region followed by the replacement of the missing teeth #16, #17, #27 with the artificial teeth.

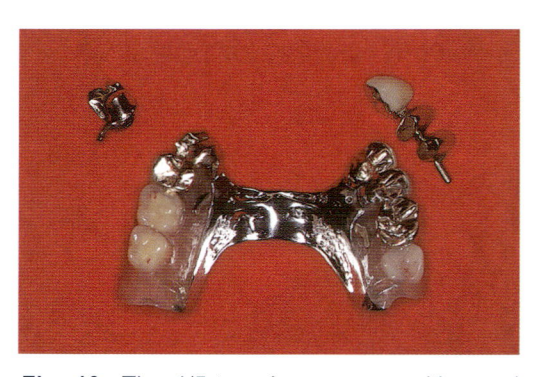

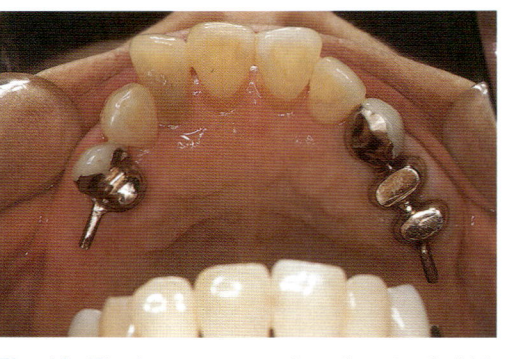

Fig. 10   The 4/5-type inner crown with a rod projection for #14 (upper left), the resin-facing crown for #23 and Cone-crown-type inner crowns for #24, #25 (with a rod projection) connected (upper right), and the Suginaka bolt telescope denture for missing teeth #15-#17, #26-#27 were completed.

Fig. 11   The inner crowns placed on teeth #14, #23-#25.

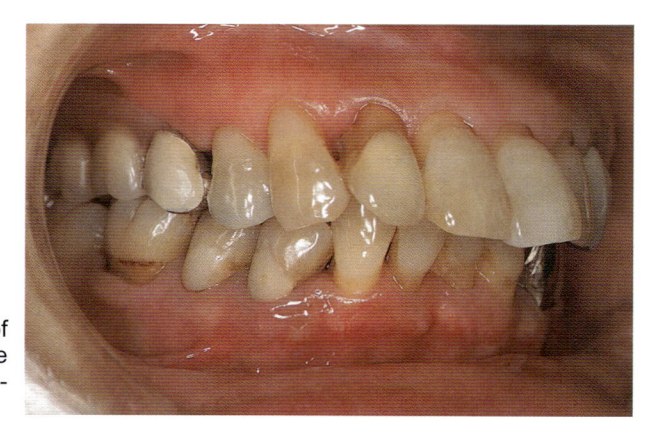

Fig. 12   Right buccal view of the Suginaka bolt telescope denture for missing teeth #15-#17, #26-#27.

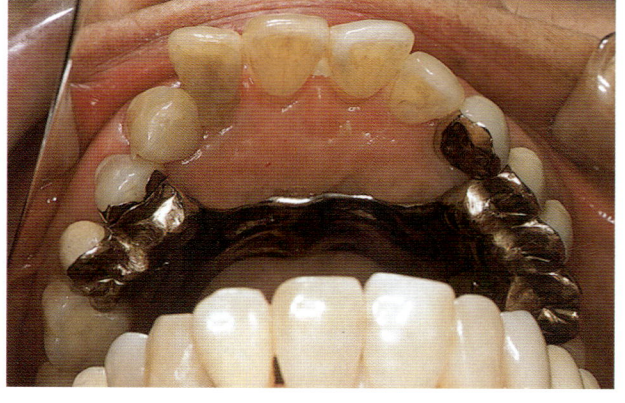

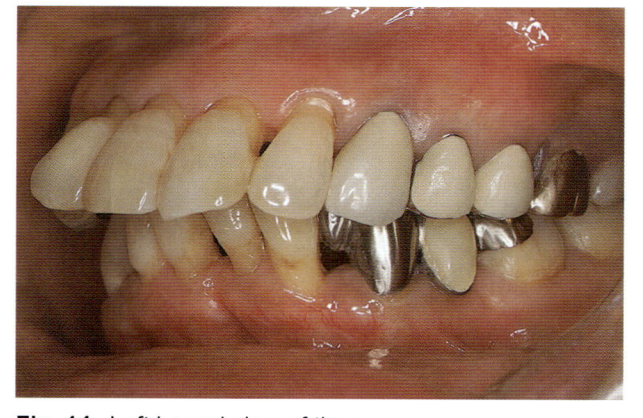

Fig. 13   Upper occlusal view of the same one.

Fig. 14   Left buccal view of the same one.

 **Key Point !**   For older patients, even for the vital tooth as tooth #14, as thicker abutment preparation is made possible, the 4/5 crown-type double crown was selected. If the Cone-crown-type double crown would be selected for tooth #23, because a great volume of tooth reduction might be required for placement of the inner crown due to the different axial inclination and lead to a decrease in retention of it, it was decided to use the resin-facing crown.

1. Suginaka bolt attachment dentures

2) Suginaka bolt telescope dentures

⑬Bilateral distal extension missing case: Missing teeth #46-#47, #35-#37; Patient: 53-year-old woman
Teeth #45, #34: 4/5 outer crown-type double crown (facing-type inner crown with a rod projection)

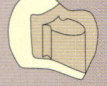

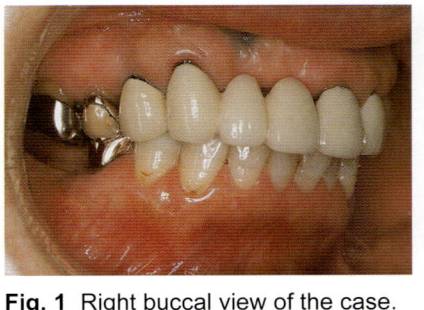

Fig. 1 Right buccal view of the case.

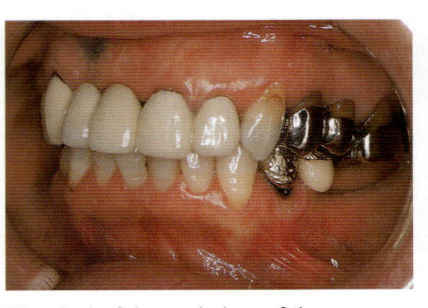

Fig. 2 Left buccal view of the case.

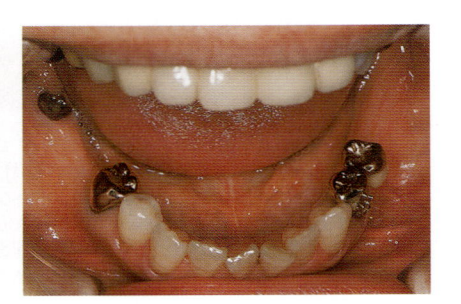

Fig. 3 Lower occlusal view of the case before extraction of tooth #38.

Fig. 4 Buccal view of the facing-type inner crown with a rod projection of 4/5 outer crown-type double crown for #45.

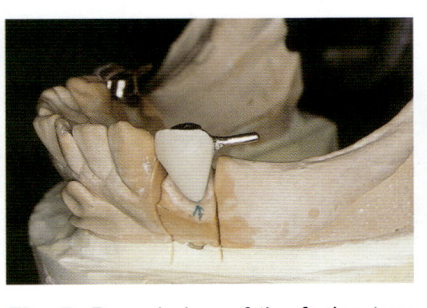

Fig. 5 Buccal view of the facing-type inner crown with a rod projection of 4/5 outer crown-type double crown for #34.

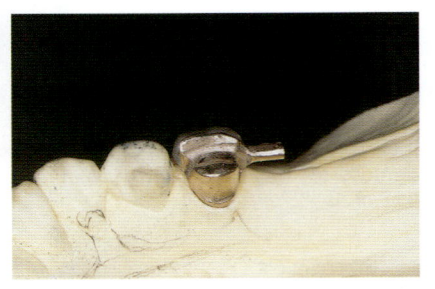

Fig. 6 Lingual view of the facing-type inner crown for #45.

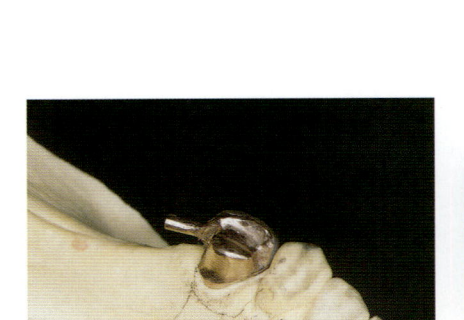

Fig. 7 Lingual view of the facing-type inner crown for #34.

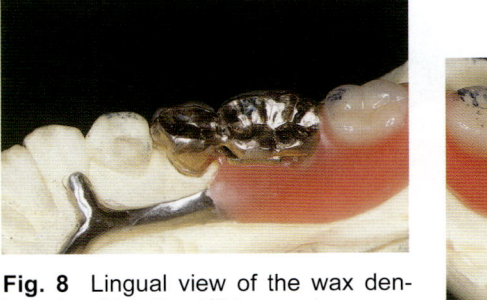

Fig. 8 Lingual view of the wax denture, in which the 4/5-type outer crown for #45 and facing-type metal tooth for missing tooth #46 involving a Suginaka bolt attachment were one-piece casted, and the missing tooth #47 was replaced with the artificial tooth.

Fig. 9 Lingual view of the wax denture, in which the 4/5-type outer crown for #34 and facing-type metal tooth for missing tooth #35 involving a Suginaka bolt attachment were one-piece casted, and the missing teeth #36-#37 were replaced with the artificial teeth.

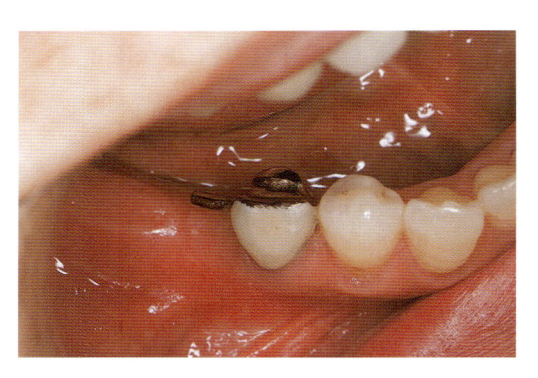

Fig. 10 Resin facing-type inner crown placed on #45.

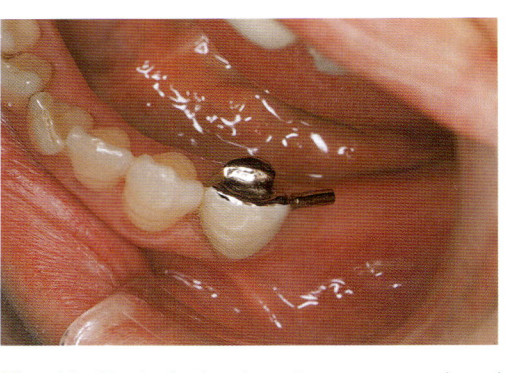

Fig. 11 Resin facing-type inner crown placed on #34.

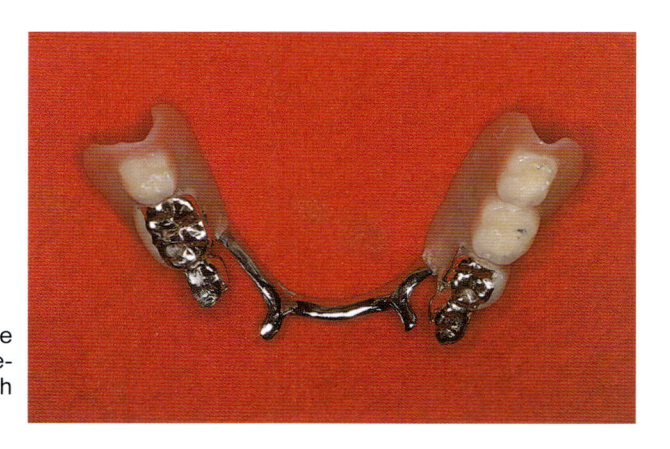

Fig. 12 Occlusal view of the completed Suginaka bolt telescope denture for missing teeth #35-#37, #46-#47.

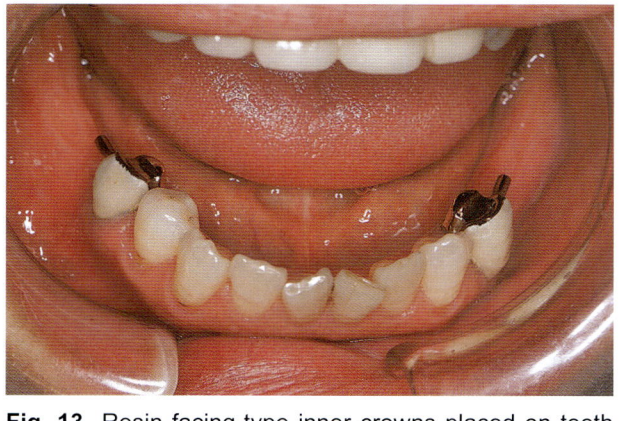

Fig. 13 Resin facing-type inner crowns placed on teeth #34 and #45, respectively.

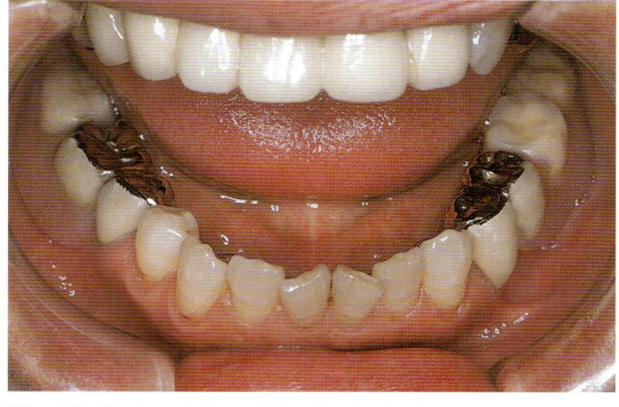

Fig. 14 Occlusal view of the Suginaka bolt telescope denture placed on the missing teeth #35-#37, #46-#47 region.

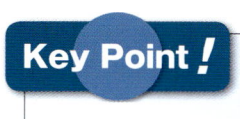
Key Point !

There are two ways of fabricating the 4/5 outer crown-type double crown; one uses the facing-type inner crown and 4/5 crown-type outer crown, and the other uses the 4/5-type crown for both inner and outer crowns.

1. Suginaka bolt attachment dentures

2) Suginaka bolt telescope dentures

⑭ Bilateral distal extension missing case: Missing teeth #45-#47, #34-#37; Patient: 70-year-old woman
Teeth #33, #44: Cone-crown-type double crown (inner crown with a plate projection)

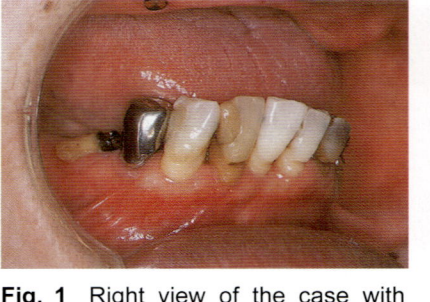

Fig. 1 Right view of the case with missing teeth #45-#47, #34-#37.

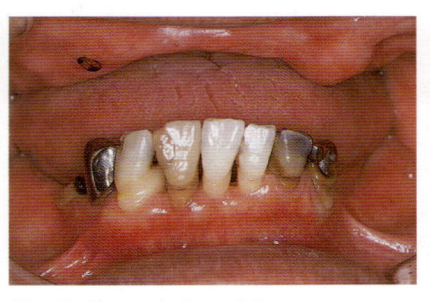

Fig. 2 Frontal view of the same none.

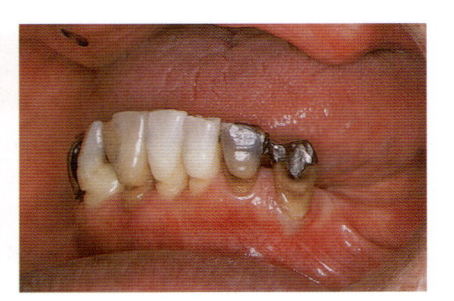

Fig. 3 Left view of the same one.

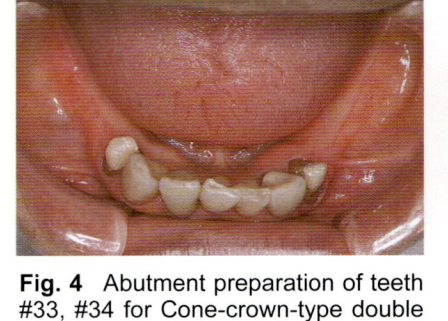

Fig. 4 Abutment preparation of teeth #33, #34 for Cone-crown-type double crown.

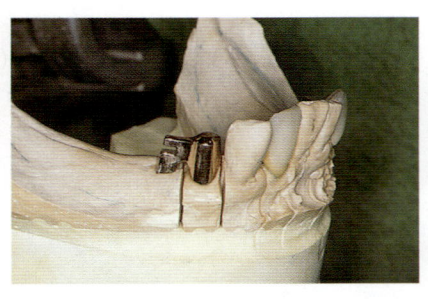

Fig. 5 Buccal view of the Cone-crown-type inner crown with a plate projection placed on #44.

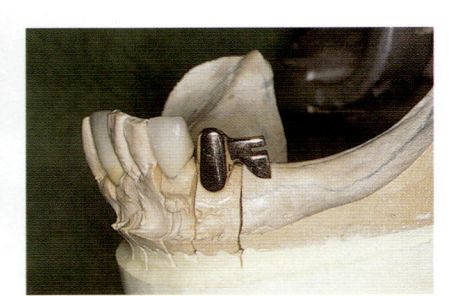

Fig. 6 Buccal view of the Cone-crown-type inner crown with a plate projection placed on #33.

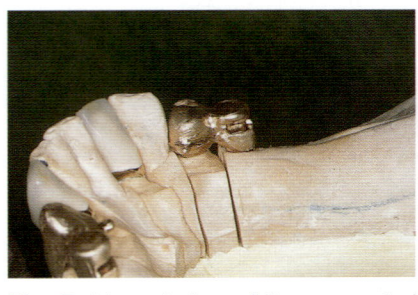

Fig. 7 Lingual view of the connected Cone-crown-type outer crown for #44 and metal tooth for missing tooth #45 involving a Suginaka bolt attachment. Both of these were planned for complete veneer restoration with hybrid resin.

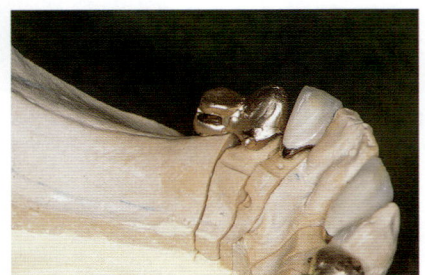

Fig. 8 Lingual view of the connected Cone-crown-type outer crown for #33 and metal tooth for missing tooth #34 involving a Suginaka bolt attachment. Both of these were planned for complete veneer restoration with hybrid resin.

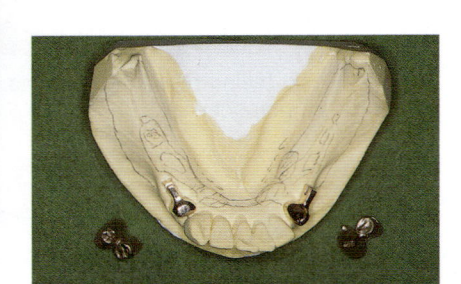

Fig. 9 The inner crowns for teeth #33, #44 returned to the working cast model.

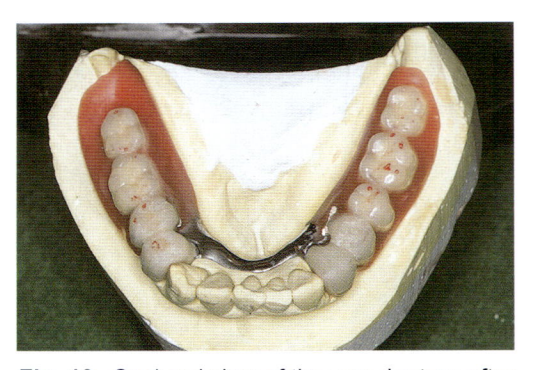

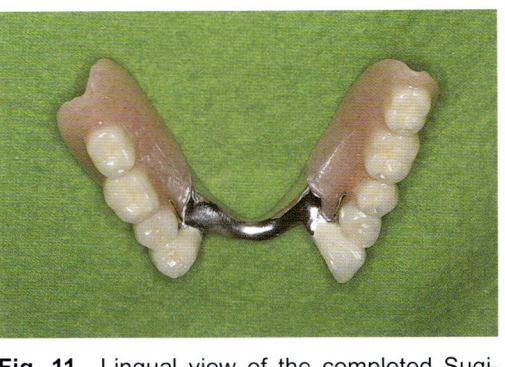

Fig. 10 Occlusal view of the wax denture after complete veneer of the outer crowns for #33, #44 and metal teeth for missing teeth #34, #45 with hybrid resin and replacement of the missing teeth #35-#37, #46-#47 with the artificial teeth.

Fig. 11 Lingual view of the completed Suginaka bolt telescope denture for missing teeth #34-#37, #45-#47.

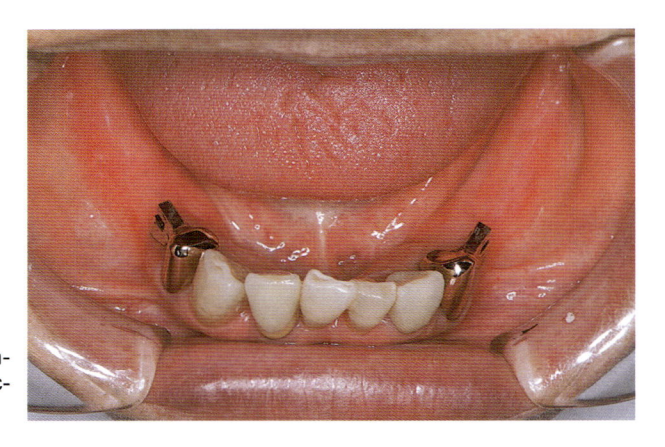

Fig. 12 Occlusal view of the inner crowns with a plate projection placed on #33, #44.

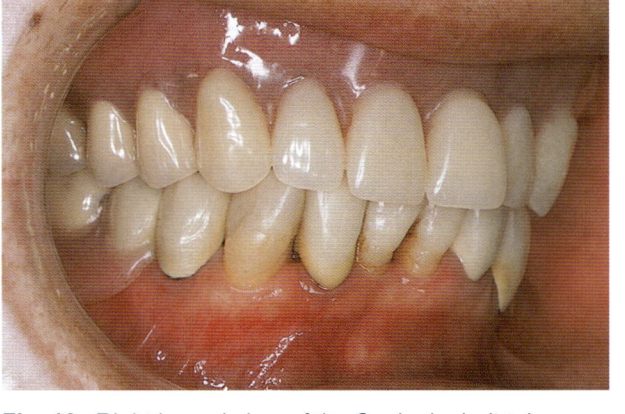

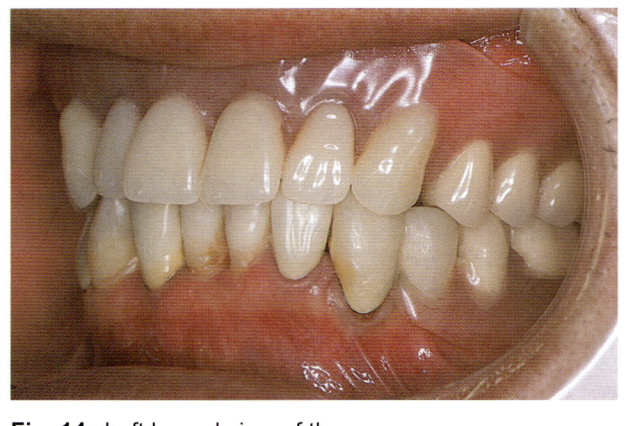

Fig. 13 Right buccal view of the Suginaka bolt telescope denture placed on the missing teeth #34-#37, #45-#47 region.

Fig. 14 Left buccal view of the same one.

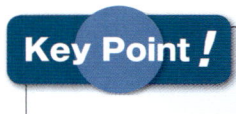 **Key Point !**

As the use of the plate projection may make contact with the denture basal surface during rotating/sinking of the denture base, it is necessary to maintain a slight space between them in the bilateral distal extension missing cases.

1. Suginaka bolt attachment dentures

2) Suginaka bolt telescope dentures

⑮ Few remaining teeth/Multiple missing teeth case: Missing teeth #11-#17, #21-#25, #27, #33-#37, #43-#47; Patient: 70-year-old woman
Teeth #26, #32, #42: Cone-crown-type double crown (inner crown with a rod projection)

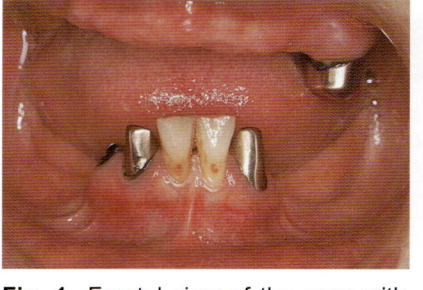

Fig. 1 Frontal view of the case with multiple missing teeth and stump of #43.

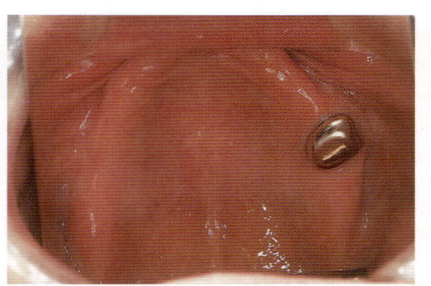

Fig. 2 Upper occlusal view of the case.

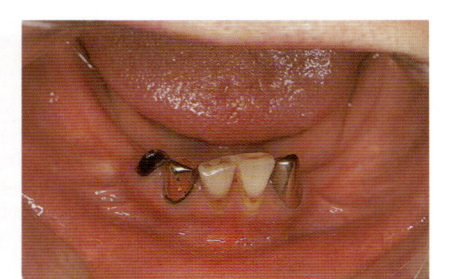

Fig. 3 Lower occlusal view of the case. The patient presented to the clinic with the chief complaint of masticatory dysfunction and a speech defect due to poor retention in the existing Cone-crown-type upper and lower dentures.

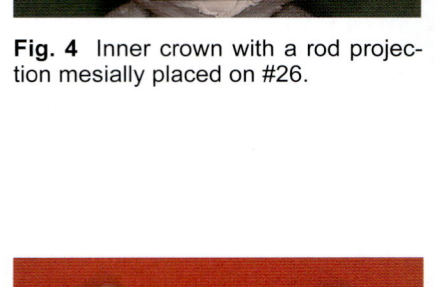

Fig. 4 Inner crown with a rod projection mesially placed on #26.

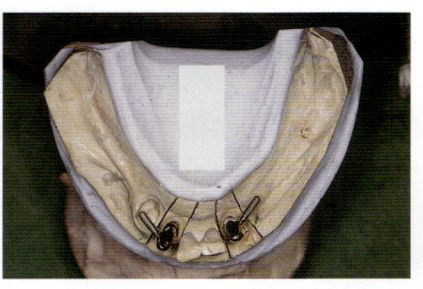

Fig. 5 Occlusal view of the inner crowns with a rod projection distally placed on #32, #42.

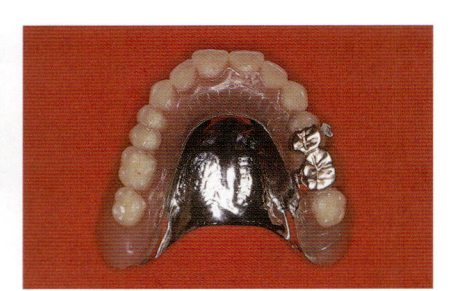

Fig. 6 Upper Suginaka bolt telescope denture with the Cone-crown-type outer crown for #26. Buccally-placed hook.

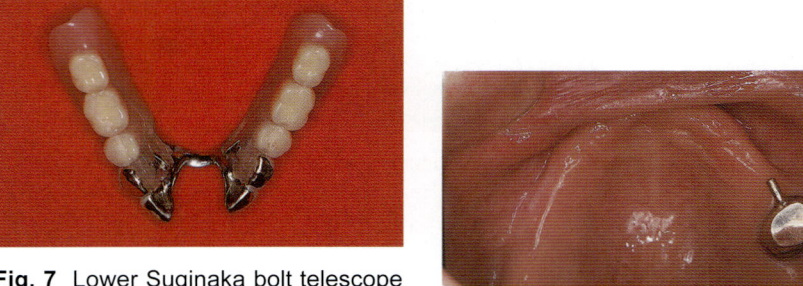

Fig. 7 Lower Suginaka bolt telescope denture with the Cone-crown-type outer crowns for #32, #42.

Fig. 8 Inner crown with a rod projection placed on #26.

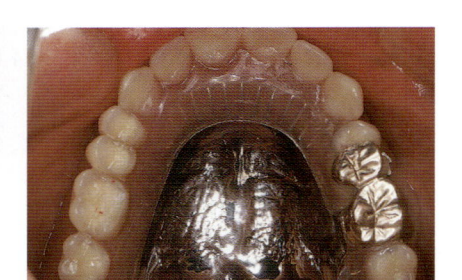

Fig. 9 Occlusal view of the Suginaka bolt telescope denture placed on the missing teeth #11-17, #21-25, #27 region.

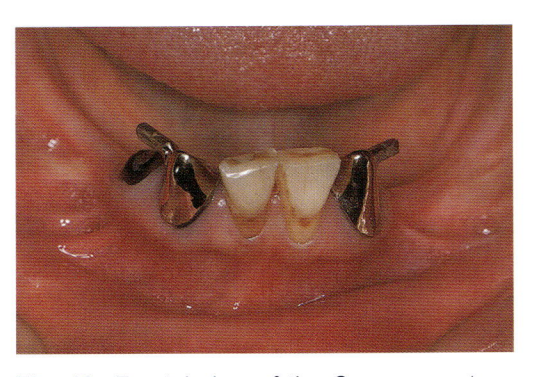

Fig. 10 Frontal view of the Cone-crown-type inner crowns with a rod projection placed on #32, #42.

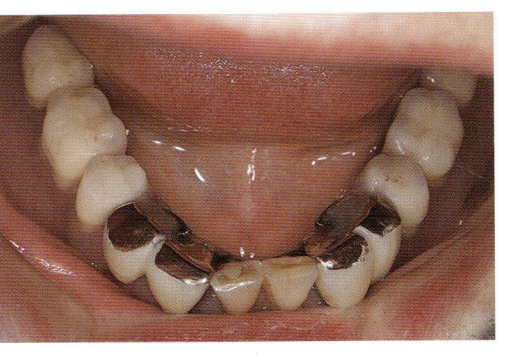

Fig. 11 Occlusal view of the Suginaka bolt telescope denture placed on the missing teeth #33-#37, #43-#47 region.

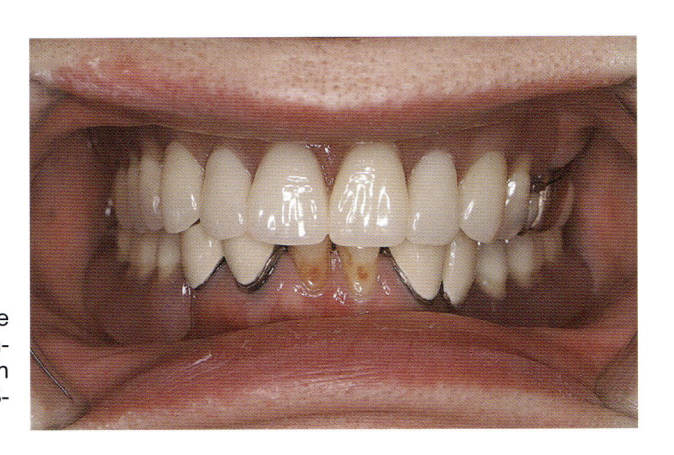

Fig. 12 Frontal view of the Suginaka bolt telescope denture placed on the missing teeth #11-#17, #21-#25, #27, #33-#37, #43-#47 region.

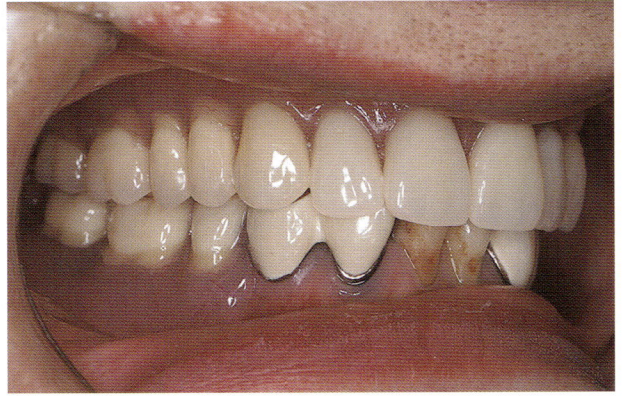

Fig. 13 Right buccal view of the same one.

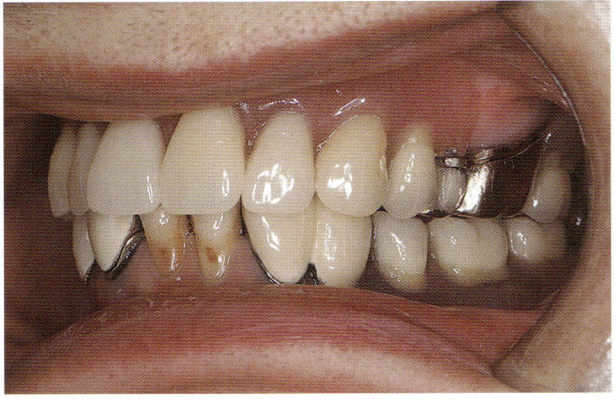

Fig. 14 Left buccal view of the same one. Buccally-placed hook.

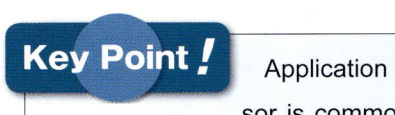

Key Point!   Application of the Cone-crown-type double crown to the lower lateral incisor is commonly difficult because the abutment tooth becomes thin, but it can be applied to patients who eat no hard food. In overdentures, under which the stump is located, even if the tooth extraction is required, just a rod projection can be used.

1. Suginaka bolt attachment dentures

2) Suginaka bolt telescope dentures

⑯Few remaining teeth/Multiple missing teeth case: Missing teeth #31-#37, #41-#42, #44-47; Patient: 66-year-old woman
Tooth #43: Cone-crown-type double crown (inner crown with a rod projection)

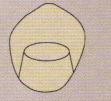
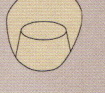

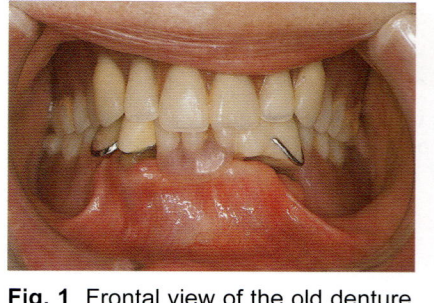

Fig. 1 Frontal view of the old denture for missing teeth #31-#37, #41-#42, #44-#47.

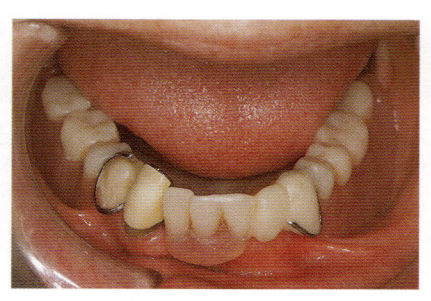

Fig. 2 Lower occlusal view of the same one.

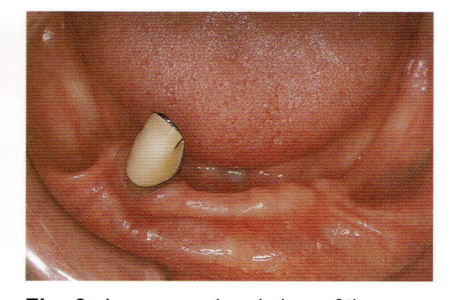

Fig. 3 Lower occlusal view of the case with the old lower denture removed.

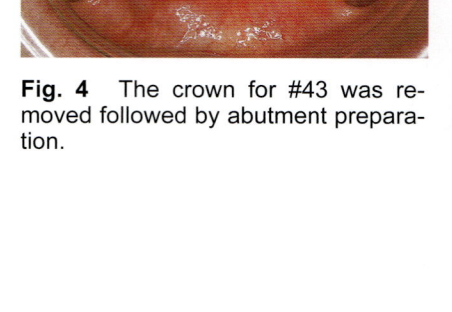

Fig. 4 The crown for #43 was removed followed by abutment preparation.

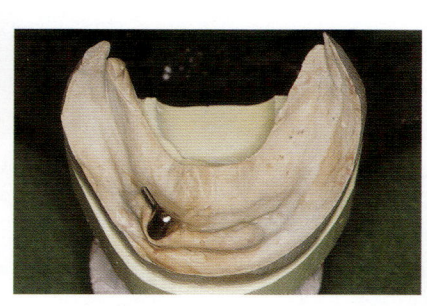

Fig. 5 Cone-crown-type inner crown with a rod projection placed on #43.

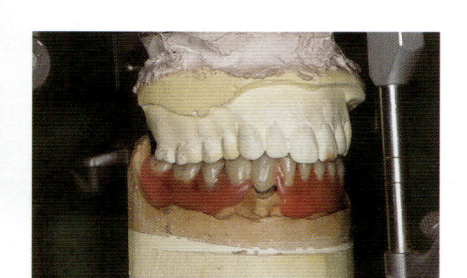

Fig. 6 One-piece casted facing-type outer crown for #43 and metal tooth for #44 involving a Suginaka bolt attachment. The missing teeth were replaced with the artificial teeth.

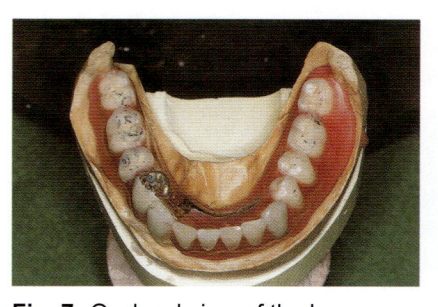

Fig. 7 Occlusal view of the lower wax denture after replacement of the missing teeth with the artificial teeth.

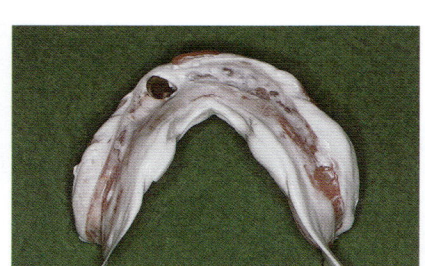

Fig. 8 Checking denture base fit of the wax denture.

Fig. 9 Bite-seating impression taking with the wax denture.

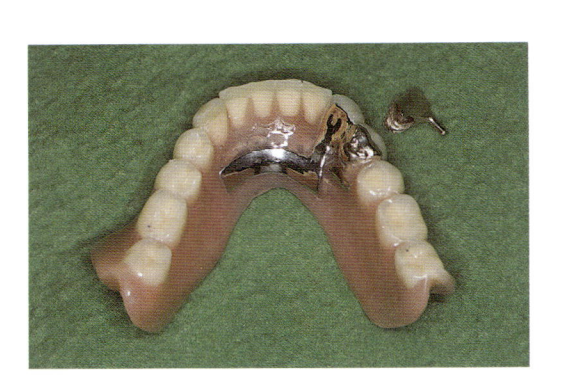

Fig. 10 Completed inner crown with a rod projection for #43 and Suginaka bolt telescope denture for missing teeth #31-#37, #41-#42, #44-#47.

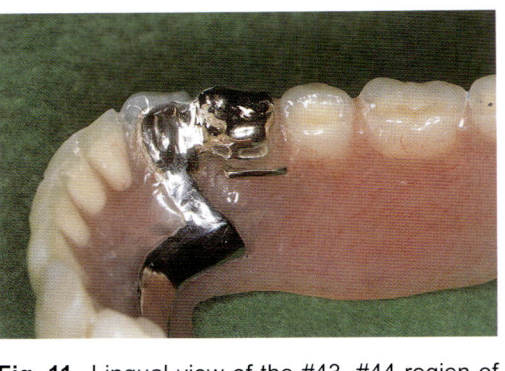

Fig. 11 Lingual view of the #43, #44 region of the completed telescope denture.

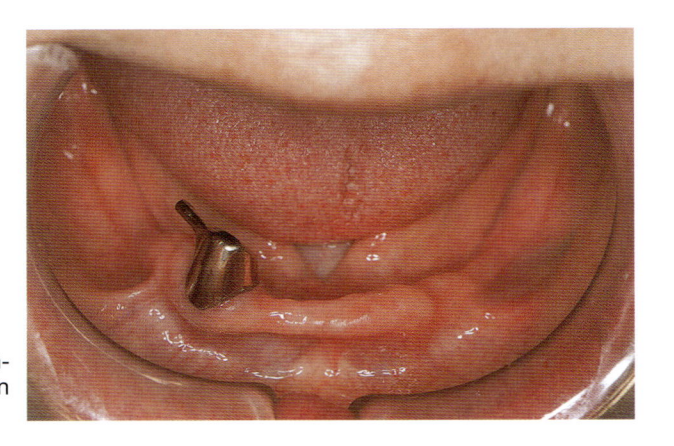

Fig. 12 Frontal view of the inner crown with a rod projection placed on #43.

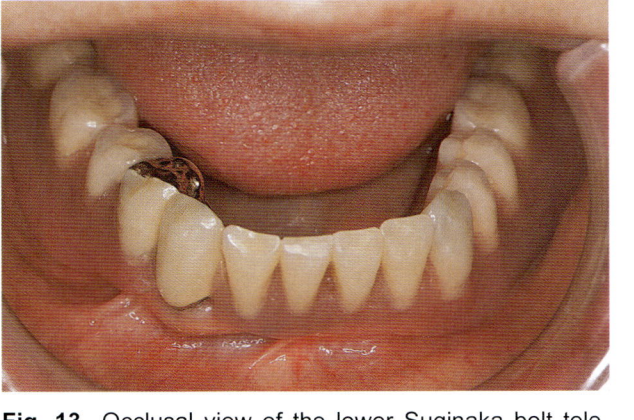

Fig. 13 Occlusal view of the lower Suginaka bolt telescope denture placed in the mouth.

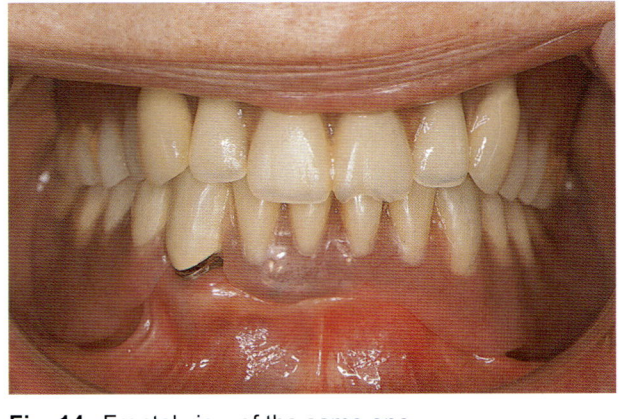

Fig. 14 Frontal view of the same one.

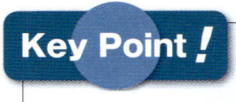
Key Point !

As the present case, in cases with the poor residual ridge, it is necessary to often check the denture base fit.

2. Suginaka bolt lock dentures

①Unilateral distal extension missing case: Missing tooth #17; Patient: 51-year-old woman
 Tooth #16: Healthy tooth; Lock retainer

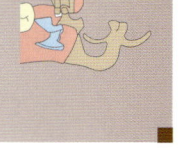

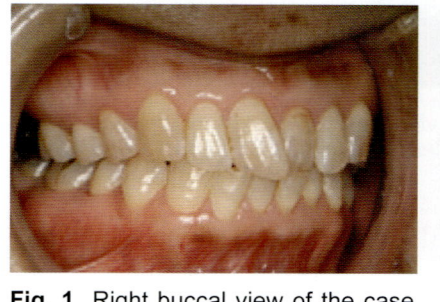

Fig. 1 Right buccal view of the case with missing tooth #17.

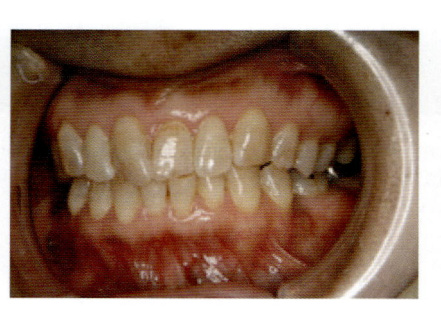

Fig. 2 Left buccal view of the same one.

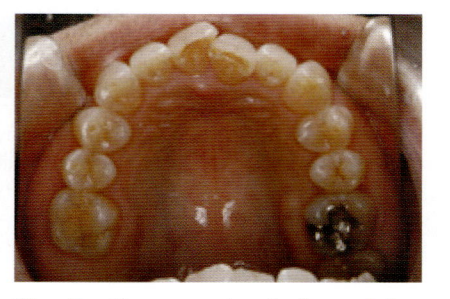

Fig. 3 Upper occlusal view of the same one.

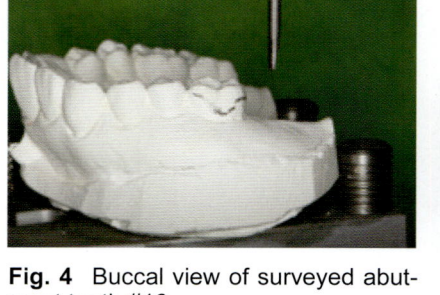

Fig. 4 Buccal view of surveyed abutment tooth #16.

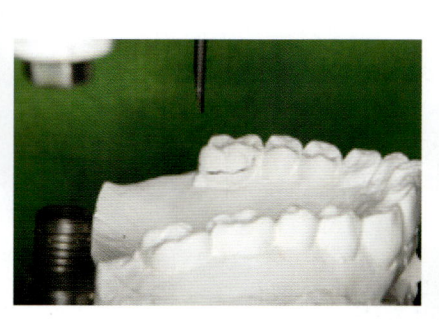

Fig. 5 Lingual view of the same one.

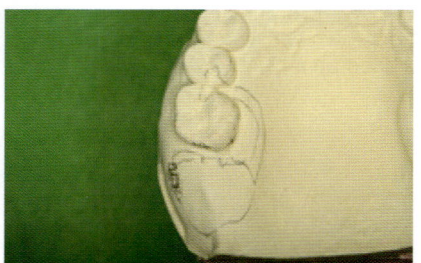

Fig. 6 Denture base outline for the lock denture for missing tooth #17.

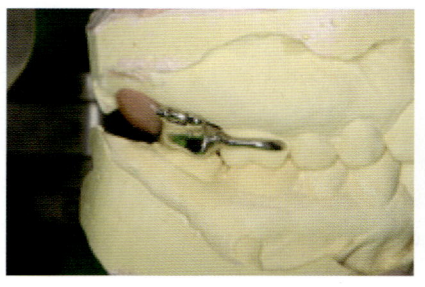

Fig. 7 Buccal view of the lock denture for missing tooth #17.

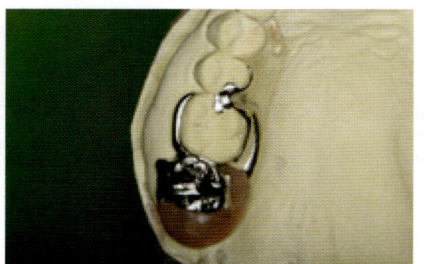

Fig. 8 Occlusal view of the lock denture, in which the temporary base (clear resin) was placed in the lingual region of teeth #14, #15.

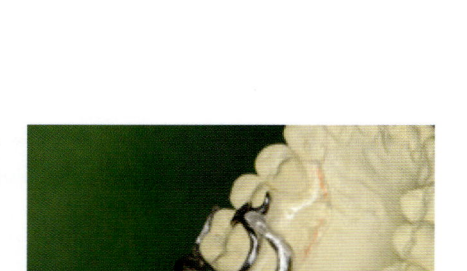

Fig. 9 Lingual view of the completed Suginaka bolt lock denture for missing tooth #17 after removal of the temporary base. The lever is opened for buccally rotating the metal tooth.

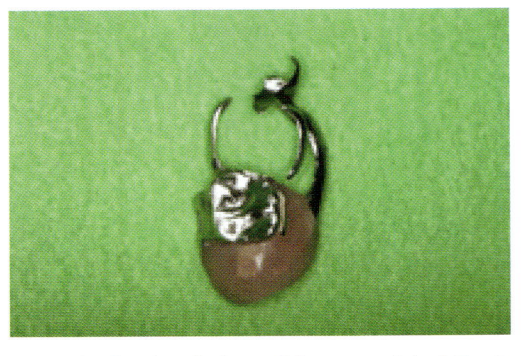

Fig. 10 Occlusal view of the completed Suginaka bolt lock denture for missing tooth #17.

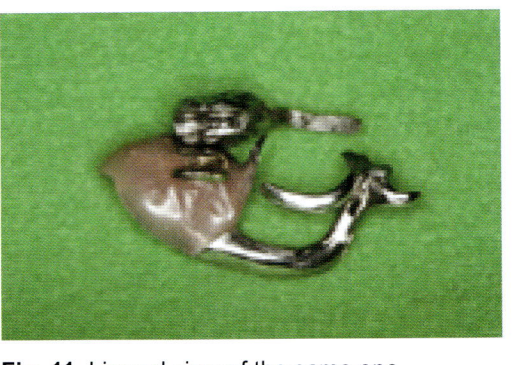

Fig. 11 Lingual view of the same one.

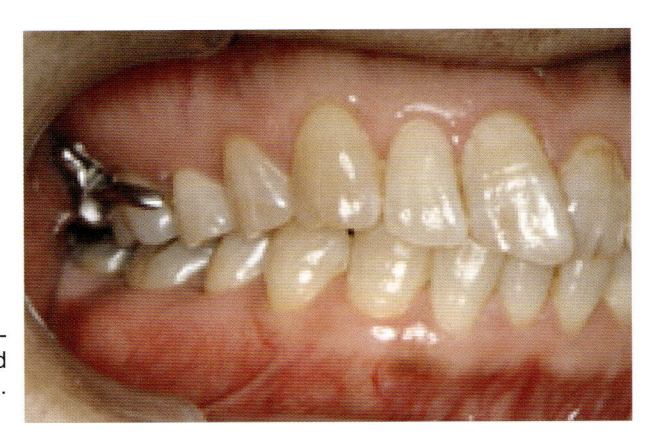

Fig. 12 Buccal view of the Suginaka bolt lock denture placed on the missing tooth #17 region.

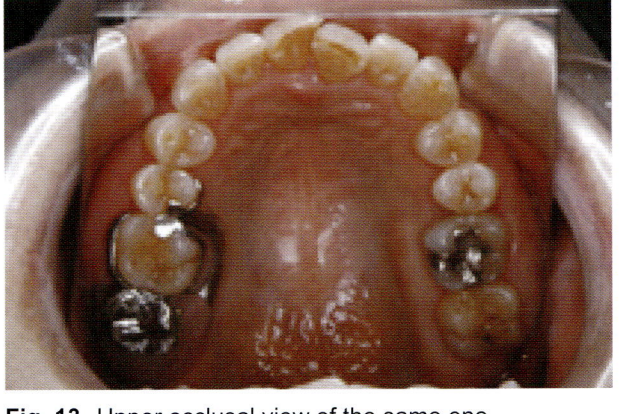

Fig. 13 Upper occlusal view of the same one.

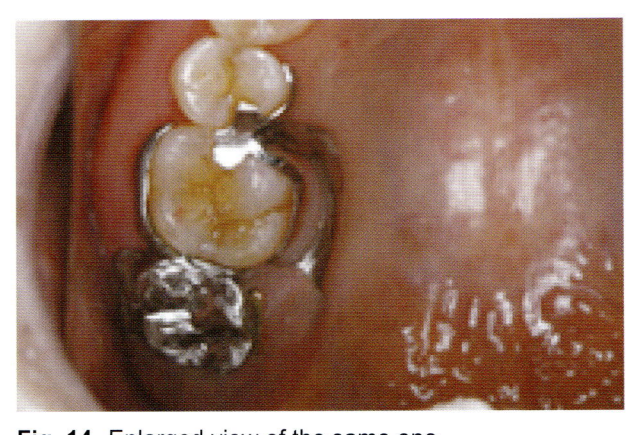

Fig. 14 Enlarged view of the same one.

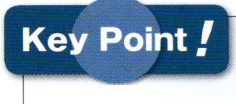 **Key Point !** It is important to allow the patient to practice sufficiently on the model with the temporary base placed as shown in Fig. 3 to be accustomed to insertion and removal of the lock denture. For unilateral distal extension lock dentures, both the buccal and lingual arms of the lock retainer should be placed within the deep undercut area below the survey line to avoid them from coming in contact with gingiva.

2. Suginaka bolt lock dentures

②Unilateral distal extension missing case: Missing tooth #37; Patient: 66-year-old man
Tooth #36: Inlay restored tooth (vital tooth); Lock retainer

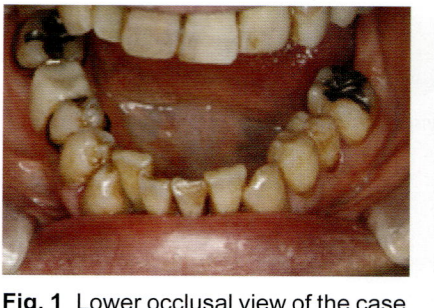

Fig. 1 Lower occlusal view of the case with missing tooth #37.

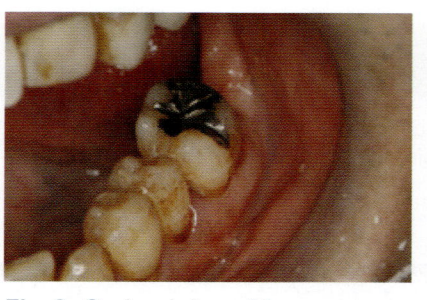

Fig. 2 Occlusal view of the same one.

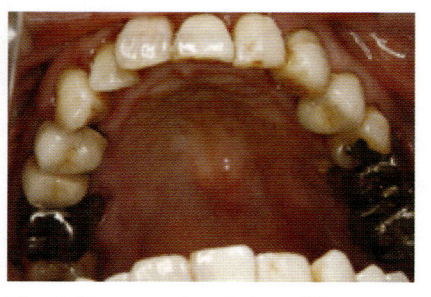

Fig. 3 Upper occlusal view of the same one.

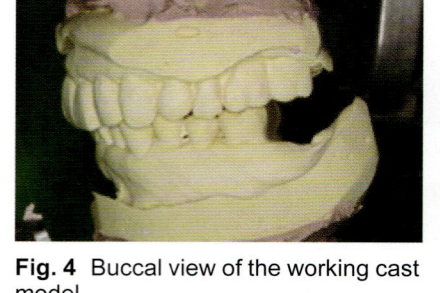

Fig. 4 Buccal view of the working cast model.

Fig. 5 Buccal view of the lock retainer for tooth #36.

Fig. 6 Lingual view of the same one.

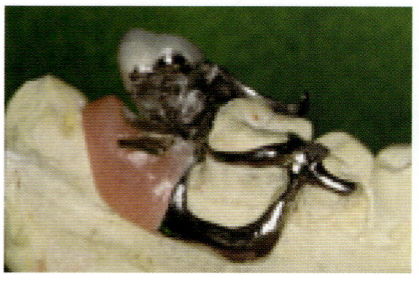

Fig. 7 Lingual view of the lock denture, in which the hook is opened for buccally rotating the metal tooth for missing tooth #37.

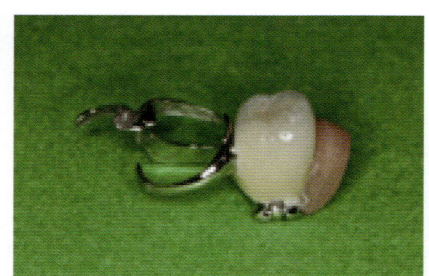

Fig. 8 Buccal view of the completed Suginaka bolt lock denture for missing tooth #37.

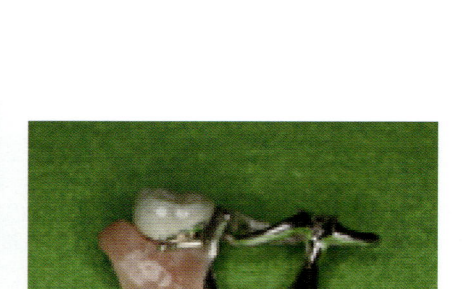

Fig. 9 Lingual view of the same one.

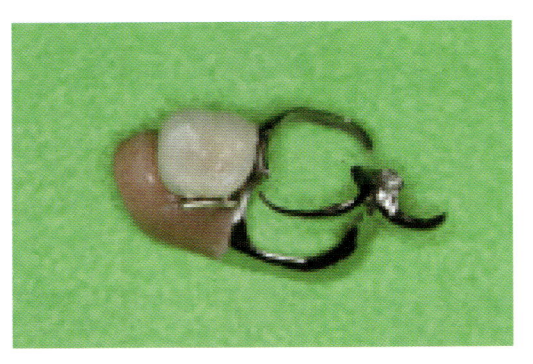

Fig. 10 Occlusal view of the same one.

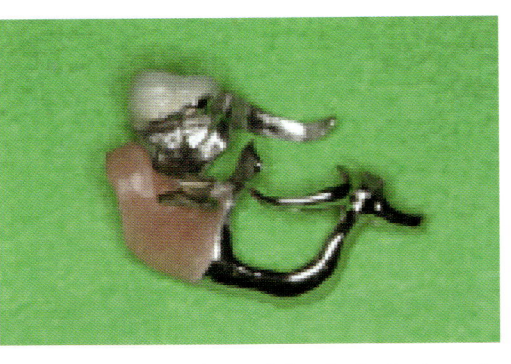

Fig. 11 Lingual view of the lock denture, in which the hook is opened for buccally rotating the metal tooth for missing tooth #37.

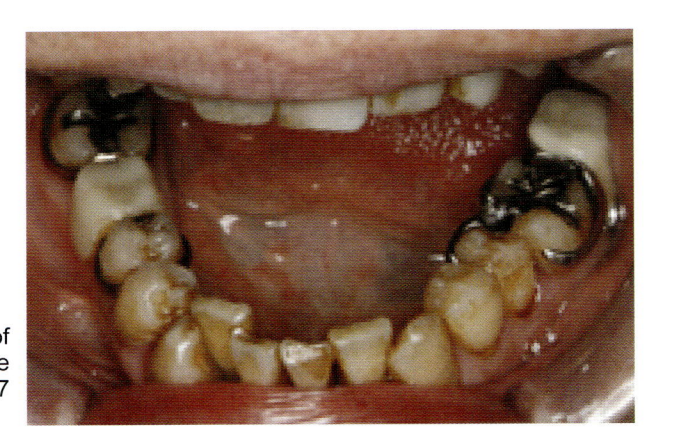

Fig. 12 Lower occlusal view of the Suginaka bolt lock denture placed on the missing tooth #37 region.

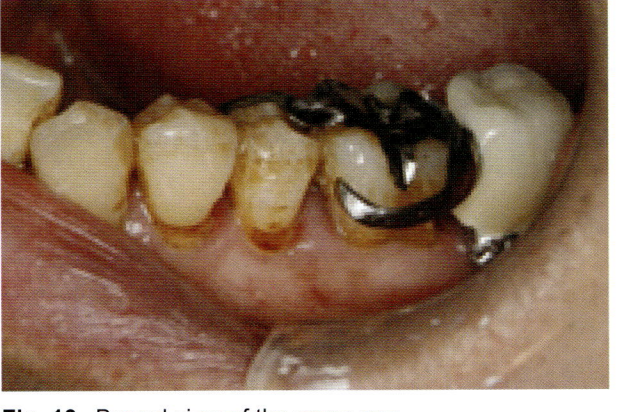

Fig. 13 Buccal view of the same one.

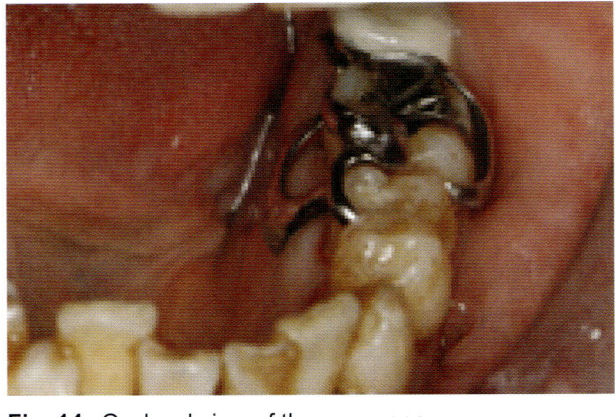

Fig. 14 Occlusal view of the same one.

Key Point ! With the longer clinical coronal length of the abutment tooth results in an increase in sinking depth/rotational angle of the denture base, the guide plane is to be shortened and the proximal plate is contacted with its lower end for facilitating rotation of the denture. The total contact a proximal plate between a long guide plane makes the same effect as a cantilever bridge and the patient may experience pain, so care must be taken to avoid danger. For unilateral distal extension lock dentures, both the buccal and lingual arms of the lock retainer should be placed within the deep undercut area below the survey line to avoid them from coming in contact with gingiva/dental root.

2. Suginaka bolt lock dentures

③Unilateral distal extension missing case: Missing teeth #37-#38; Patient: 74-year-old man
Teeth #35, #36: Healthy teeth (vital teeth); Lock retainer

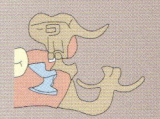

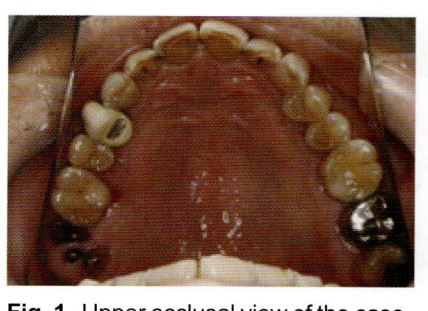

Fig. 1 Upper occlusal view of the case.

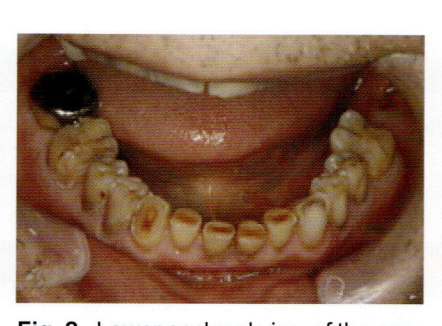

Fig. 2 Lower occlusal view of the case with missing teeth #37-#38.

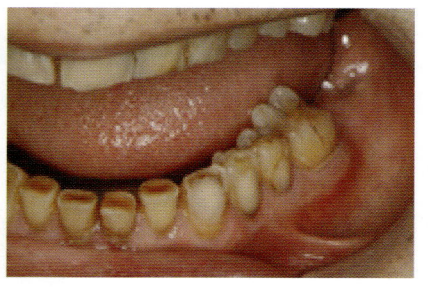

Fig. 3 Occlusal view of the same one.

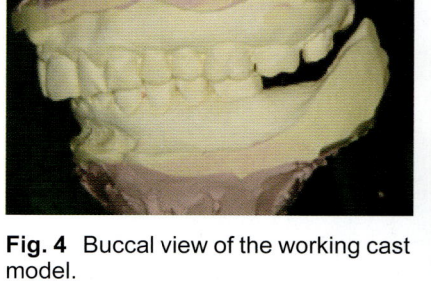

Fig. 4 Buccal view of the working cast model.

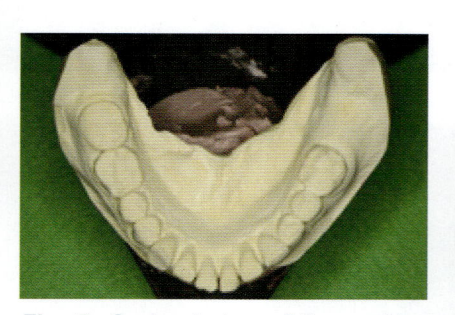

Fig. 5 Occlusal view of the working cast model. Denture base outline of lock denture for missing teeth #37-#38.

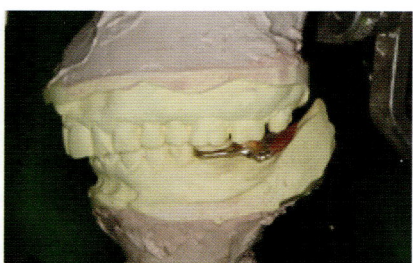

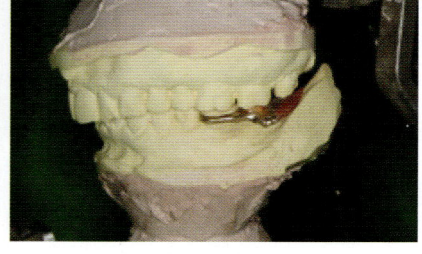

Fig. 6 Buccal view of the lock denture after replacement of the missing teeth #37-#38 with the artificial teeth.

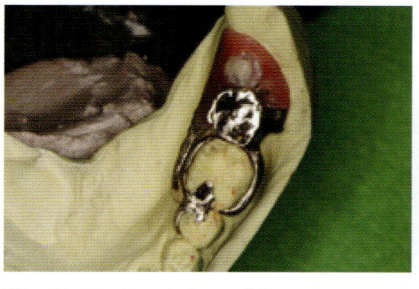

Fig. 7 Occlusal view of the same one.

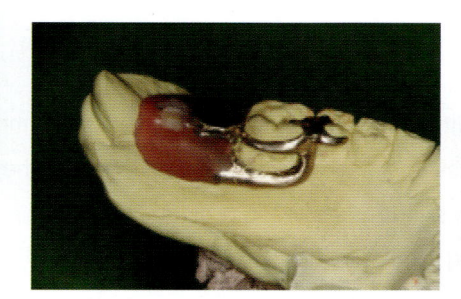

Fig. 8 Lingual view of the same one.

Fig. 9 Lingual view of the lock denture, in which the lever is opened for buccally rotating the metal tooth.

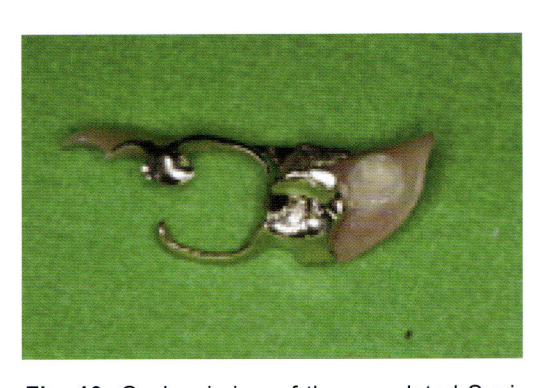

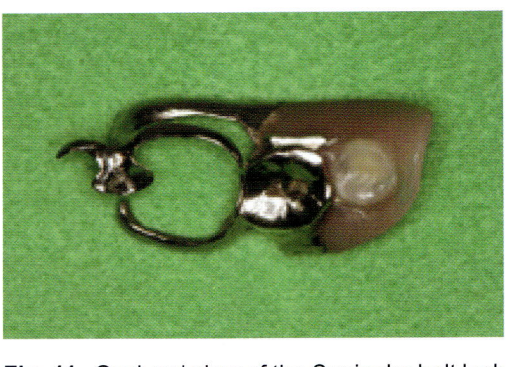

Fig. 10 Occlusal view of the completed Suginaka bolt lock denture with the temporary base.

Fig. 11 Occlusal view of the Suginaka bolt lock denture without the temporary base for missing teeth #37-#38 .

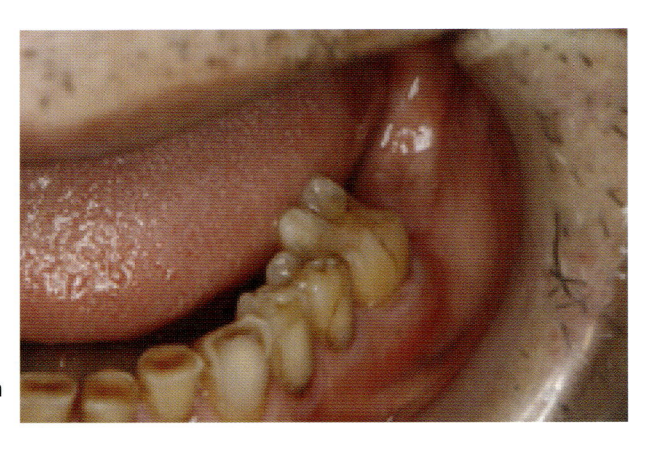

Fig. 12 Rest seats formed on abutment teeth #35, #36.

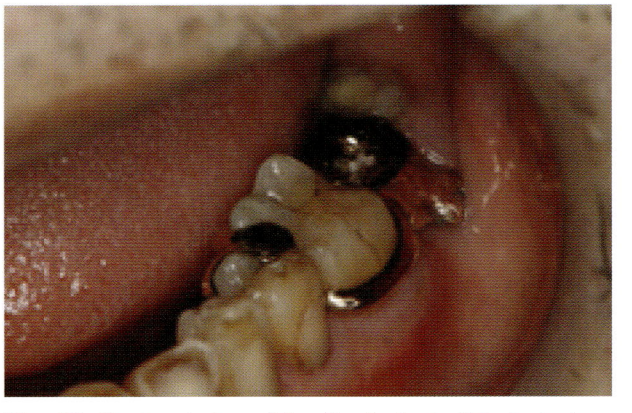

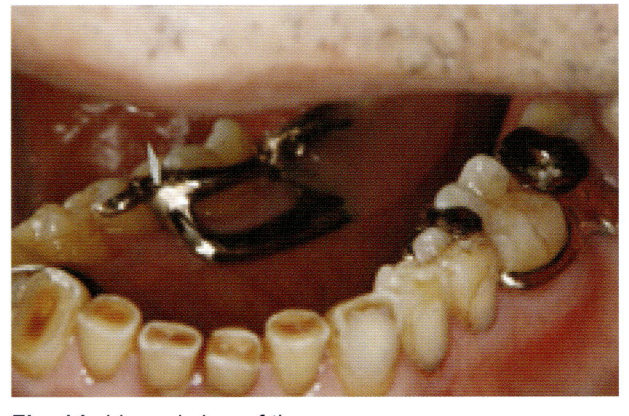

Fig. 13 Occlusal view of the Suginaka bolt lock denture placed on the missing teeth #37-#38 region.

Fig. 14 Lingual view of the same one.

 **Key Point !** The lock retainer can be used even in the distal extension missing cases of the second and third molars. It is necessary to allow the patient to practice sufficiently on the model using the lock denture with the temporary base to be accustomed to insertion and removal of the lock denture. As a matter of course, both the buccal and lingual arms of the lock retainer should be placed within the deep undercut area below the survey line to avoid them from coming in contact with gingiva/dental root.

2.Suginaka bolt lock dentures

④Unilateral distal extension missing case: Missing teeth #26-#27; Patient: 69-year-old woman
Tooth #25: Healthy tooth (vital teeth); Lock retainer

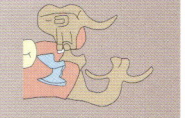

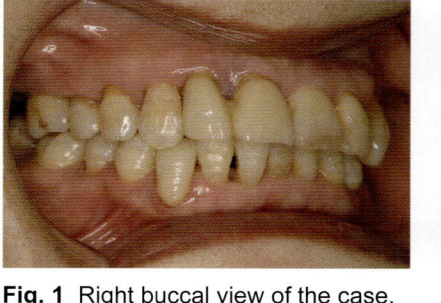

Fig. 1 Right buccal view of the case.

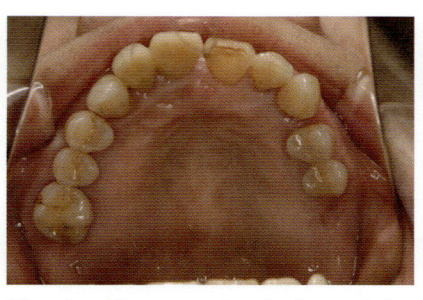

Fig. 2 Upper occlusal view of the case with missing teeth #26-#27.

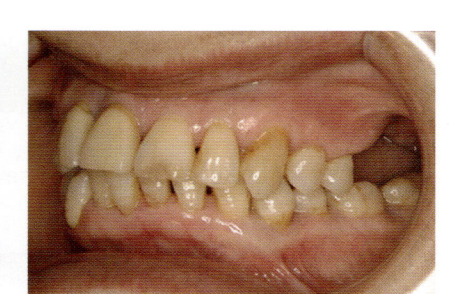

Fig. 3 Left buccal view of the same one.

Fig. 4 Buccal view of the wax denture after the missing teeth #26-#27 were replaced with the metal tooth covered fully with a hybrid resin and artificial tooth, respectively.

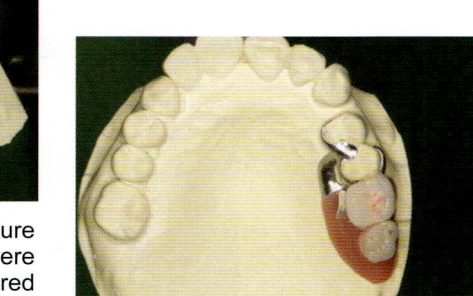

Fig. 5 Occlusal view of the same one.

Fig. 6 Lingual view of the same one.

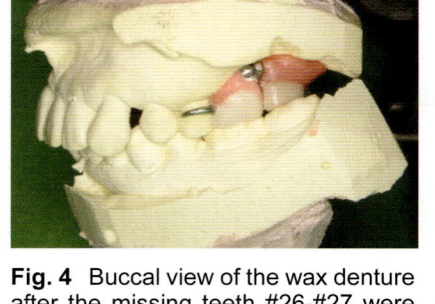

Fig. 7 Lingual view of the lock denture, in which the hook is opened for buccally rotating the metal tooth for missing tooth #26.

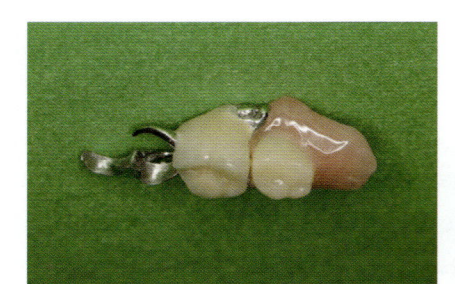

Fig. 8 Buccal view of the completed Suginaka bolt lock denture for missing teeth 26-#27.

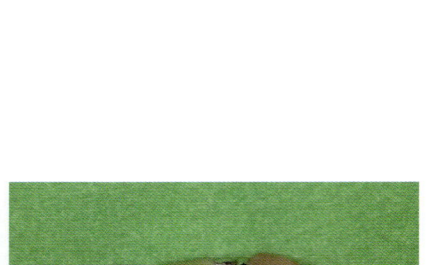

Fig. 9 Occlusal view of the same one.

114

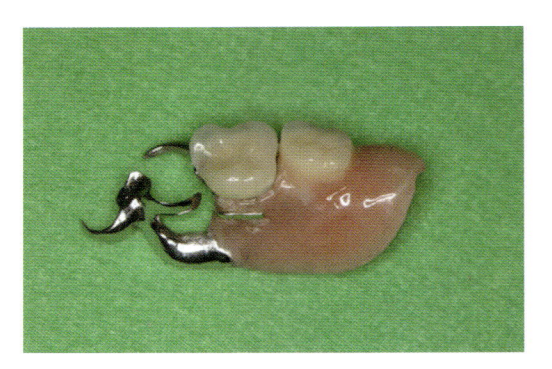

Fig. 10 Lingual view of the same one.

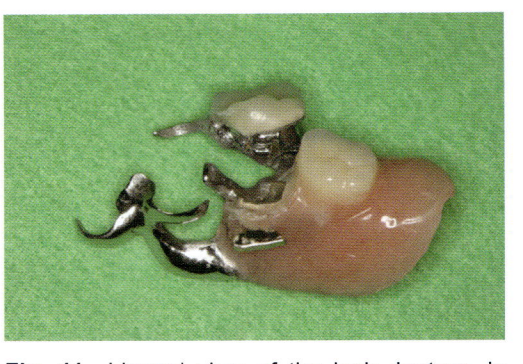

Fig. 11 Lingual view of the lock denture, in which the hook is opened for buccally rotating the metal tooth for missing tooth #26.

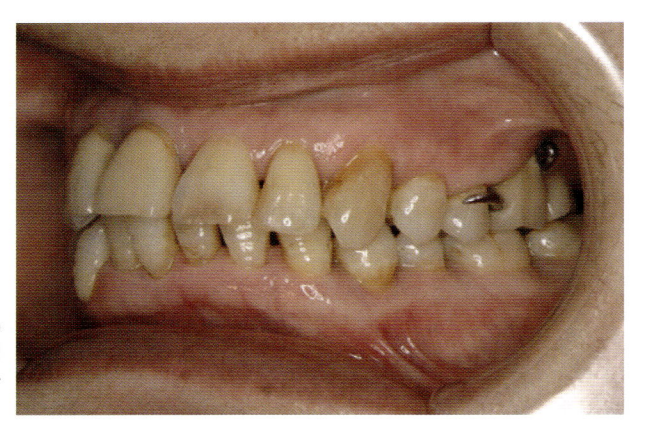

Fig. 12 Left buccal view of the Suginaka bolt lock denture placed on the missing teeth #26-#27 region.

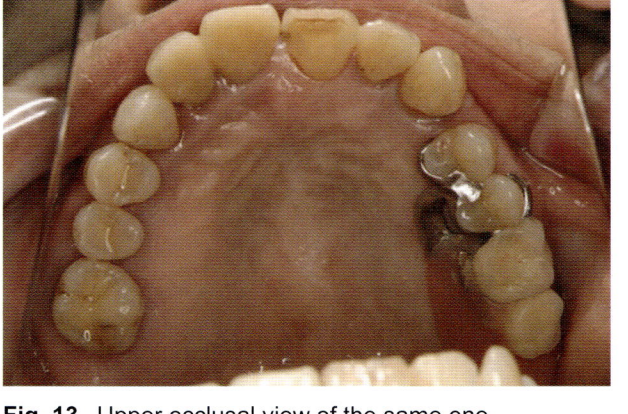

Fig. 13 Upper occlusal view of the same one.

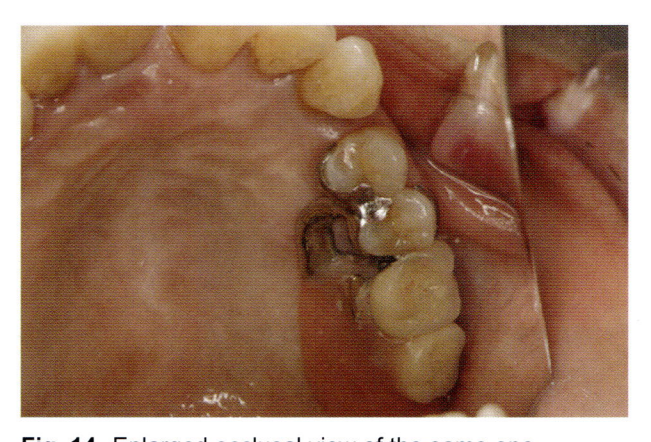

Fig. 14 Enlarged occlusal view of the same one.

Key Point !　Before treatment planning, since the sinking depth/rotational angle of the denture base could increase due to significant edentulous ridge resorption, although it seemed impossible to treat the case unilaterally, the lock denture could be used without any trouble. As a matter of course, both the buccal and lingual arms of the lock retainer should be placed within the deep undercut area below the survey line for reducing a burden on the abutment tooth.

2. Suginaka bolt lock dentures

⑤ Unilateral distal extension missing case: Missing teeth #36-#37; Patient: 68-year-old woman
Tooth #35: Crown restored tooth; Lock retainer

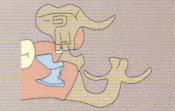

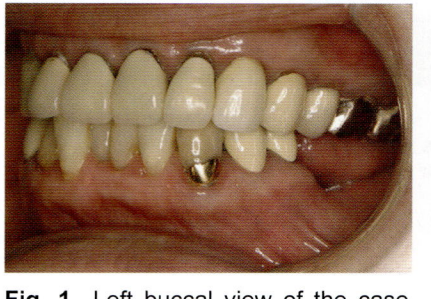

Fig. 1 Left buccal view of the case with missing teeth #36, #37.

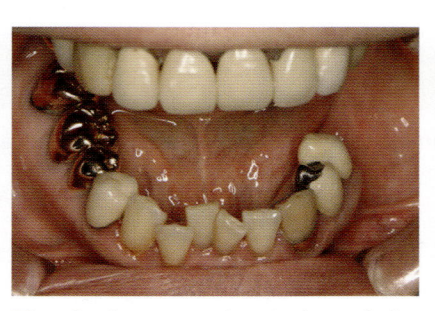

Fig. 2 Lower occlusal view of the same one.

Fig. 3 Upper occulusal view of the same one.

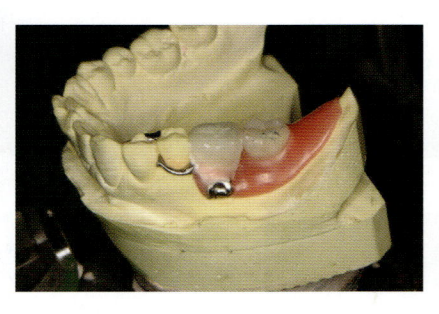

Fig. 4 Buccal view of the working cast model for fabricating the Suginaka bolt lock denture for missing teeth #36, #37.

Fig. 5 Buccal view of the wax denture after the missing teeth #36-#37 were replaced with the metal tooth covered fully with a hybrid resin and dental tooth, respectively.

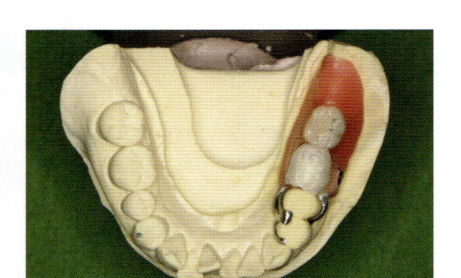

Fig. 6 Occlusal view of the same one.

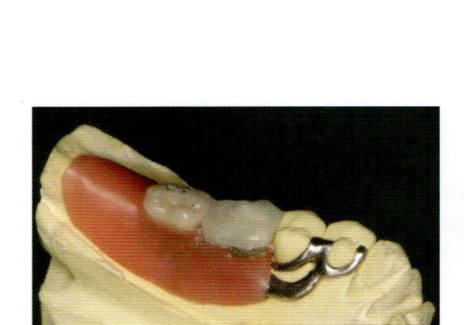

Fig. 7 Lingual view of the wax denture, in which the Suginaka bolt was embedded in the missing tooth #36 region.

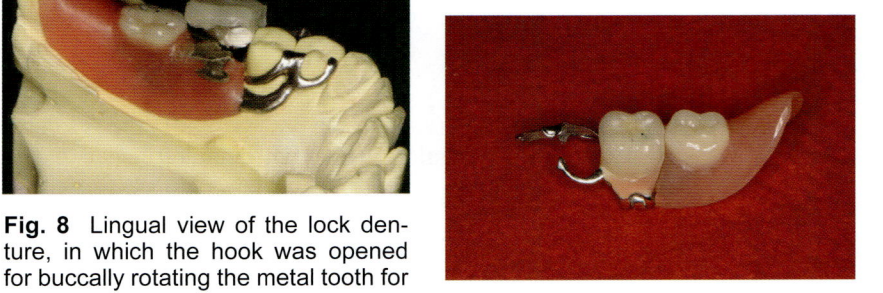

Fig. 8 Lingual view of the lock denture, in which the hook was opened for buccally rotating the metal tooth for missing tooth #36.

Fig. 9 Buccal view of the completed Suginaka bolt lock denture for missing teeth #36-#37.

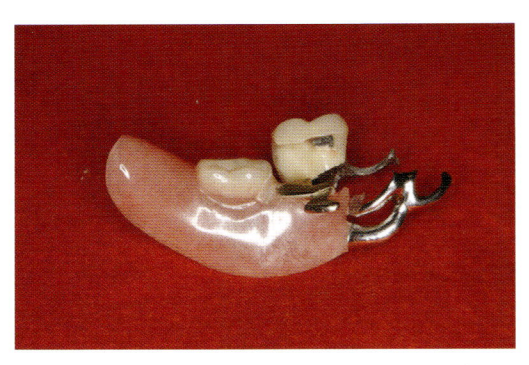

Fig. 10 Lingual view of the completed Suginaka bolt lock denture, in which the hook was opened for buccally rotating the metal tooth. In this condition, the lock denture should be inserted/removed.

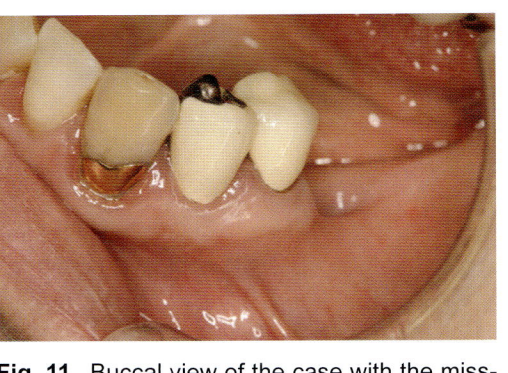

Fig. 11 Buccal view of the case with the missing teeth #36-#37 before delivery of the lock denture.

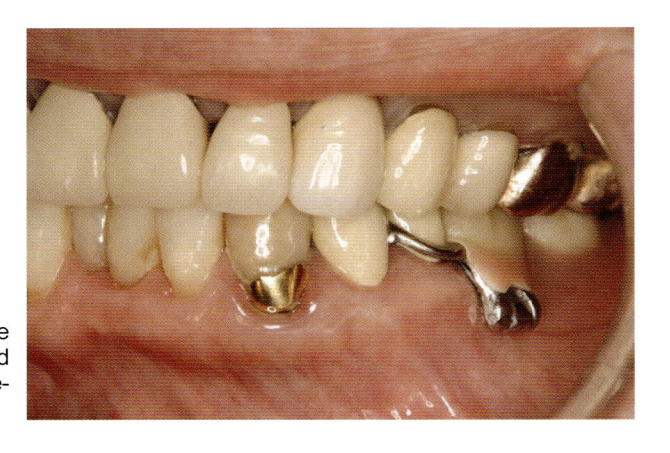

Fig. 12 Left buccal view of the Suginaka bolt lock denture placed on the missing teeth #36-#37 region.

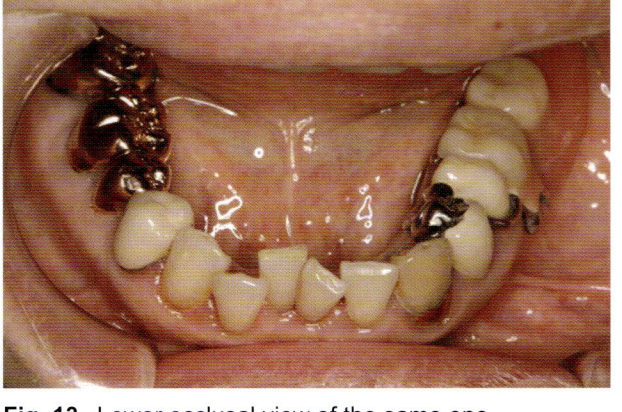

Fig. 13 Lower occlusal view of the same one.

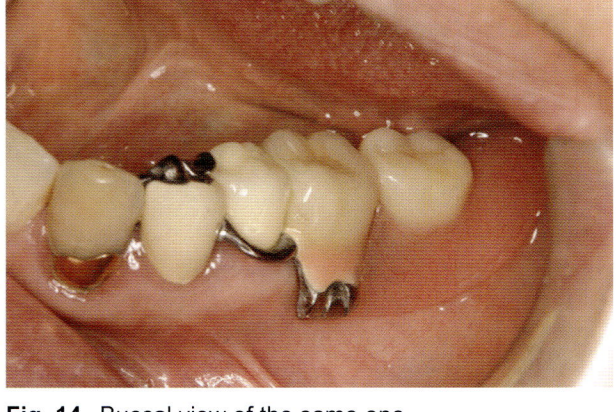

Fig. 14 Buccal view of the same one.

 **Key Point !**

Suginaka bolt lock retainers can be applied without the need of any restoration on the abutment tooth, as it is now. The undercut amount in the present case was less, so the clasp tip was extended to the interproximal area between teeth #34 and #35.

2. Suginaka bolt lock dentures

⑥Unilateral distal extension missing case: Missing teeth #45-#47; Patient:
43-year-old woman
Tooth #44: Healthy tooth; Lock retainer

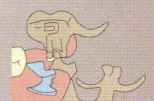
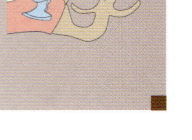

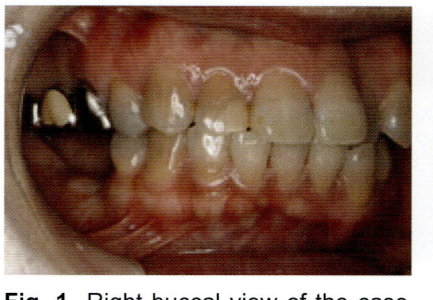

Fig. 1 Right buccal view of the case with missing teeth #45-#47.

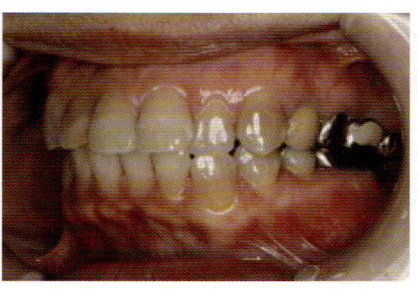

Fig. 2 Left buccal view of the same one.

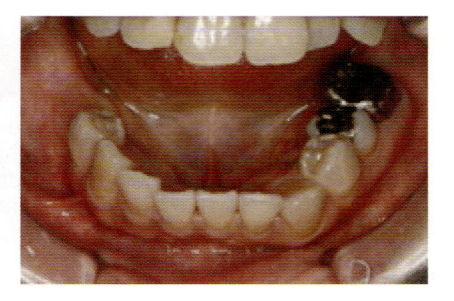

Fig. 3 Lower occlusal view of the same one.

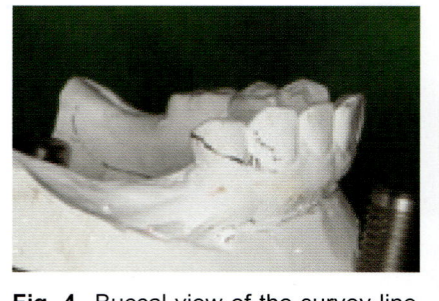

Fig. 4 Buccal view of the survey line drawn on the coronal surface of tooth #45.

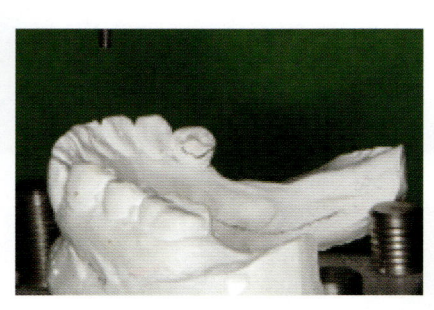

Fig. 5 Lingual view of the same one.

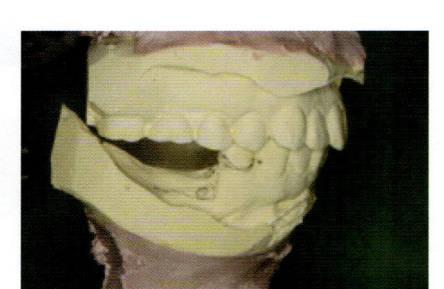

Fig. 6 Buccal view of the denture base outline of the lock denture for missing teeth #45-#47.

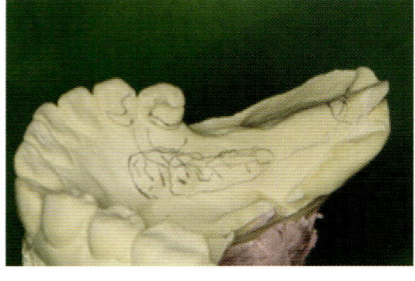

Fig. 7 Lingual view of the same one.

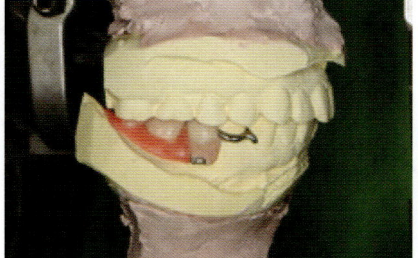

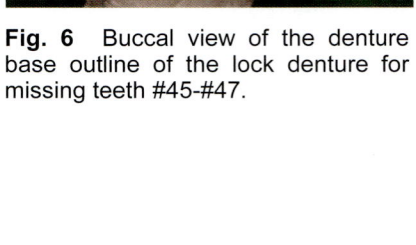
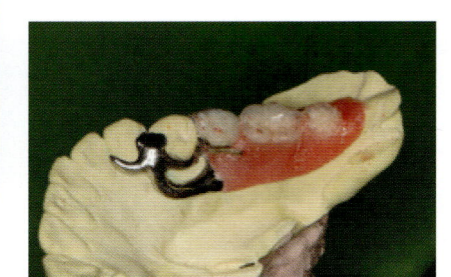

Fig. 8 Buccal view of the wax denture at the completion of replacement of the missing teeth #45-#47 with the artificial teeth. The buccal arm is extended to tooth #43 due to insufficient undercuts.

Fig. 9 Lingual view of the same one.

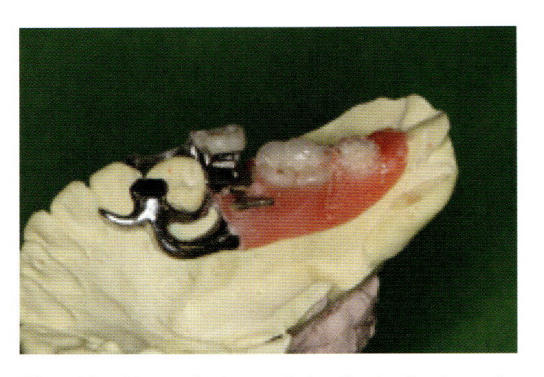

Fig. 10 Lingual view of the lock denture, in which the lever was opened for buccally rotating the metal tooth.

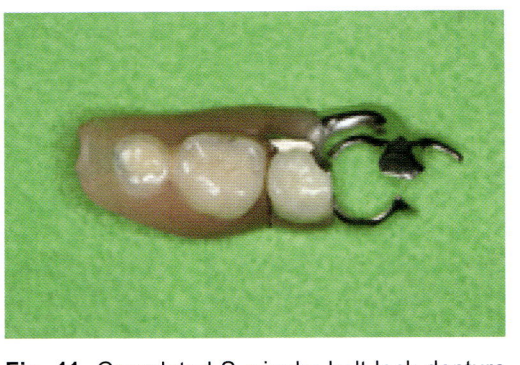

Fig. 11 Completed Suginaka bolt lock denture for missing teeth #45-#47.

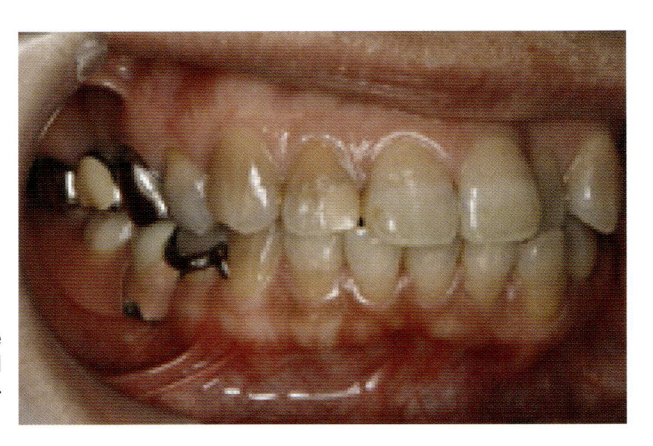

Fig. 12 Right buccal view of the Suginaka bolt lock denture placed on the missing teeth #45-#47 region.

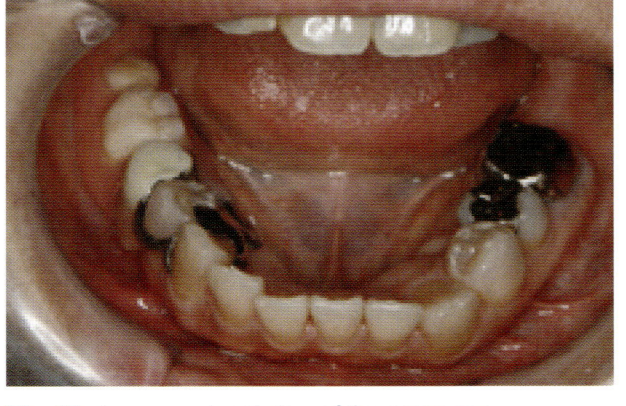

Fig. 13 Lower occlusal view of the same one.

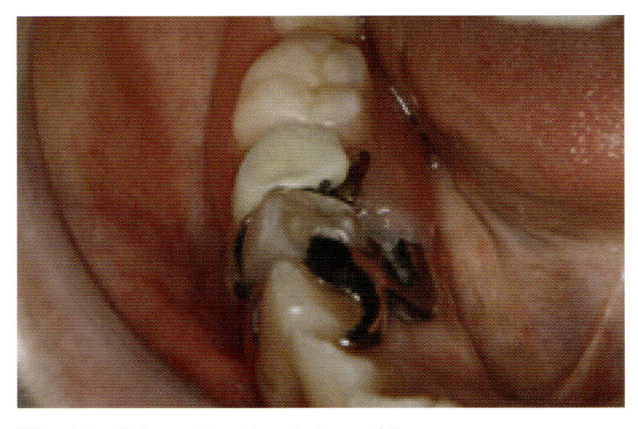

Fig. 14 Enlarged occlusal view of the same one.

Key Point !

As the present case, even 3 missing teeth in distal extension cases, if the residual ridge has larger width, hard mucosa, and the clinical crown length of the abutment tooth is not long, prosthetic treatment can be performed unilaterally with a single abutment tooth; however, prosthetic treatment should be performed with cross-arch design under the opposite conditions. For your information, prosthetic treatment in the maxill is always performed with cross-arch design.

2. Suginaka bolt lock dentures

⑦Unilateral distal extension missing case: Missing teeth #25-#27, #16-#17; Patient: 80-year-old woman
Tooth #15: Full metal crown restored tooth; Lock retainer
Tooth #24: Worn tooth; Lock retainer

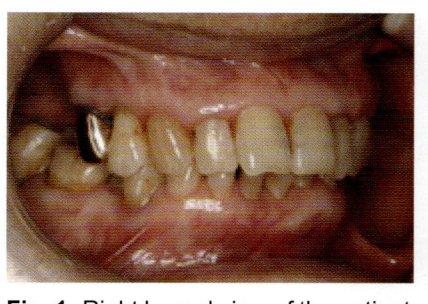

Fig. 1 Right buccal view of the patient with missing teeth #25-#27, #16-#17.

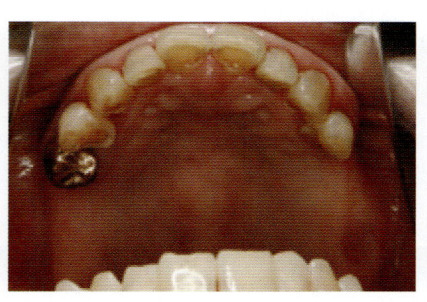

Fig. 2 Upper occlusal view of the same one.

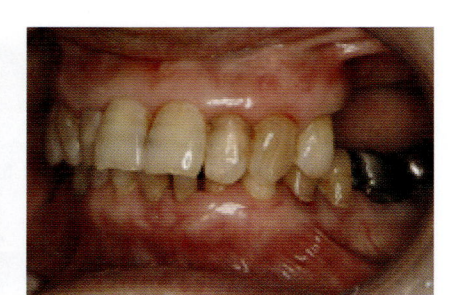

Fig. 3 Left buccal view of the same one.

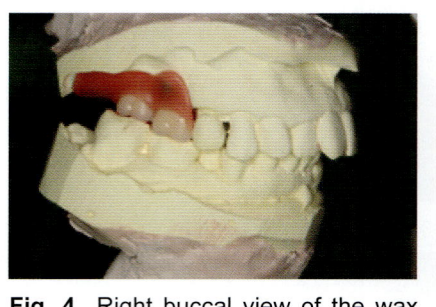

Fig. 4 Right buccal view of the wax denture, the missing teeth #16-#17 are replaced with the artificial teeth. A hinge is involved in the buccal gingival region of the metal tooth replacing the missing tooth #16 region.

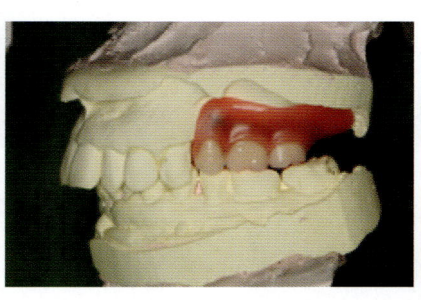

Fig. 5 Left buccal view of the wax denture, the missing teeth #25-#27 are replaced with the artificial teeth. A hinge is involved in the buccal gingival region of the metal tooth replacing the missing tooth #25 region.

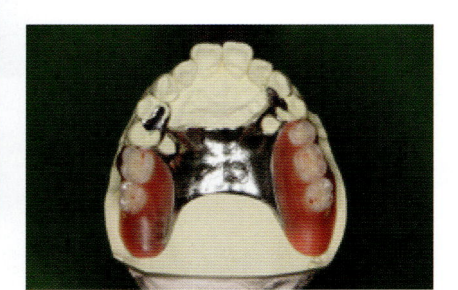

Fig. 6 Occlusal view of the wax lock denture after arangement of the missing teeth #25-#27, #16-#17 with the artificial teeth (before replacement of the missing teeth #16, #25 with the metal teeth).

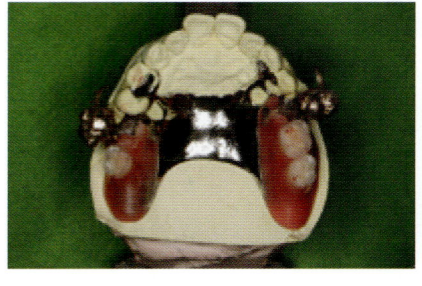

Fig. 7 Occlusal view of the wax lock denture with completed buccally rotating metal teeth for missing teeth #16, #25.

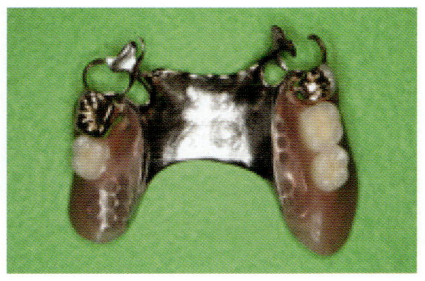

Fig. 8 Occlusal view of the completed Suginaka bolt lock denture for missing teeth #25-#27, #16-#17.

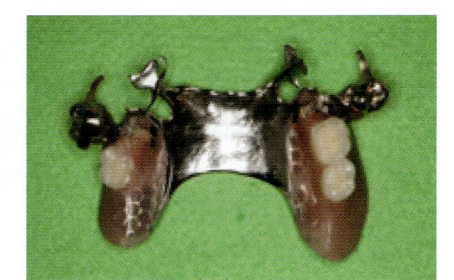

Fig. 9 Occlusal view of the completed Suginaka bolt lock denture with buccally rotating metal teeth for missing teeth #16, #25.

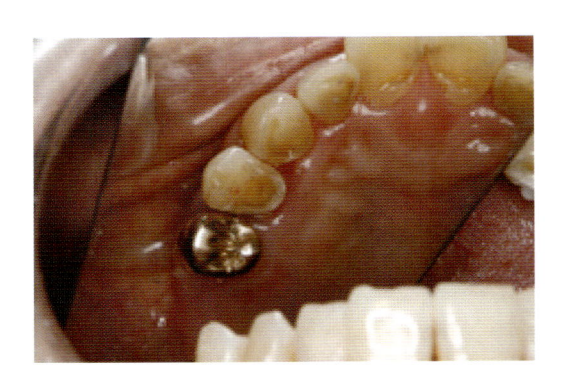

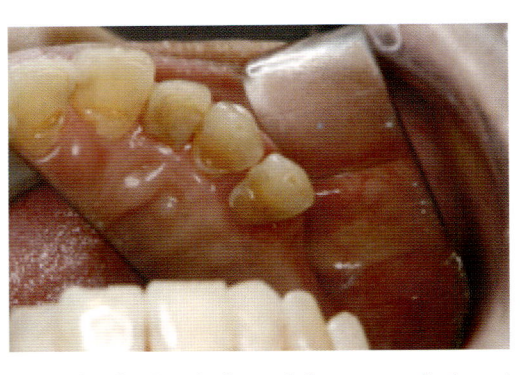

Fig. 10 Occlusal view of the full metal crown on abutment tooth #15.

Fig. 11 Occlusal view of the worn abutment tooth #24.

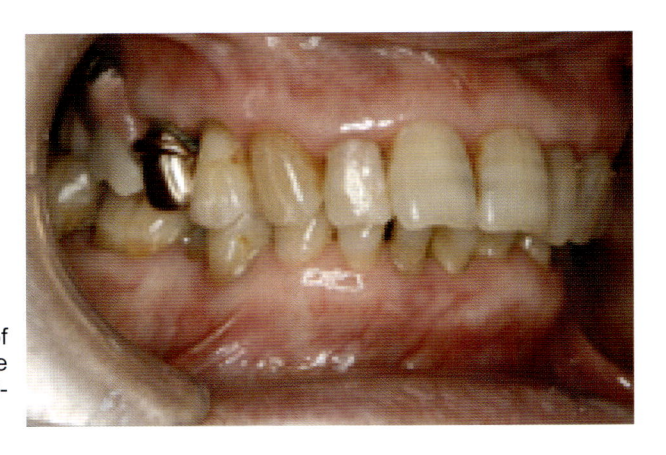

Fig. 12 Right occlusal view of the Suginaka bolt lock denture placed on the missing teeth #25-#27, #16-#17 region.

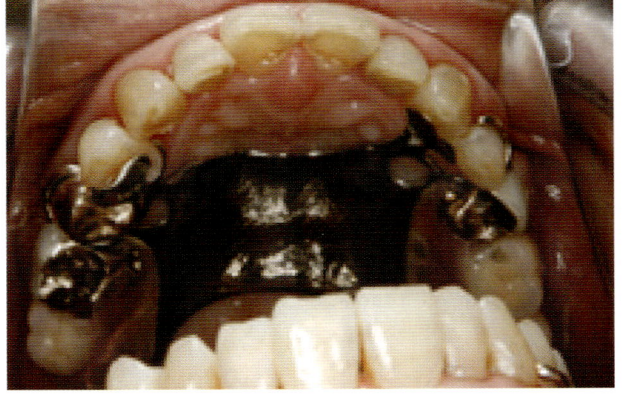

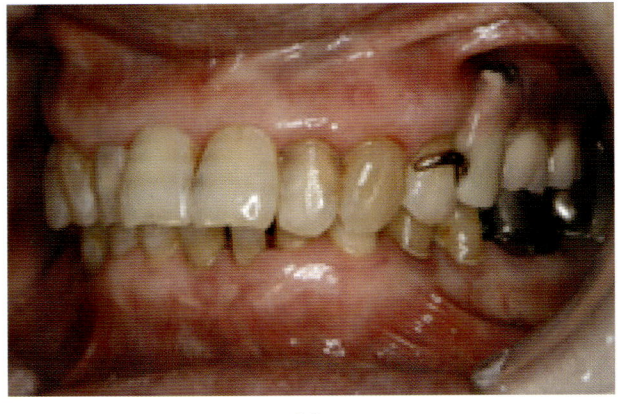

Fig. 13 Upper occlusal view of the same one.

Fig. 14 Left buccal view of the same one.

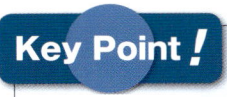 **Key Point !**

Regardless of significant wear of the lingual cusp of tooth #24, the formation of the mesial rest seat and achievement of lingual bracing through the lingual rest formed on tooth #23 allowed the lock retainer to function.

2. Suginaka bolt lock dentures

⑧Bilateral distal extension missing case: Missing teeth #35-#37, #46-#47; Patient: 64-year-old woman
Teeth #34, #45: Restored teeth; Lock retainer

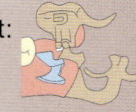

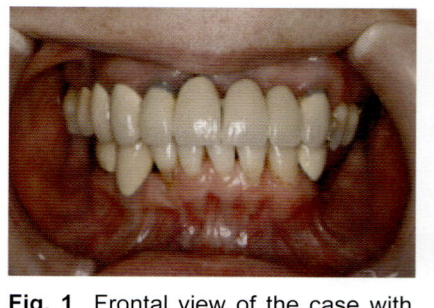

Fig. 1 Frontal view of the case with missing teeth #35-#37, #46-#47.

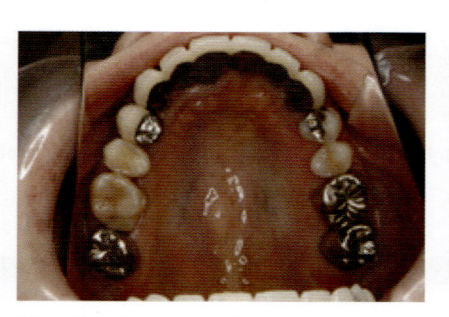

Fig. 2 Upper occlusal view of the same one.

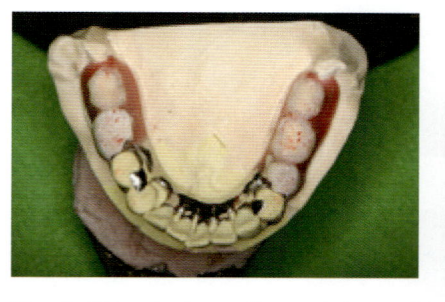

Fig. 3 Lower occlusal view of the same one.

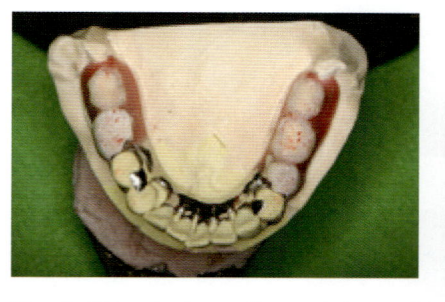

Fig. 4 Wax denture after replacement of the missing teeth #35-#37, #46-#47 with the artificial teeth.

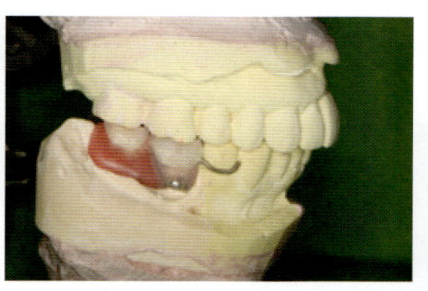

Fig. 5 Buccal view of the lock retainer for missing tooth #46 with the artificial tooth.

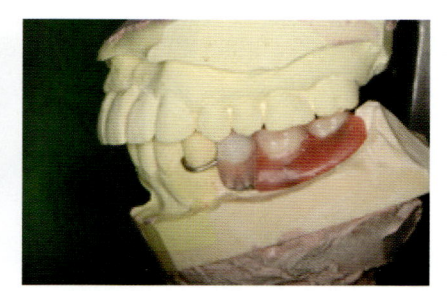

Fig. 6 Buccal view of the lock retainer for missing tooth #35 with the artificial tooth.

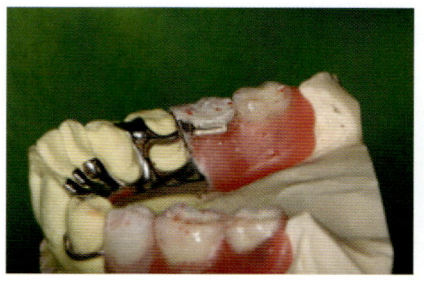

Fig. 7 Lingual view of the lock retainer for missing tooth #46 with the artificial tooth.

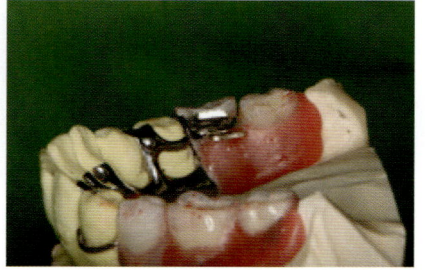

Fig. 8 Lingual view of the lock retainer, in which the lever was opened on buccally rotating metal tooth for the missing tooth #46.

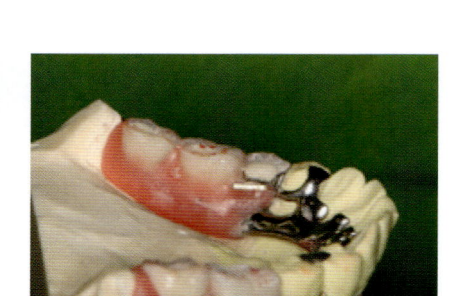

Fig. 9 Lingual view of the lock retainer for missing tooth #35 with the artificial tooth.

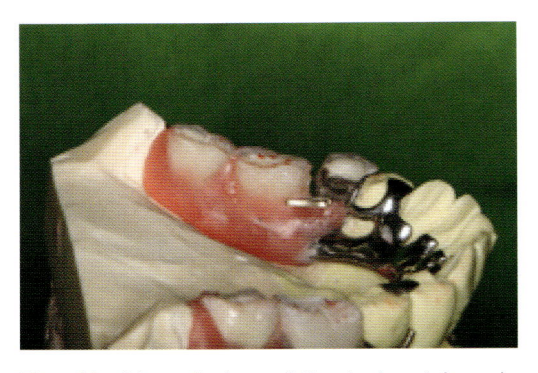

Fig. 10 Lingual view of the lock retainer, in which the lever was opened on buccally rotating metal tooth for the missing tooth #35.

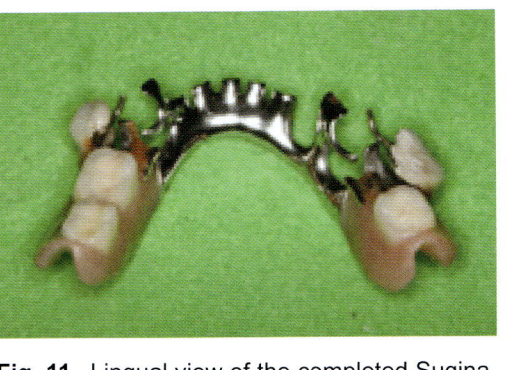

Fig. 11 Lingual view of the completed Suginaka bolt lock denture for missing teeth #35-#27, #46-#47 with buccally rotating metal teeth for #34, #45.

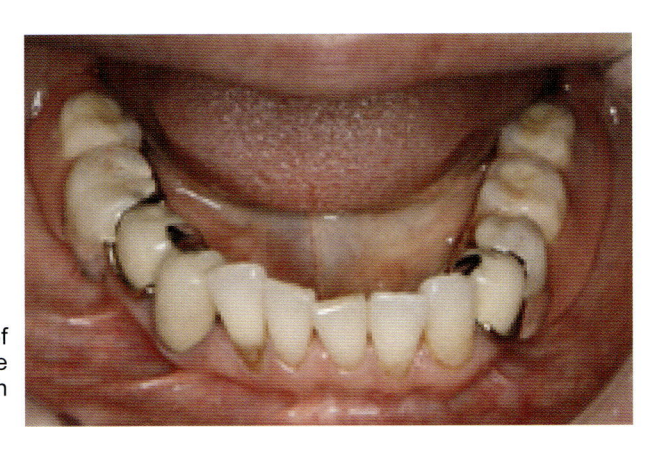

Fig. 12 Lower occlusal view of the Suginaka bolt lock denture placed on the missing teeth #35-#37, #46-#47 region.

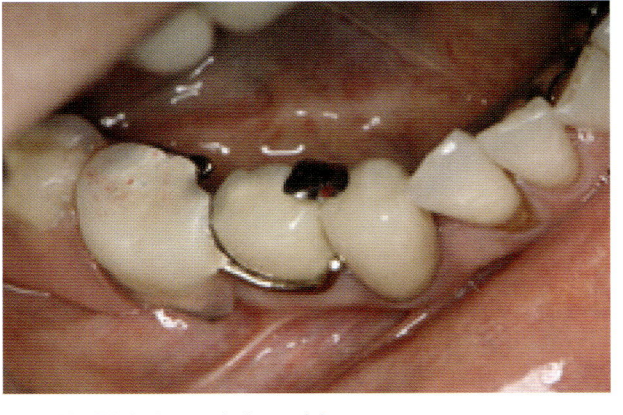

Fig. 13 Right buccal view of the same one.

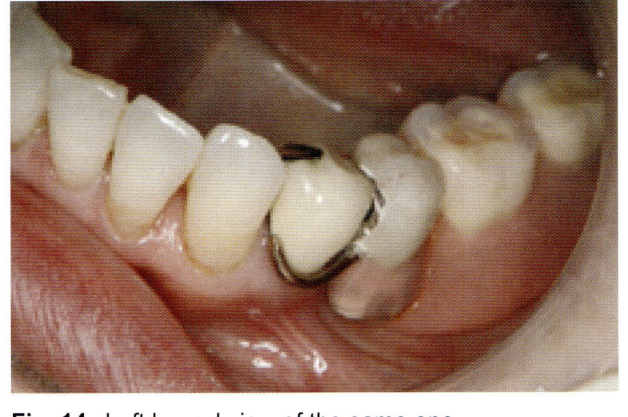

Fig. 14 Left buccal view of the same one.

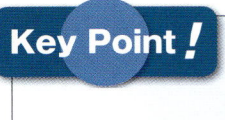

Key Point !   Teeth #34, #45 had already been restored with PFM crowns, but if they cannot be used as abutment teeth of RPD due to the inadequate coronal contour, it is necessary to restore them as abutment teeth. However, the use of Suginaka bolt lock retainers is no longer necessary for it and the existing restorations can be used as they are now.

2. Suginaka bolt lock dentures

⑨Bilateral distal extension missing case: Missing teeth #34-#37, #44-#47; Patient: 79-year-old woman
Teeth #33, #43: Healthy teeth; Lock retainer
Tooth #44: Overdenture

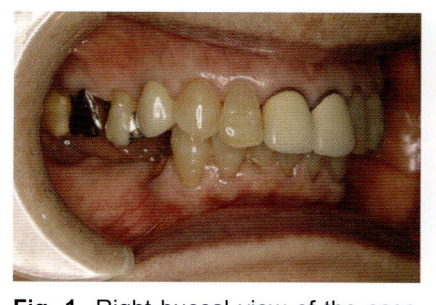

Fig. 1　Right buccal view of the case with missing teeth #34-#37, #44-#47.

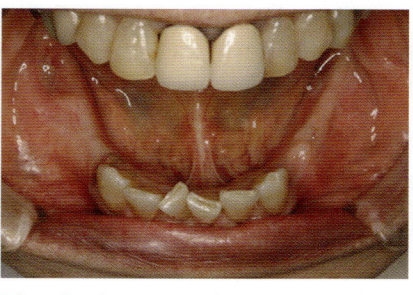

Fig. 2　Lower occlusal view of the same one.

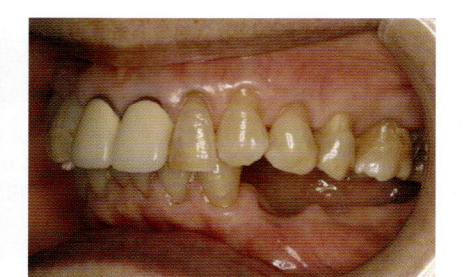

Fig. 3　Left buccal view of the same one.

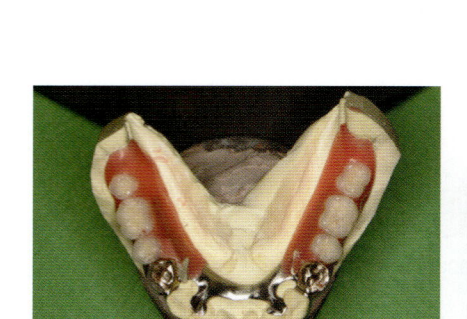

Fig. 4　Stump of tooth #44.

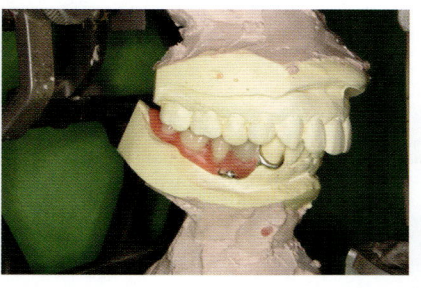

Fig. 5　Right buccal view of the wax denture after replacement of the missing teeth #34-#37, #44-#47 with the artificial teeth, in which the teeth #33, #43 was used as lock retainers.

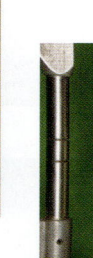

Fig. 6　Left buccal view of the same one.

Fig. 7　Occlusal view of the same one.

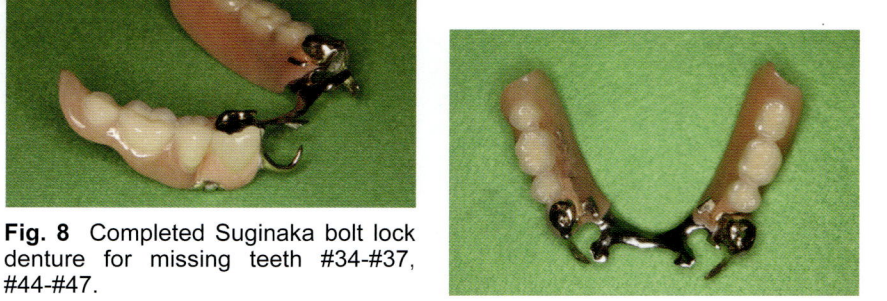

Fig. 8　Completed Suginaka bolt lock denture for missing teeth #34-#37, #44-#47.

Fig. 9　Occlusal view of the same one, in which the metal teeth for missing teeth #34, #44 were rotated buccally.

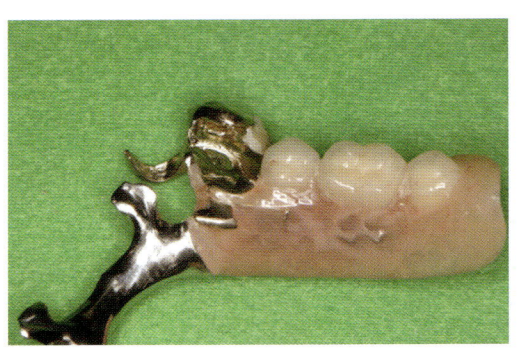

Fig. 10 Lingual view of the lock denture with the metal tooth for missing tooth #44 rotated buccally.

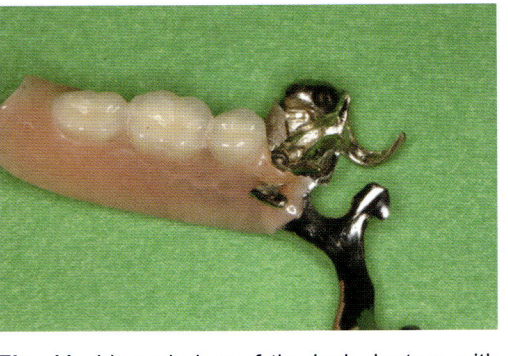

Fig. 11 Lingual view of the lock denture with the metal tooth for missing tooth #34 rotated buccally.

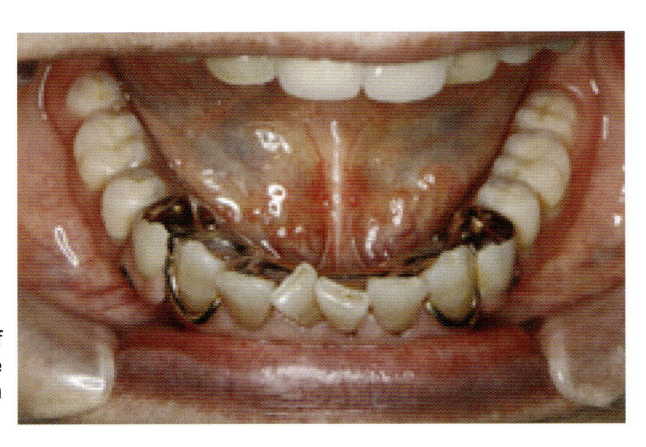

Fig. 12 Lower occlusal view of the Suginaka bolt lock denture placed on the missing teeth #34-#37, #44-#47 region.

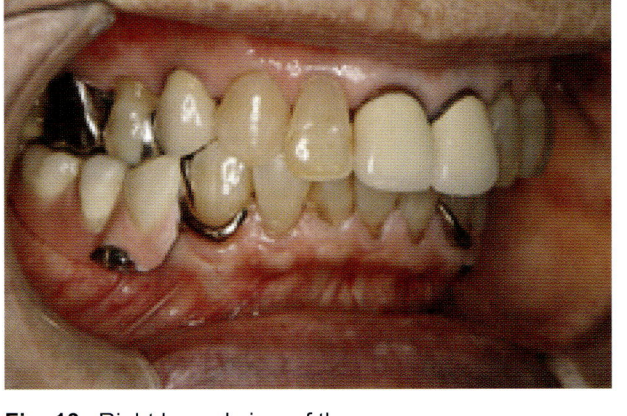

Fig. 13 Right buccal view of the same one.

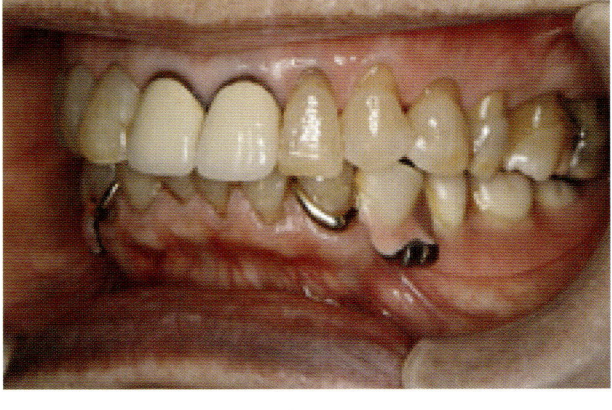

Fig. 14 Left buccal view of the same one.

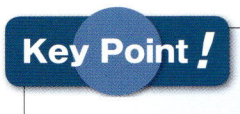

Key Point !

Commonly, it is often impossible to set the hinge for the lock retainer due to creation of undercuts in the buccal alveolar region of the stump. However, in the present case, no undercuts were created in its buccal region, thus allowing hinge setting.

2. Suginaka bolt lock dentures

⑩Few remaining teeth/Multiple missing teeth case: Missing teeth #31-#37, #41-#42, #44-47;Patient: 72-year-old woman
　　Tooth #43: Healthy tooth; Lock retainer

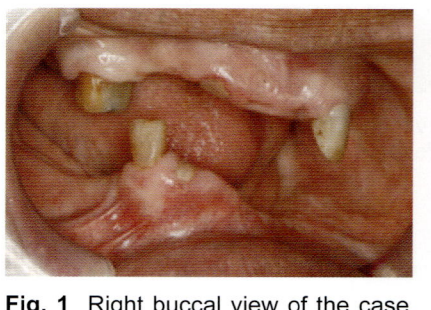

Fig. 1 Right buccal view of the case with missing teeth #31-#37, #41-#42, #44-47.

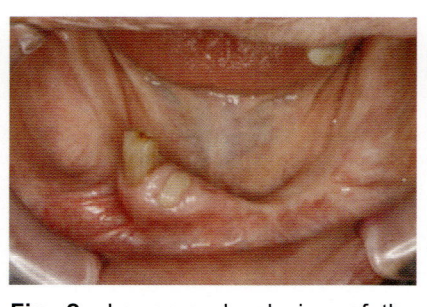

Fig. 2 Lower occlusal view of the same one. The overdenture will be placed on the stump of tooth # 42.

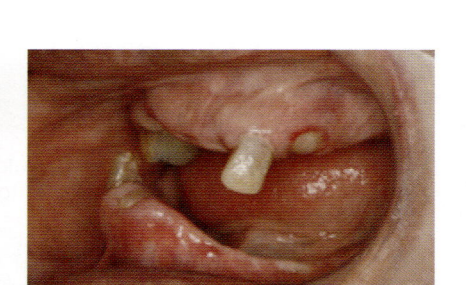

Fig. 3 Left buccal view of the same one.

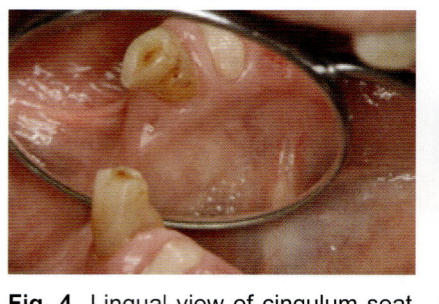

Fig. 4 Lingual view of cingulum seat formed on tooth #43. As there are little undercuts labially, undercuts were created in the rest seat.

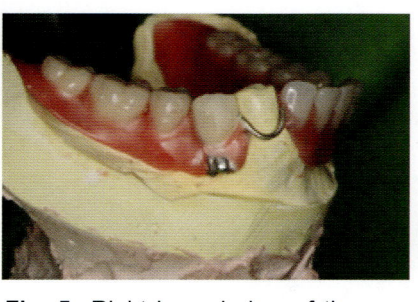

Fig. 5 Right buccal view of the wax denture, in which tooth #43 was used as a lock retainer and the missing teeth #31-#37, #41-#42, #44-47 were replaced with the artificial teeth.

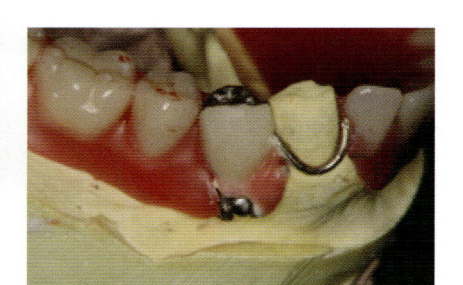

Fig. 6 Buccal view of the buccal arm placed on tooth #43 and the metal tooth for missing tooth #44.

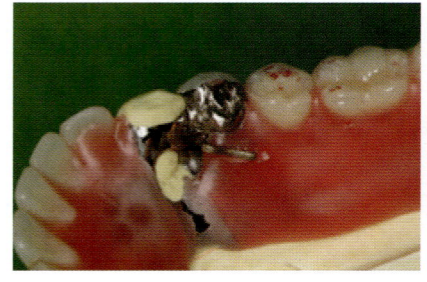

Fig. 7 Lingual view of the cingulum rest on the tooth #43 and metal tooth for missing tooth #44.

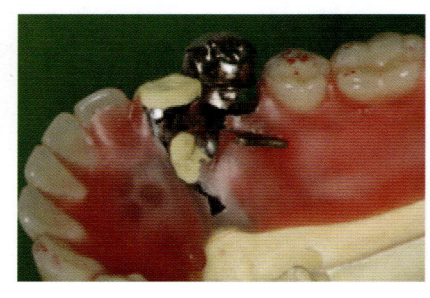

Fig. 8 Lingual view of the wax denture, in which the hook was opened for buccally rotating the metal tooth for missing tooth #44.

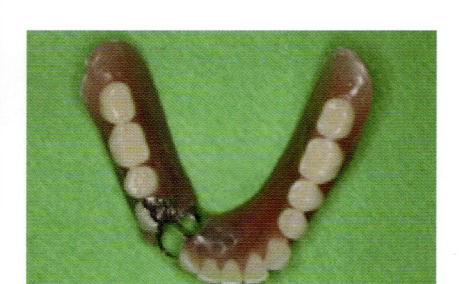

Fig. 9 Occlusal view of the completed Suginaka bolt lock denture for missing teeth #31-#37, #41-#42, #44-47.

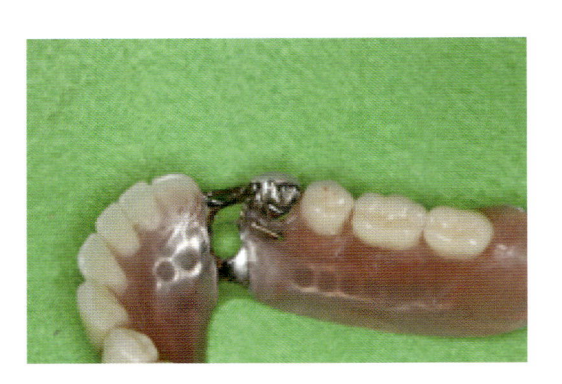

Fig. 10 Lingual view of the lock retainer for tooth #43.

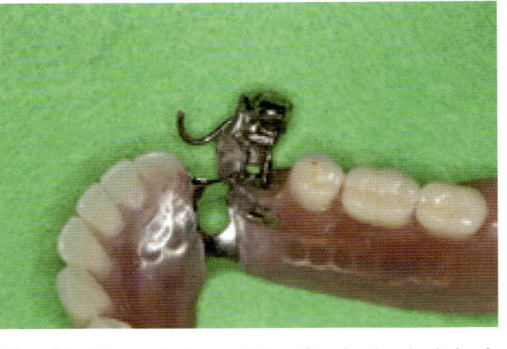

Fig. 11 Lingual view of the Suginaka bolt lock denture with the metal tooth for missing tooth #44 rotated buccally.

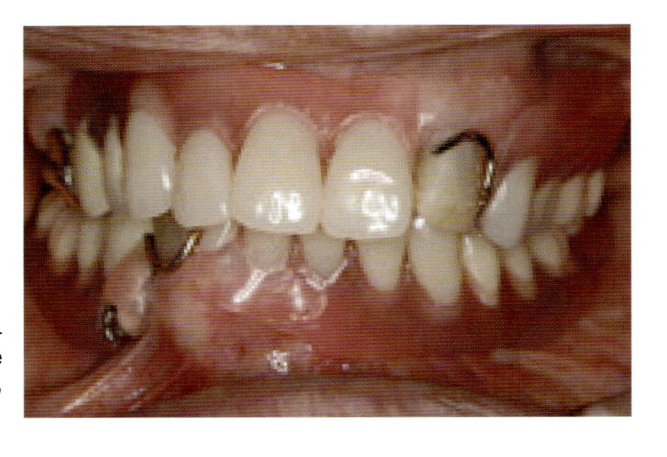

Fig. 12 Frontal view of the Sugina-ka bolt lock denture placed on the missing teeth #31-#37, #41-#42, #44-47 region.

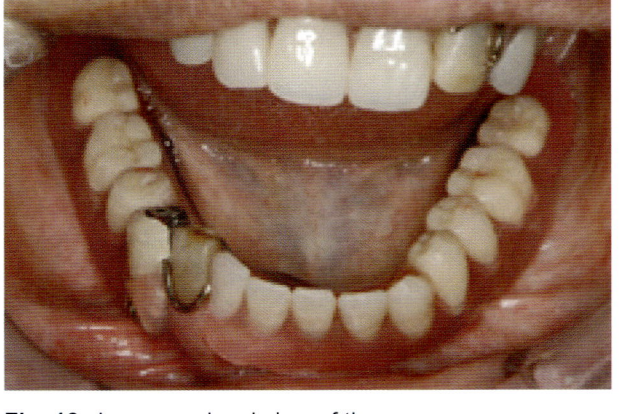

Fig. 13 Lower occlusal view of the same one.

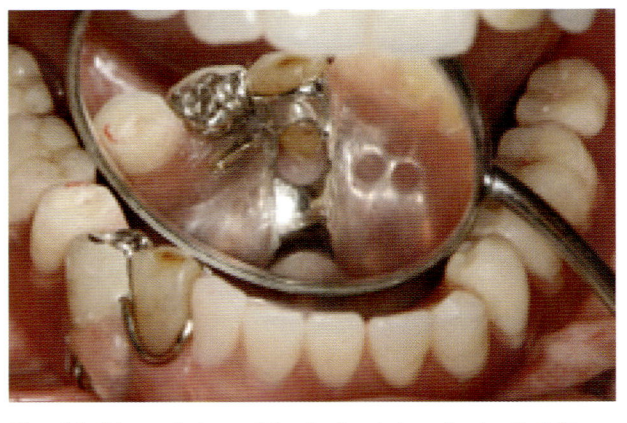

Fig. 14 Lingual view of the lock retainer for tooth #43.

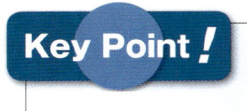 **Key Point !**

When placing Suginaka bolt lock retainer on the canine, it is probably best to form the cingulum rest.

3. Suginaka bolt dentures

①Tooth bounded missing case: Missing teeth #36-#37; Patient: 58-year-old woman
Tooth #35: Cone-crown-type double crown (inner crown with a rod projection)
Tooth #38: Rest

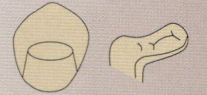

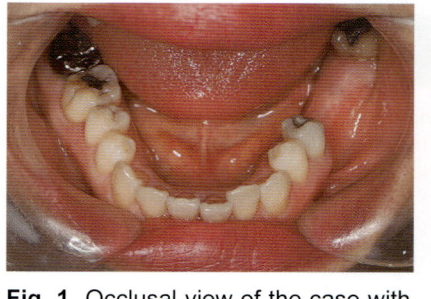

Fig. 1 Occlusal view of the case with missing teeth #36-#37.

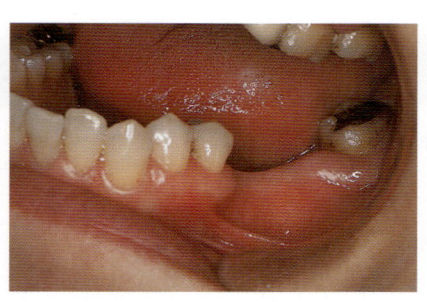

Fig. 2 Buccal view of the same one.

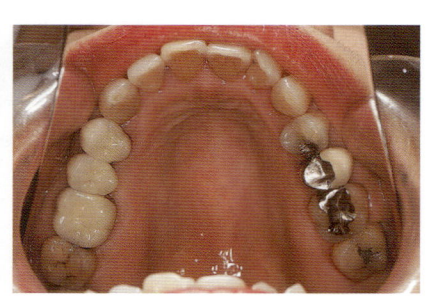

Fig. 3 Upper occlusal view of the case.

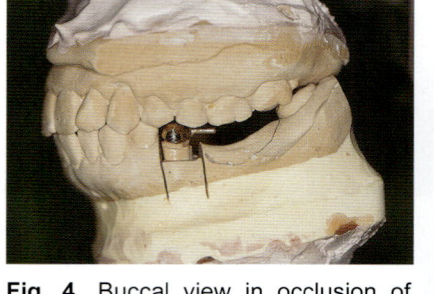

Fig. 4 Buccal view in occlusion of the inner crown with a rod projection placed on tooth #35.

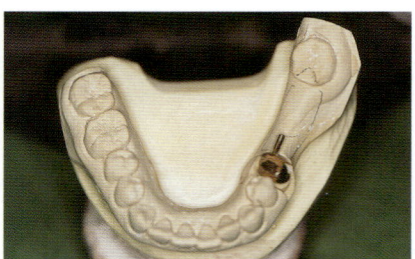

Fig. 5 Buccal view of the inner crown with a rod projection for tooth #35.

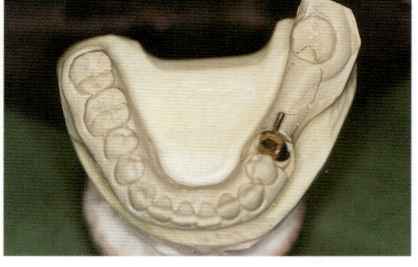

Fig. 6 Occlusal view of the same one.

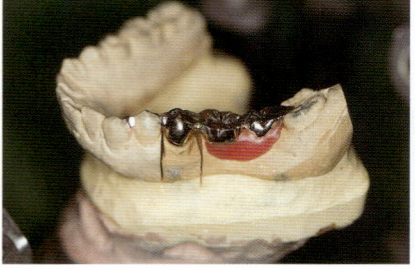

Fig. 7 Buccal view of the Suginaka bolt denture with the outer crown for tooth #35, the lingual arm with a marginal rest for tooth #34, a rest for tooth #38, and the metal teeth for missing teeth #36-#37.

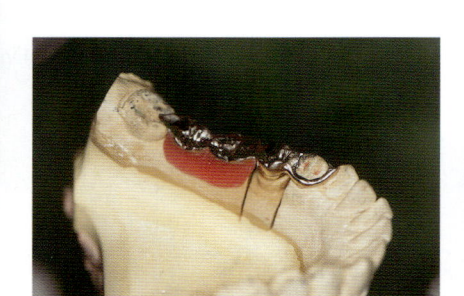

Fig. 8 Lingual view of the same one.

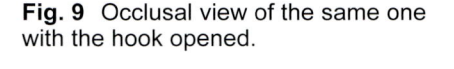

Fig. 9 Occlusal view of the same one with the hook opened.

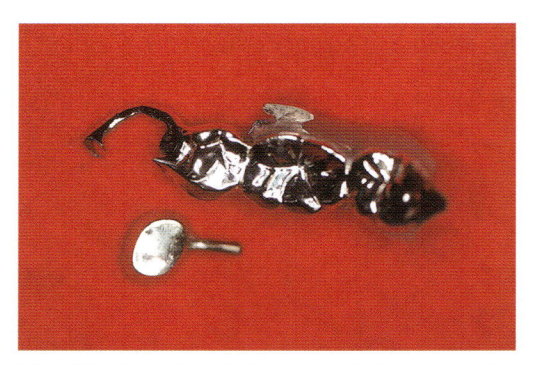

Fig. 10 Completed Suginaka bolt denture for missing teeth #36-#37 and inner crown with a rod projection for tooth #35.

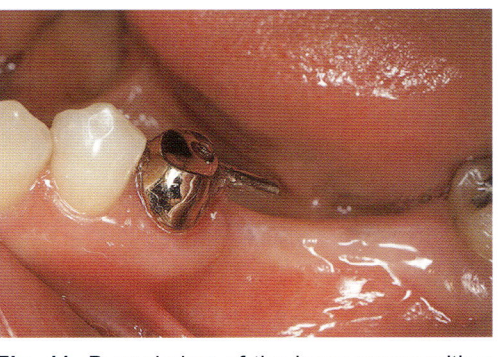

Fig. 11 Buccal view of the inner crown with a rod projection placed on tooth #35.

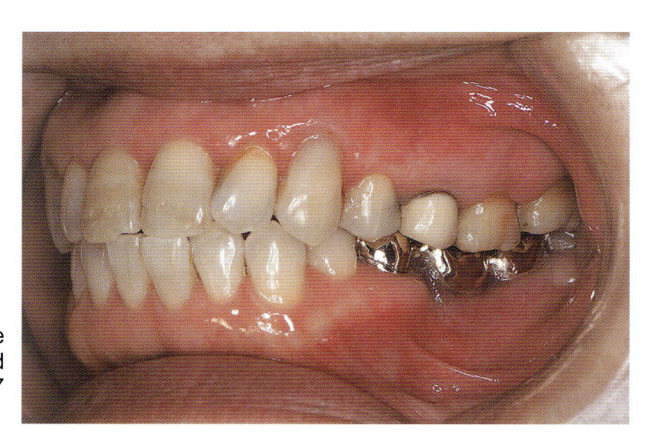

Fig. 12 Left buccal view of the Suginaka bolt denture placed on the missing teeth #36-#37 region.

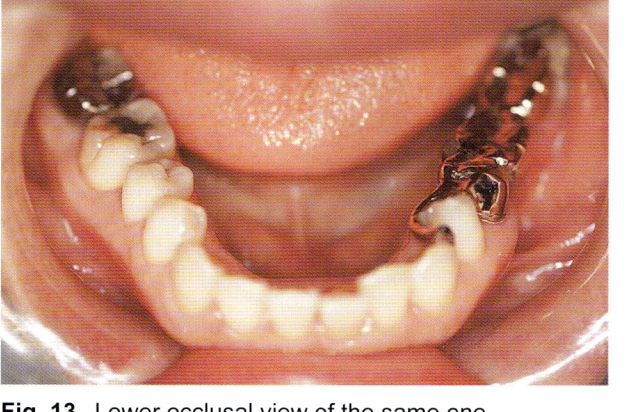

Fig. 13 Lower occlusal view of the same one.

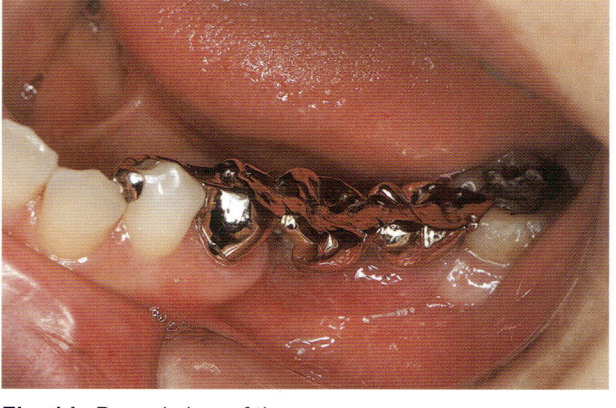

Fig. 14 Buccal view of the same one.

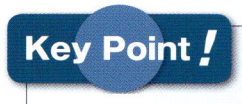
Key Point !

Even though the tooth #38 should be lost, this telescope denture could be used under these conditions.

3. Suginaka bolt dentures

②Tooth bounded missing case: Missing teeth #35-#37; Patient: 59-year-old woman
　Tooth #34: Lingual arm with a marginal rest
　Tooth #38: Cone-crown-type double crown (inner crown with a rod projection)

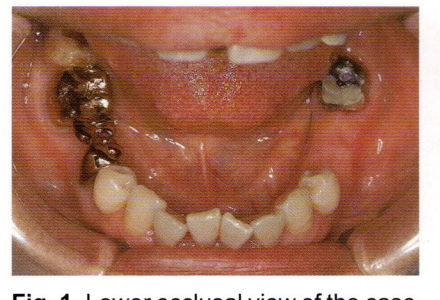

Fig. 1 Lower occlusal view of the case with missing teeth #35-#37.

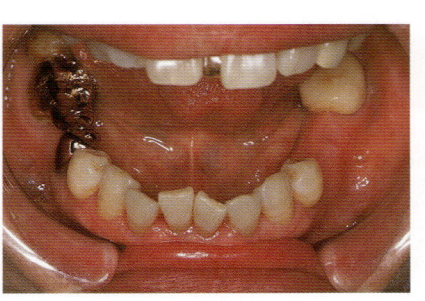

Fig. 2 Lower occlusal view of the case with preparation of tooth #38 for the Cone-crown-type double crown followed by cementation of the temporary crown.

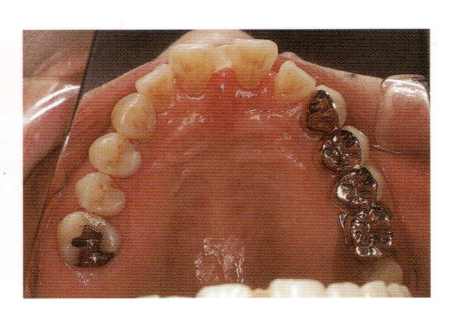

Fig. 3 Upper occlusal view of the same case.

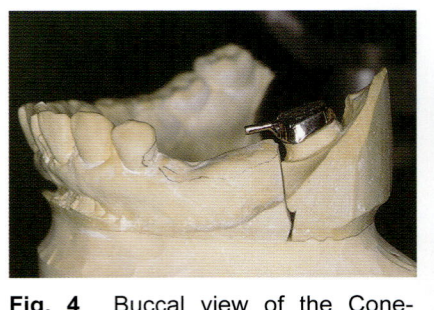

Fig. 4 Buccal view of the Cone-crown-type inner crown with a rod projection provided on the mesial surface of tooth #38.

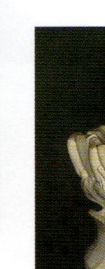

Fig. 5 Occlusal view of the same one.

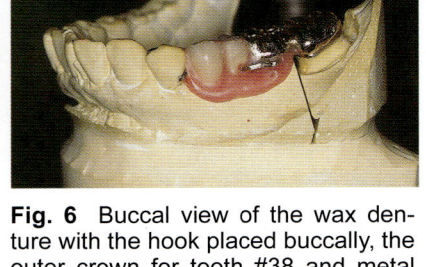

Fig. 6 Buccal view of the wax denture with the hook placed buccally, the outer crown for tooth #38 and metal tooth for missing tooth #37 one-piece casted, and the missing teeth #35-#36 replaced with the artificial teeth.

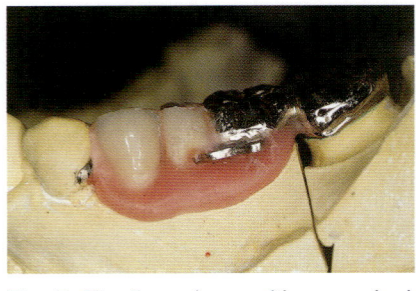

Fig. 7 The lingual arm with a marginal rest placed on tooth #34 through the use of distoproximal and buccocervical undercuts.

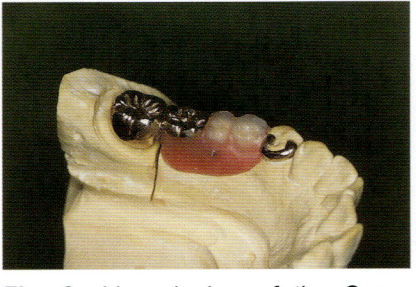

Fig. 8 Lingual view of the Cone-crown-type outer crown for tooth #38 and lingual arm with a marginal rest for tooth #34.

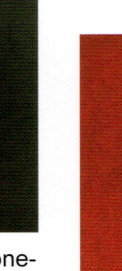

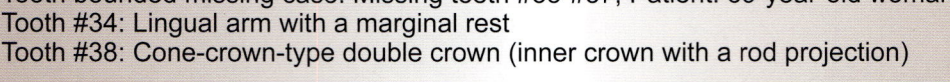

Fig. 9 Completed Suginaka bolt denture for missing teeth #35-#37 with the hook opened.

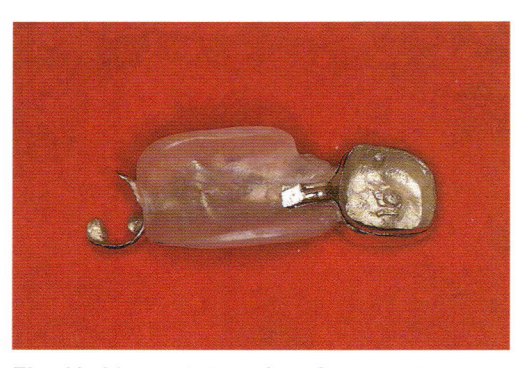

Fig. 10 Mucosal view of the Suginaka bolt denture with the inner crown for tooth #38 set in the outer crown and the hook closed.

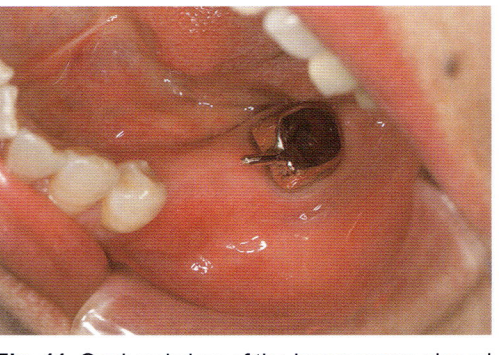

Fig. 11 Occlusal view of the inner crown placed on tooth #38, in which a rod projection is provided mesially.

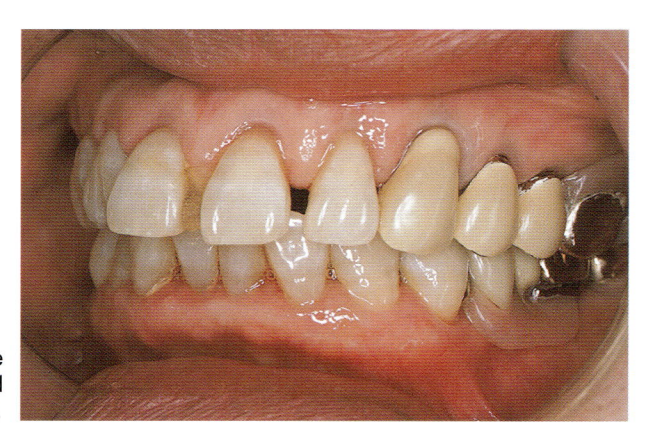

Fig. 12 Left buccal view of the Suginaka bolt denture placed on the missing #35-#37 region.

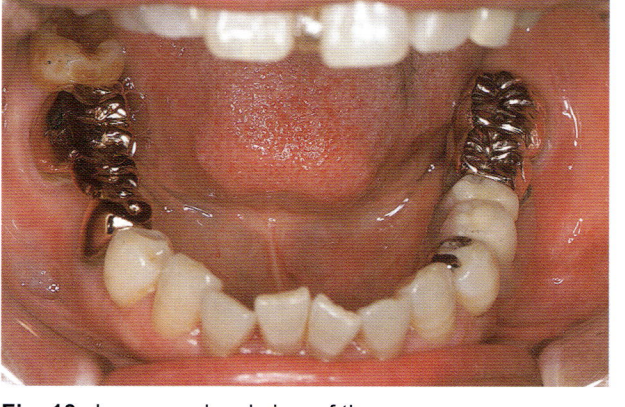

Fig. 13 Lower occlusal view of the same one.

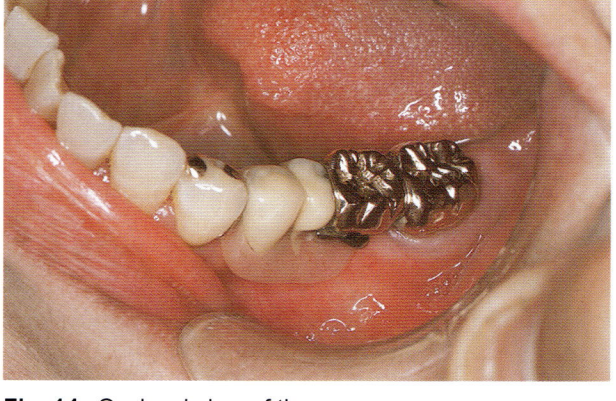

Fig. 14 Occlusal view of the same one.

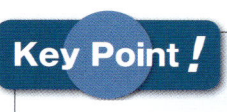

Key Point !

When using distoproximal and buccocervical undercuts for retention of the retainer for tooth #34, attention must be paid to allow the metal to avoid contact with the dental root due to placement in the deeper cervical area.

3. Suginaka bolt dentures

③Tooth bounded missing case: Missing teeth #14-#16; Patient: 67-year-old woman
    Tooth #17: Ring clasp
    Tooth #13: Cone-crown-type double crown (inner crown with a rod projection)

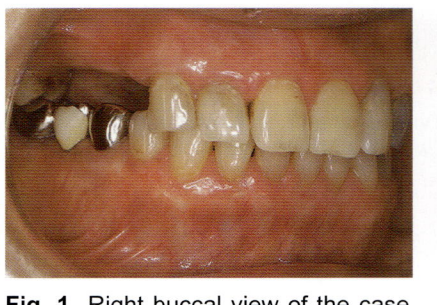

Fig. 1 Right buccal view of the case with missing teeth #14-#16.

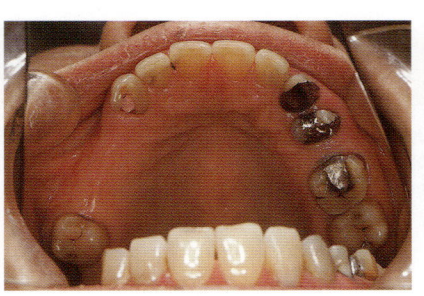

Fig. 2 Upper occlusal view of the same case.

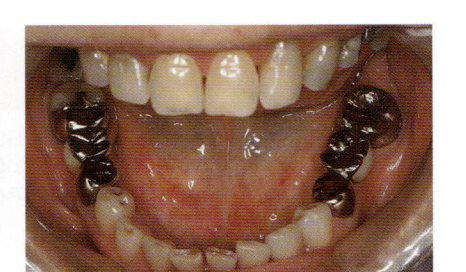

Fig. 3 Lower occlusal view of the same case.

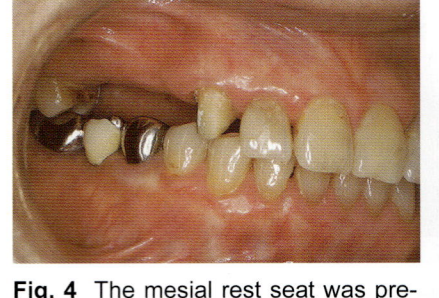

Fig. 4 The mesial rest seat was prepared on tooth #17. Buccal view of the prepared tooth #13 for Cone-crown-type inner crown.

Fig. 5 Buccal view of the working cast with teeth #13, #17 prepared.

Fig. 6 Occlusal view of the Cone-crown-type inner crown with a rod projection placed on tooth #13.

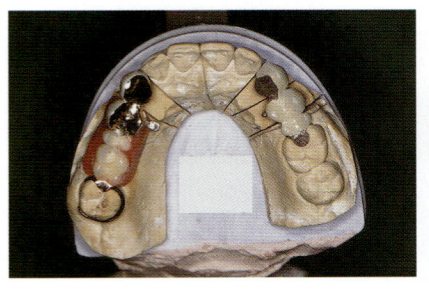

Fig. 7 Occlusal view of the wax denture with the facing-type outer crown placed on tooth #13, the ring clasp placed on tooth #17, the facing-type metal tooth (involving a Suginaka bolt attachment) replaced for missing tooth #14, and the artificial teeth replaced for missing teeth #15, #16. A prototype hook was used.

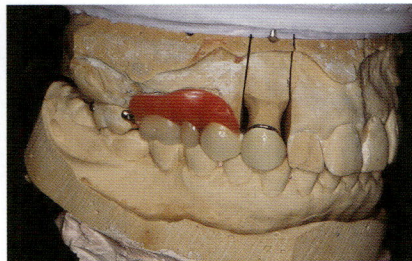

Fig. 8 Buccal view of the wax denture with the missing teeth #14-#16 replaced with the artificial teeth.

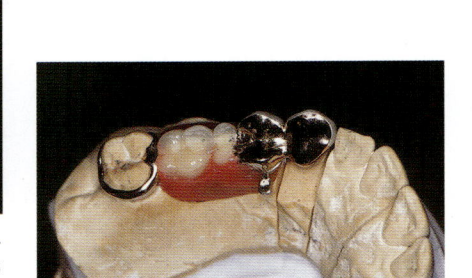

Fig. 9 Occlusal or lingual view of the same one.

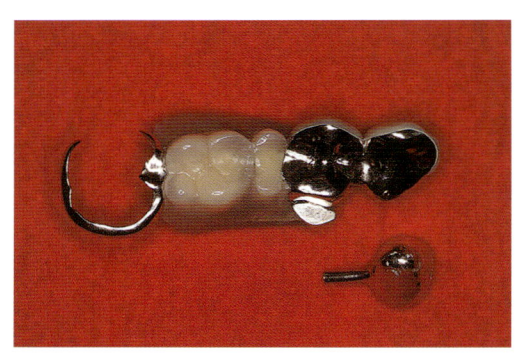

Fig. 10 Occlusal view of the completed Cone-crown-type inner crown with a rod projection for tooth #13 and Suginaka bolt denture for missing teeth #14-#16.

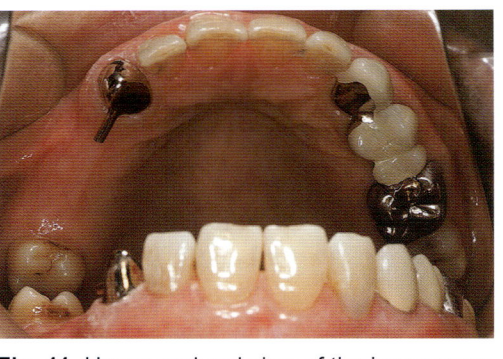

Fig. 11 Upper occlusal view of the inner crown placed on tooth #13.

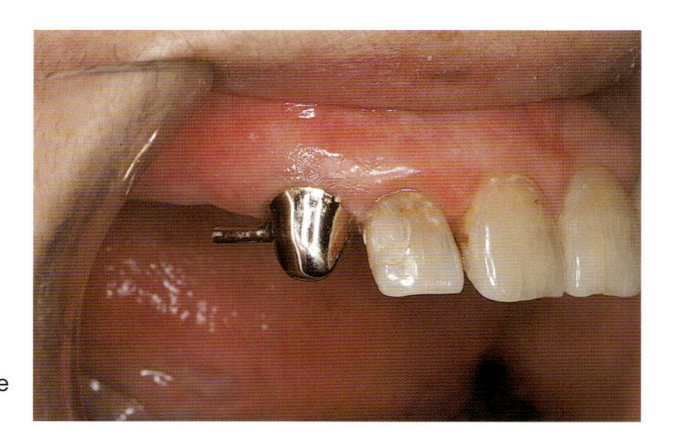

Fig. 12 Buccal view of the same one.

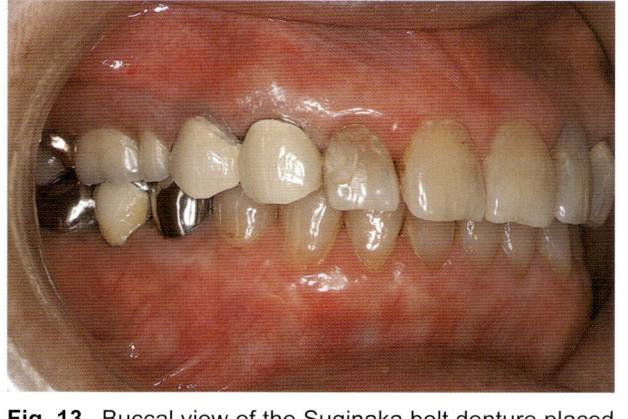

Fig. 13 Buccal view of the Suginaka bolt denture placed on the missing teeth #14-#16 region.

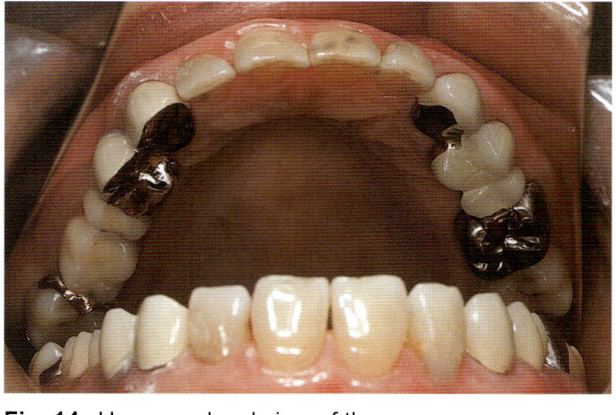

Fig. 14 Upper occlusal view of the same one.

 **Key Point !**

Because of insufficient mesial proximal undercuts of tooth #17, a ring clasp was selected for utilizing undercuts in the bucco-distally proximal corner.

3. Suginaka bolt dentures

④Bilateral distal extension missing case: Missing teeth #15-#17, #27;
Patient: 77-year-old man
Tooth #13: Porcelain fused to metal crown (PFM crown)
Tooth #14: 4/5 outer crown-type double crown (porcelain-faced inner crown with a plate projection)
Tooth #17: Ring clasp

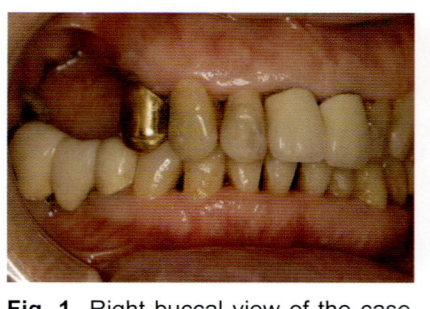

Fig. 1 Right buccal view of the case with missing teeth #15-#17, #27.

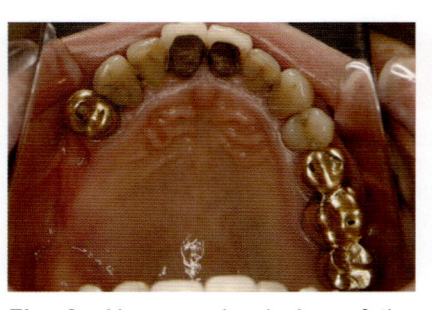

Fig. 2 Upper occlusal view of the same one.

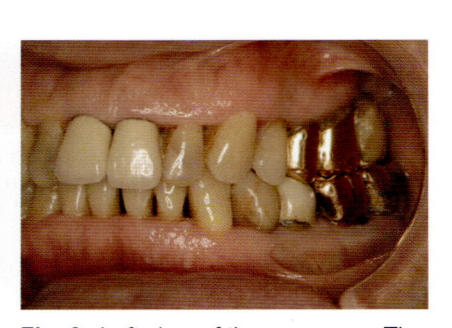

Fig. 3 Left view of the same one. The missing tooth #17 was replaced with the extension pontic.

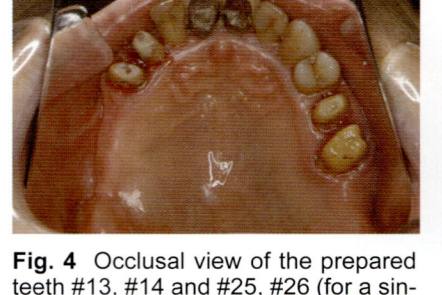

Fig. 4 Occlusal view of the prepared teeth #13, #14 and #25, #26 (for a single crown).

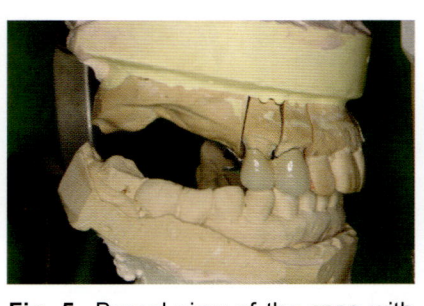

Fig. 5 Buccal view of the case with the porcelain-faced inner crown with a plate projection for tooth #14 connected to the PFM crown for tooth #13.

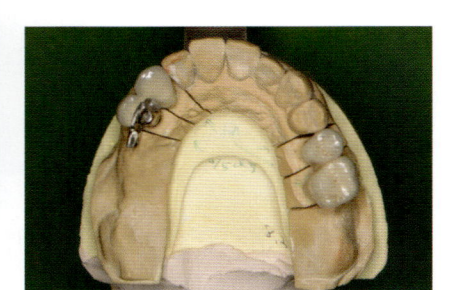

Fig. 6 Occurusal view of the same one and the PFM crowns placed on teeth #25, #26.

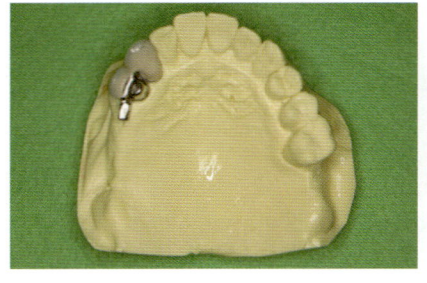

Fig. 7 Occlusal view of the case with the PFM crown for tooth #13 and the porcelain-faced inner crown for tooth #14 replaced on the working cast.

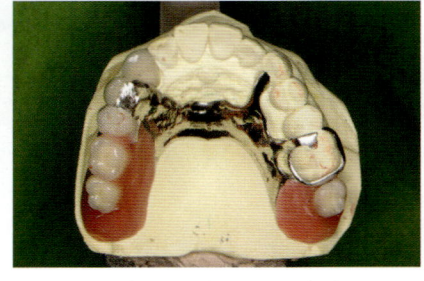

Fig. 8 Occlusal view of the wax denture, in which the 4/5 crown-type outer crown, spar, and ring clasp were placed on #14, #23, and #26, respectively and the missing teeth #15-#17, #27 were replaced with the dental teeth.

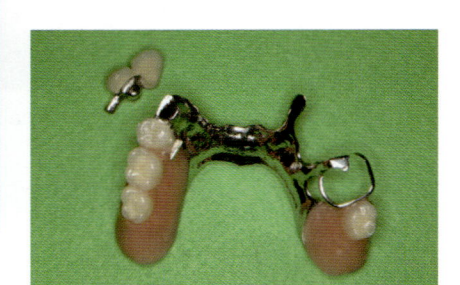

Fig. 9 Connected porcelain-faced inner crown with a plate projection for #14 and PFM crown for #13. Occlusal view of the Suginaka bolt denture for missing teeth #15-#17, #27 with 4/5 crown-type outer crown for #14 and ring clasp for #26.

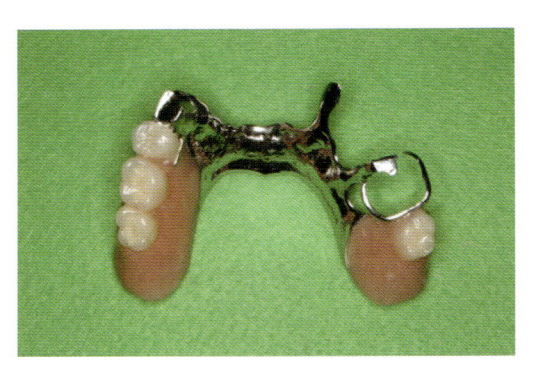

Fig. 10 Occlusal view of the completed Suginaka bolt denture for missing teeth #15-#17, #27.

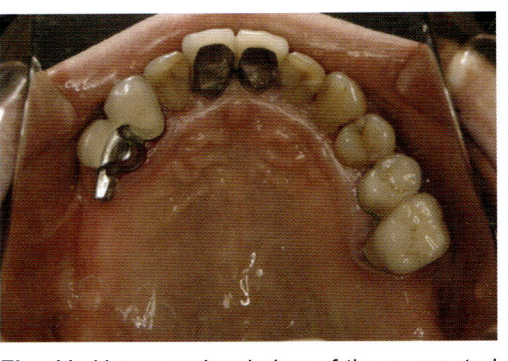

Fig. 11 Upper occlusal view of the connected porcelain-faced inner crown with a plate projection and PFM crown placed on teeth #14, #13.

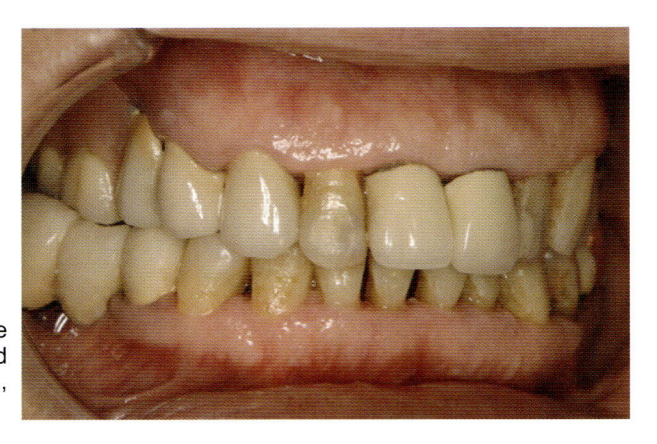

Fig. 12 Right buccal view of the Suginaka bolt denture placed on the missing teeth #15-#17, #27 region.

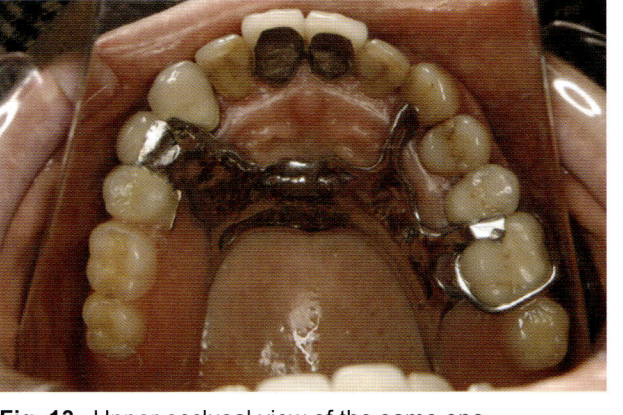

Fig. 13 Upper occlusal view of the same one.

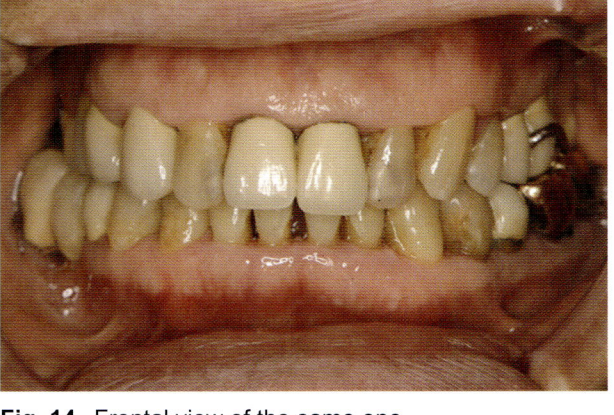

Fig. 14 Frontal view of the same one.

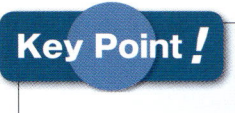

Key Point !

As the path of insertion of the denture is same as the axial surface direction of the bar projection provided to the inner crown for tooth #14, surveying for tooth #26 should be performed according to this direction. Thus, it is important to pre-determine the axial surface direction of the plate projection considering surveying of tooth #26 when waxing it.

3. Suginaka bolt dentures

⑤ Bilateral distal extension missing case: Missing teeth #17, #24–#27;
   Patient: 70-year-old woman
   Tooth #23: Cone-crown-type double crown (inner crown with a plate projection)
   Tooth #16: Akers clasp

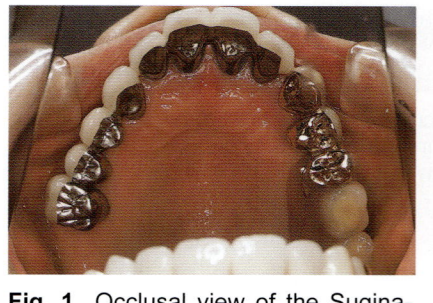

Fig. 1 Occlusal view of the Suginaka bolt telescope denture for missing teeth #25–#27 with abutment teeth #23, #24.

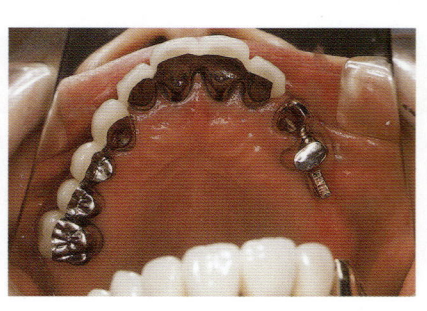

Fig. 2 Occlusal view of the connected inner crowns for teeth #23, #24.

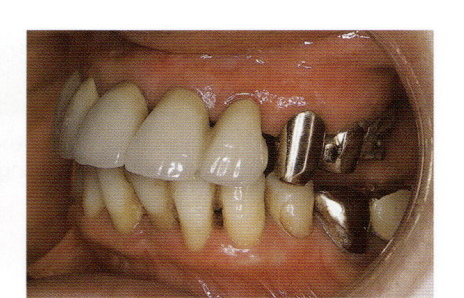

Fig. 3 Root fracture of tooth #24 8 years after insertion of the denture.

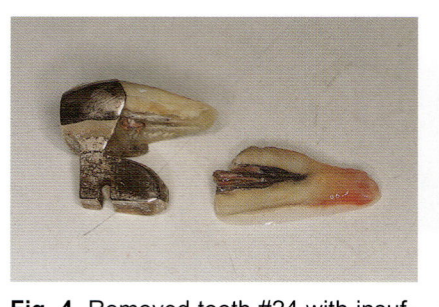

Fig. 4 Removed tooth #24 with insufficient dowel core construction.

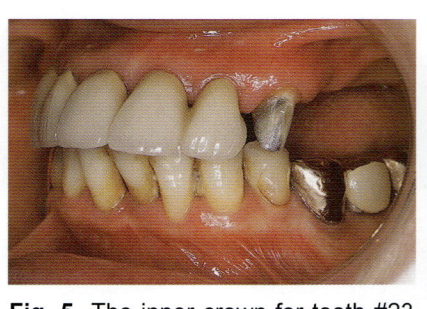

Fig. 5 The inner crown for tooth #23 was removed followed by abutment preparation again.

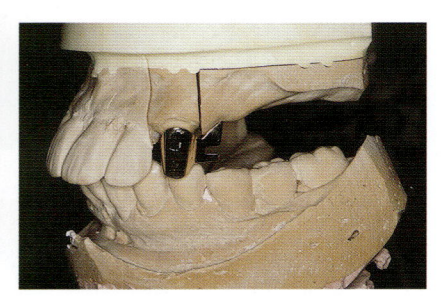

Fig. 6 Buccal view of the inner crown with a plate projection for tooth #23.

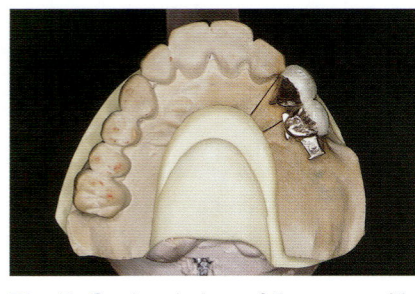

Fig. 7 Occlusal view of the case with the facing-type outer crown for tooth #23 and facing-type metal tooth for missing tooth #24 one-piece casted.

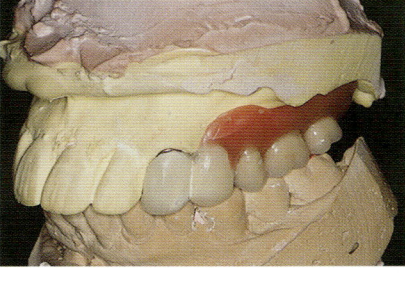

Fig. 8 Buccal view of the wax denture after replacement of the missing teeth #17, #24–#27 with the artificial teeth.

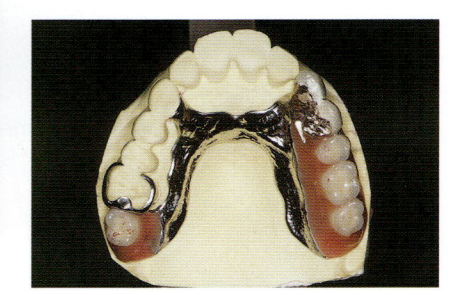

Fig. 9 Occlusal view of the wax denture with the spar placed on #13, Akers clasp placed on #16, and missing teeth #17, #24–#27 replaced with the artificial teeth, in which the facing-type metal tooth involving a Suginaka bolt attachment was arranged in the #24 region.

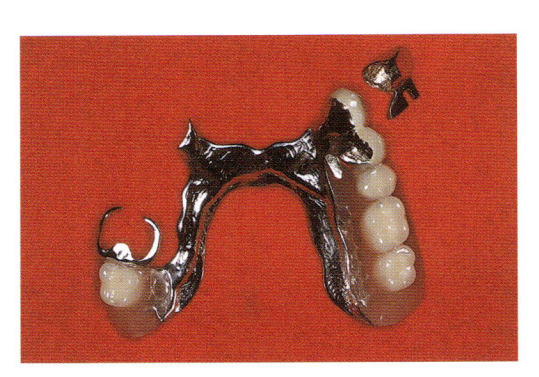

Fig. 10 Occlusal view of the completed inner crown with a plate projection for tooth #23 and Suginaka bolt denture for missing teeth #17, #24-#27.

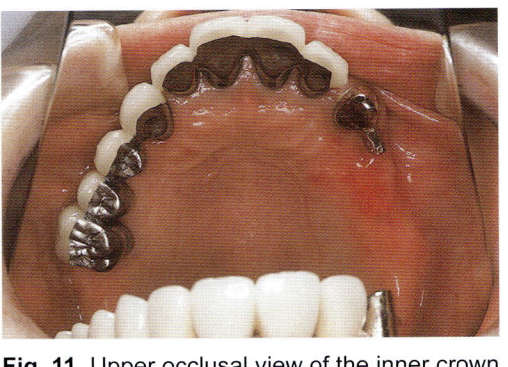

Fig. 11 Upper occlusal view of the inner crown with a plate projection placed on tooth #23.

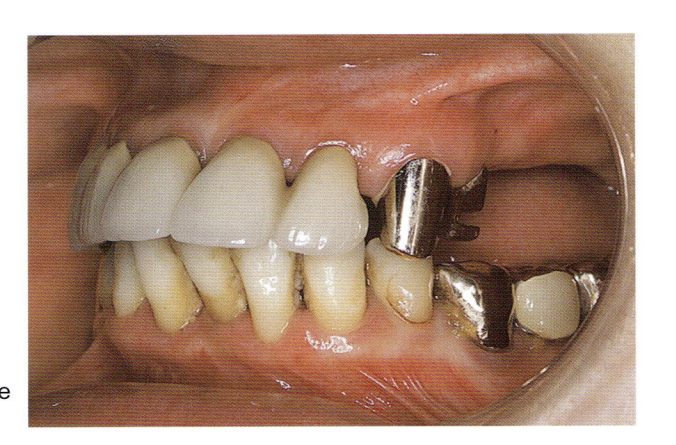

Fig. 12 Left buccal view of the same one.

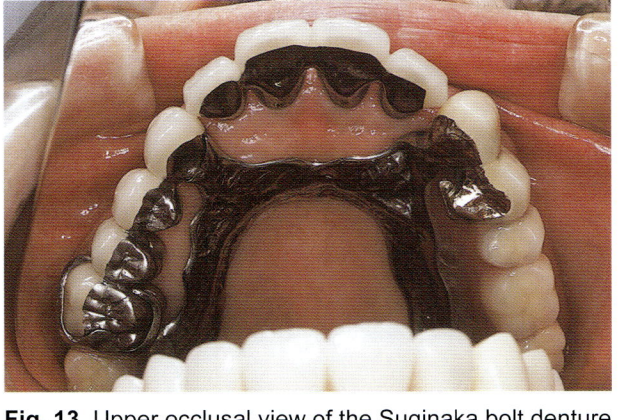

Fig. 13 Upper occlusal view of the Suginaka bolt denture placed on the missing teeth #17, #24-#27 region.

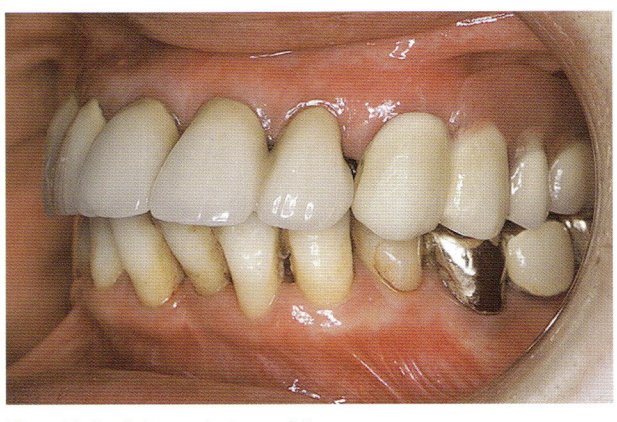

Fig. 14 Left buccal view of the same one.

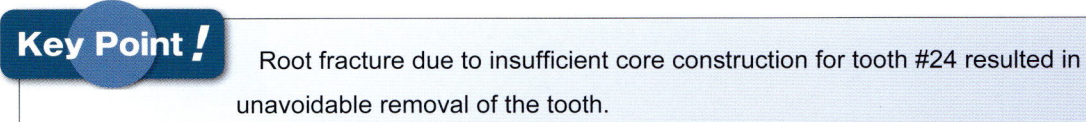

Key Point ! Root fracture due to insufficient core construction for tooth #24 resulted in unavoidable removal of the tooth.

With or without connection, you should pay careful attention to core construction.

3. Suginaka bolt dentures

⑥Tooth bounded missing case: Missing teeth #14-#16; Patient: 62-year-old woman
Tooth #13: Lock retainer
Tooth #17: Akers clasp

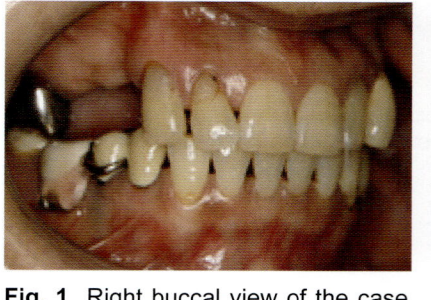

Fig. 1 Right buccal view of the case with missing teeth #14-#16.

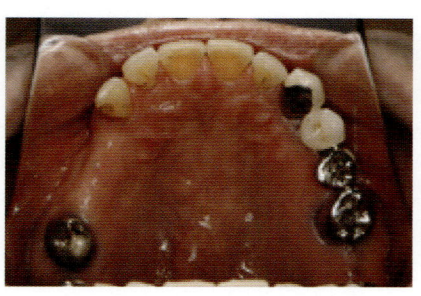

Fig. 2 Upper occlusal view of the same case.

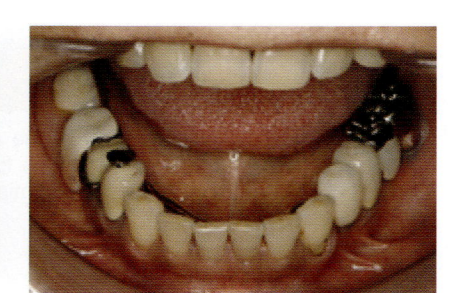

Fig. 3 Lower occlusal view of the same case.

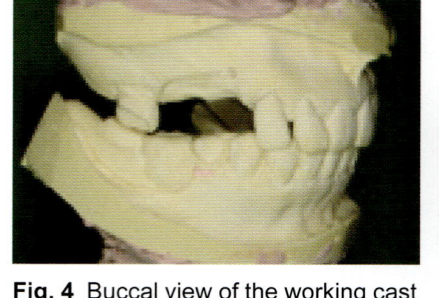

Fig. 4 Buccal view of the working cast with missing teeth #14-#16.

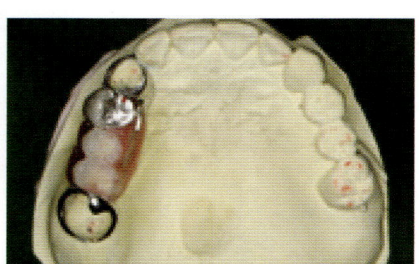

Fig. 5 Occlusal view of the same one.

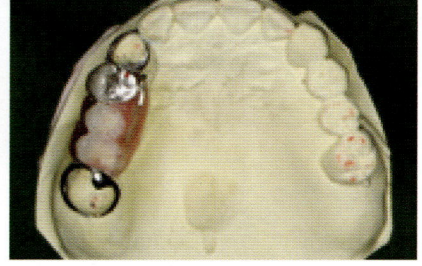

Fig.6 Occlusal view of the wax denture with the Akers clasp placed on tooth #17, lock retainer placed on tooth #13, and missing teeth #14-#17 replaced with the artificial teeth.

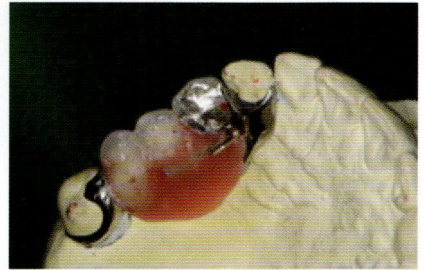

Fig. 7 Buccal view of the same one.

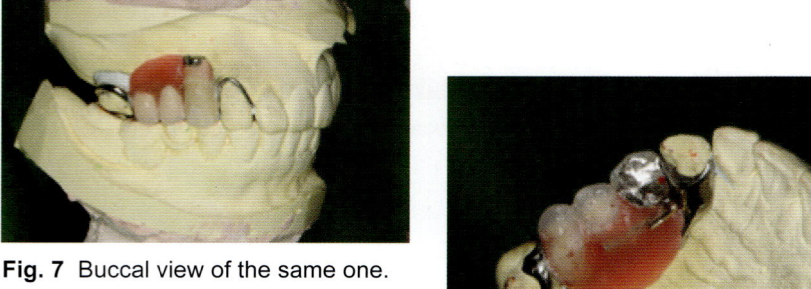

Fig. 8 Lingual view of the same one.

Fig. 9 Occlusal view of the wax denture with the metal tooth for missing tooth #14 rotated buccally through opening the hook.

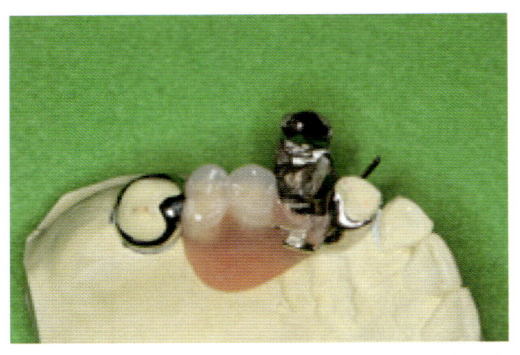

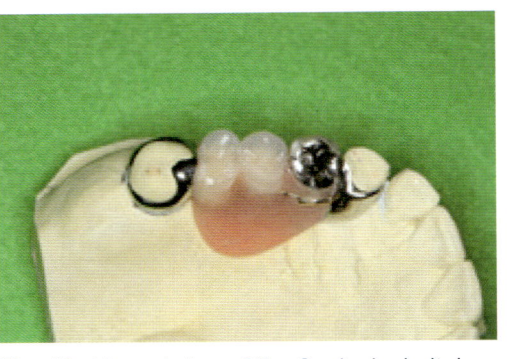

Fig. 10 Occlusal view of the completed Suginaka bolt denture for missing teeth #14-#16 with the metal tooth for missing tooth #14 rotated buccally.

Fig. 11 Lingual view of the Suginaka bolt denture with the metal tooth for missing tooth #14 replaced to the original position through closing the hook.

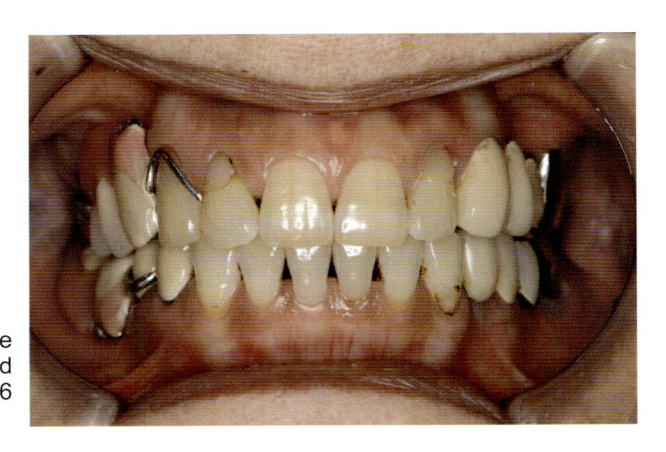

Fig. 12 Frontal view of the Suginaka bolt denture placed on the missing teeth #14-#16 region.

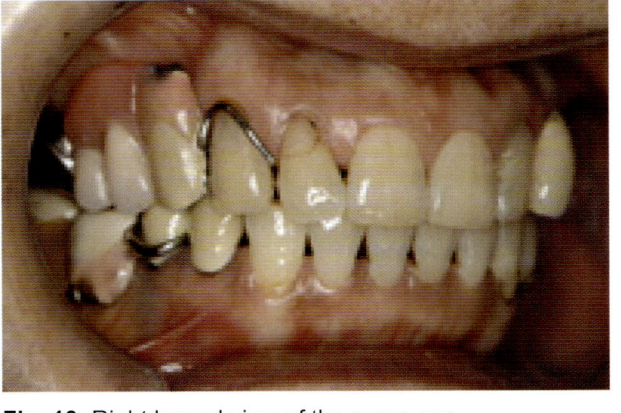

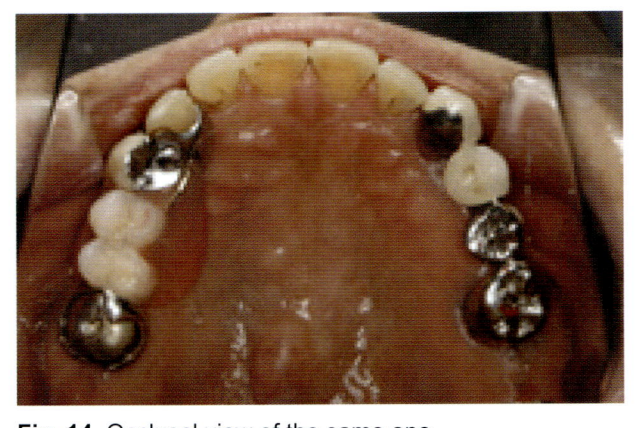

Fig. 13 Right buccal view of the same one.

Fig. 14 Occlusal view of the same one.

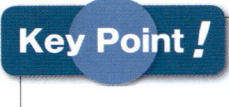
Key Point !

The lock retainer for tooth #13 appears to have contact with gingiva in figures but has no contact actually. However, attention should be taken to avoid contact with the dental root due to placement of the buccal arm in the deeper cervical area.

3. Suginaka bolt dentures

⑦Unilateral distal extension missing case with tooth bounded missing:
Missing teeth #36-#37, #45-#46; Patient: 70-year-old woman
Teeth #35, #44: Lock retainer
Tooth #47: Akers clasp

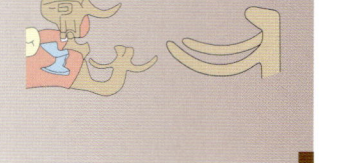

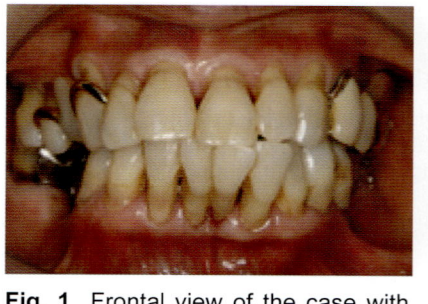

Fig. 1 Frontal view of the case with missing teeth #36-#37, #45-#46.

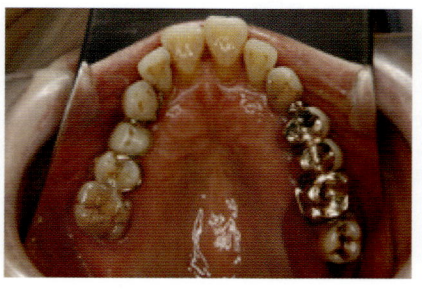

Fig. 2 Upper occlusal view of the same case.

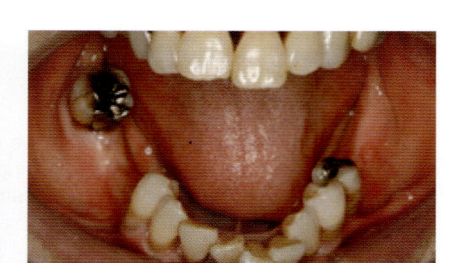

Fig. 3 Lower occlusal view of the same case.

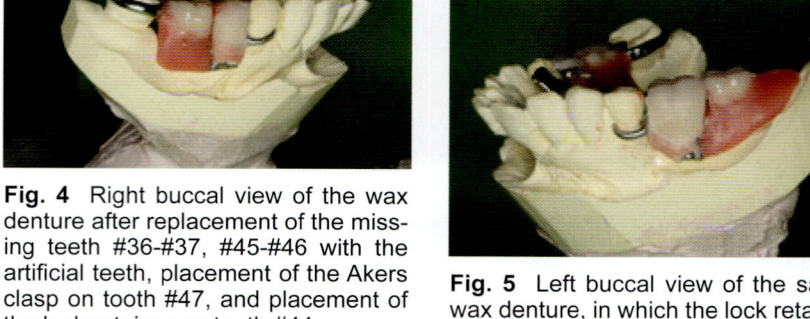

Fig. 4 Right buccal view of the wax denture after replacement of the missing teeth #36-#37, #45-#46 with the artificial teeth, placement of the Akers clasp on tooth #47, and placement of the lock retainer on tooth #44.

Fig. 5 Left buccal view of the same wax denture, in which the lock retainer was placed on tooth #35.

Fig. 6 Occlusal view of the same one. No retention is required for the Akers clasp placed on tooth #47.

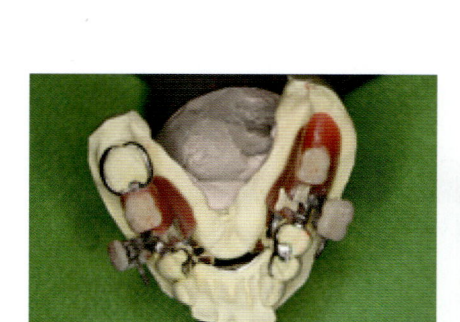

Fig. 7 Occlusal view of the wax denture with the metal teeth covered fully with a hybrid resin for missing teeth #36, #45 rotated buccally.

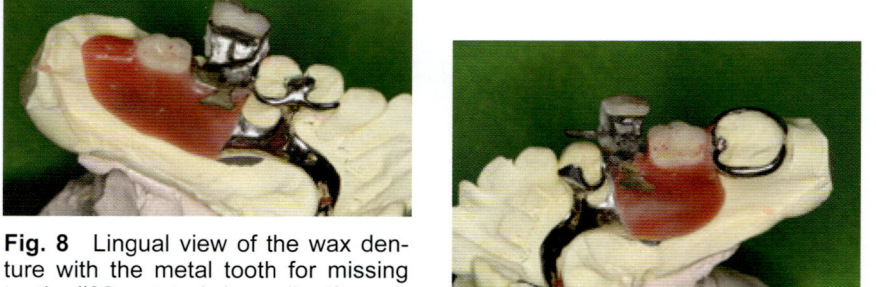

Fig. 8 Lingual view of the wax denture with the metal tooth for missing tooth #36 rotated buccally through opening the hook.

Fig. 9 Lingual view of the wax denture with the metal tooth for missing tooth #45 rotated buccally through opening the hook.

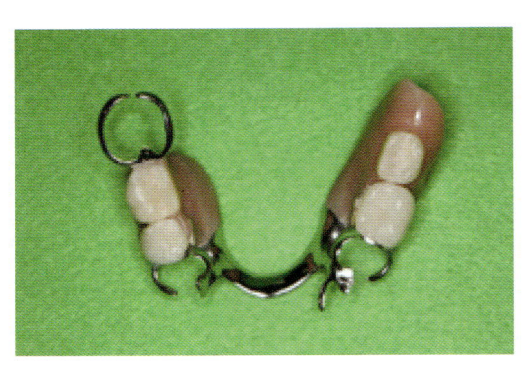

Fig. 10 Occlusal view of the completed Suginaka bolt denture for missing teeth #36-#37, #45-#46.

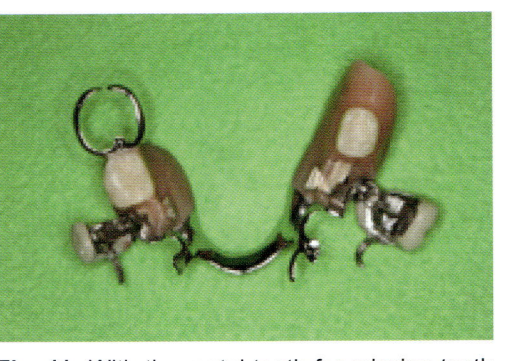

Fig. 11 With the metal teeth for missing teeth #36, #45 shown in Fig. 10 rotated buccally.

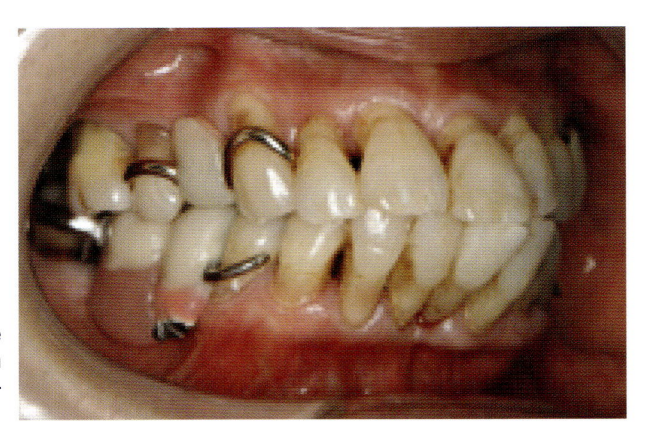

Fig. 12 Right buccal view of the Suginaka bolt denture placed on the missing teeth #36-37, #45-#46 region.

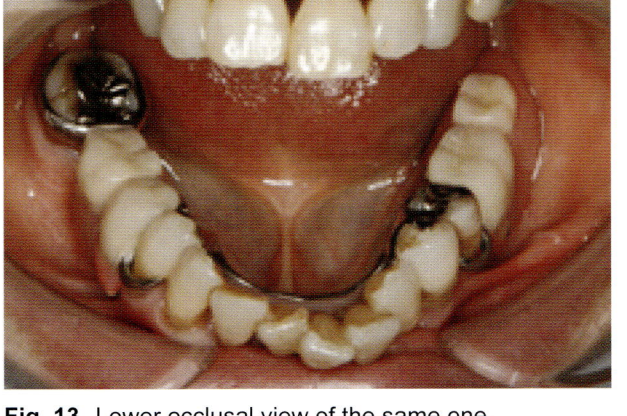

Fig. 13 Lower occlusal view of the same one.

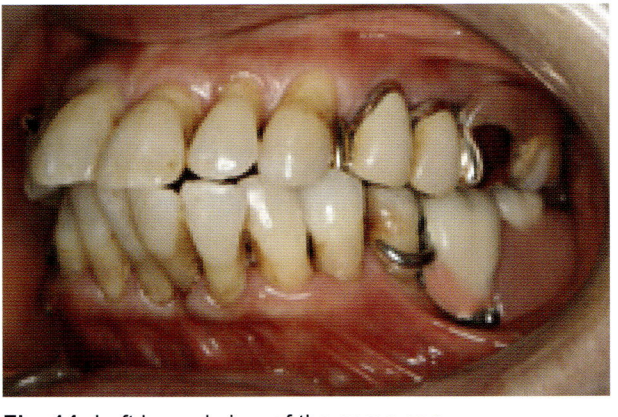

Fig. 14 Left buccal view of the same one.

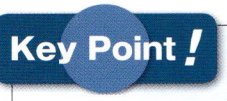
Key Point !

Filling was performed for wedge-shaped defects found in the cervical region of tooth #35, #44. Originally, the buccal arm of the lock retainer never have contact with the dental root. However, this allows lowering the buccal arm to the dental root.

3. Suginaka bolt dentures

⑧Bilateral distal extension missing case: Missing teeth #35-#37, #46-#47;
Patient: 63-year-old woman
Tooth #34: Lock retainer
Tooth #44: Porcelain fused to metal crown (PFM crown)
Tooth #45: PFM with a plate projection, Lingual arm with a marginal rest

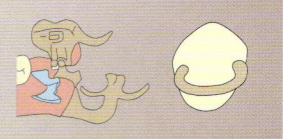

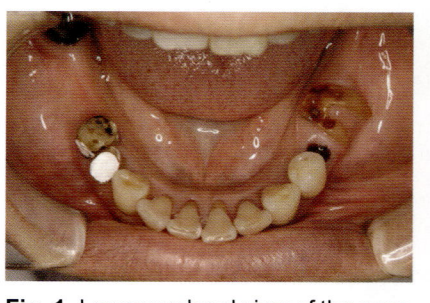

Fig. 1 Lower occlusal view of the case on initial examination. The teeth #35-#36, #48 are to be extracted.

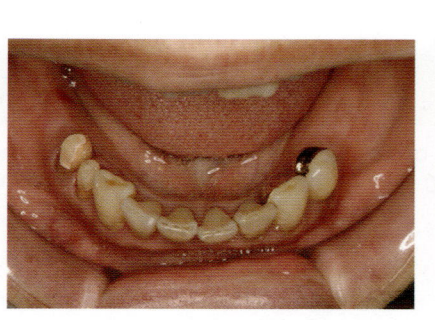

Fig. 2 Core construction in teeth #44, #45. The connected inlays placed in the teeth #33, #34 splinting the mobile teeth.

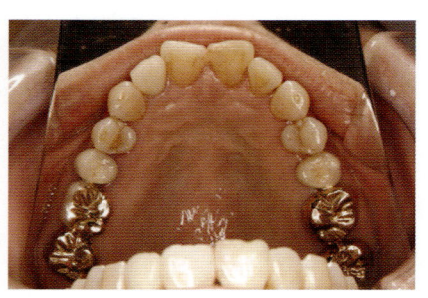

Fig. 3 Upper occlusal view of the case.

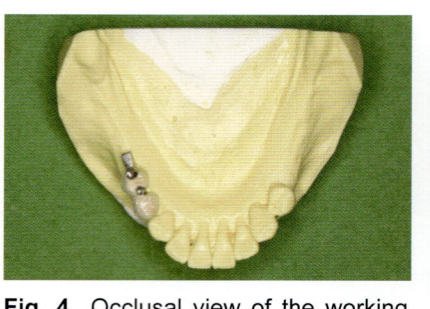

Fig. 4 Occlusal view of the working cast with PFM crowns with a plate projection for teeth #44, #45 to the original position.

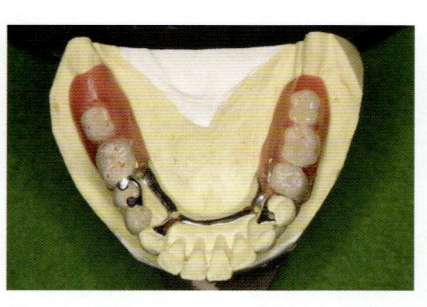

Fig. 5 Occlusal view of the wax denture after placement of the lingual arm with a marginal rest on tooth #45, lock retainer on tooth #34, and the artificial teeth on the missing teeth #35-#37, #46-#47 region.

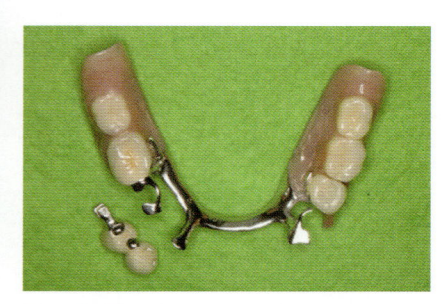

Fig. 6 The Suginaka bolt denture for missing teeth #35-#37, #46-#47 and the connected PFM crowns with the bar projection for teeth #44, #45 were completed.

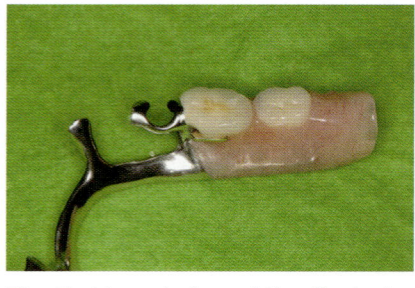

Fig. 7 Lingual view of the Suginaka bolt attachment placed in the missing tooth #46 region and lingual arm with a marginal rest for tooth #45.

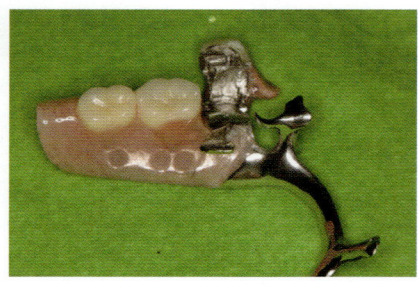

Fig. 8 Lingual view of the Suginaka bolt denture with the metal tooth for missing tooth #46 rotated buccally through opening the hook. In case, only undercuts in the bucco-distally proximal corner are used through resin as retention without use of the buccal arm.

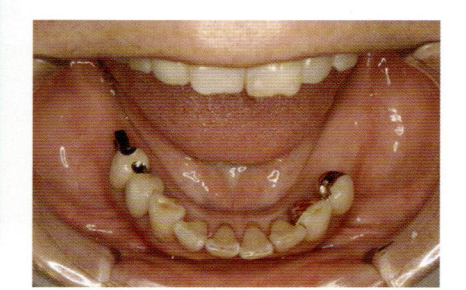

Fig. 9 Connected PFM crowns with a plate projection placed on teeth #44, #45.

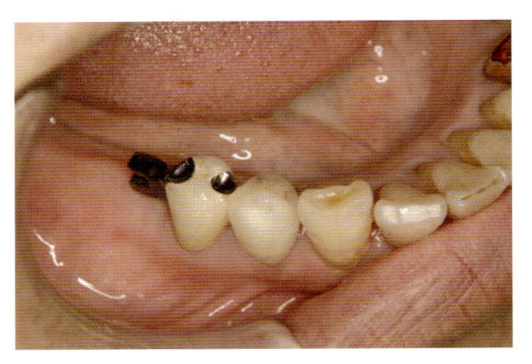

Fig. 10 Buccal view of the same one.

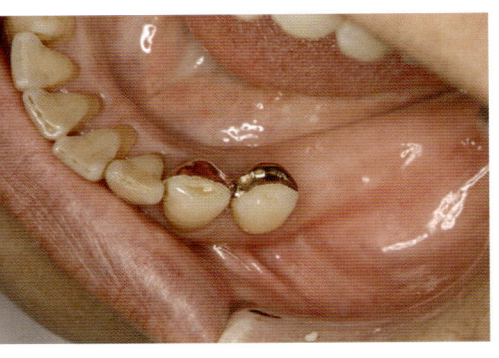

Fig. 11 Occlusal view of the teeth #33, #34 splinted with inlays.

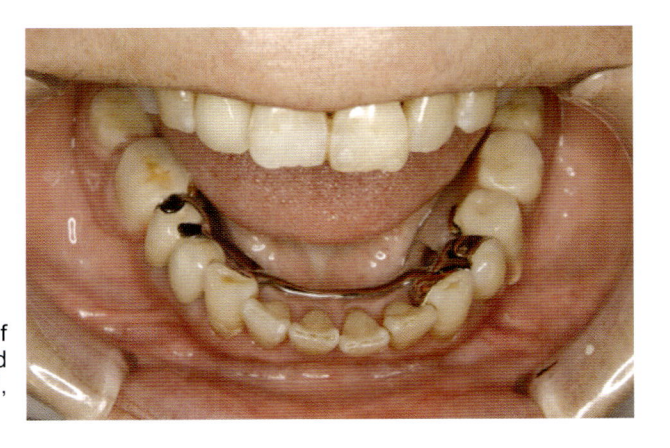

Fig. 12 Lower occlusal view of the Suginaka bolt view placed on the missing teeth #35-#37, #46-#47 region.

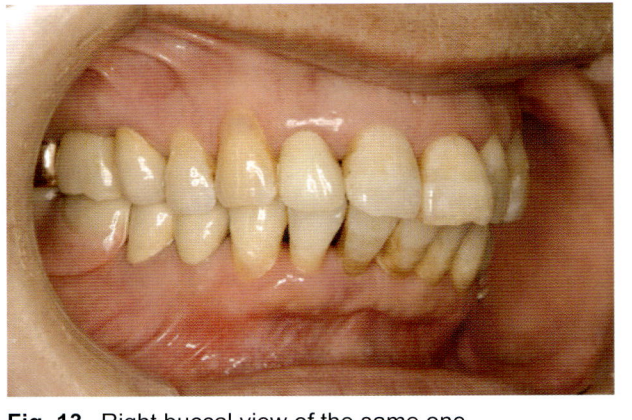

Fig. 13 Right buccal view of the same one.

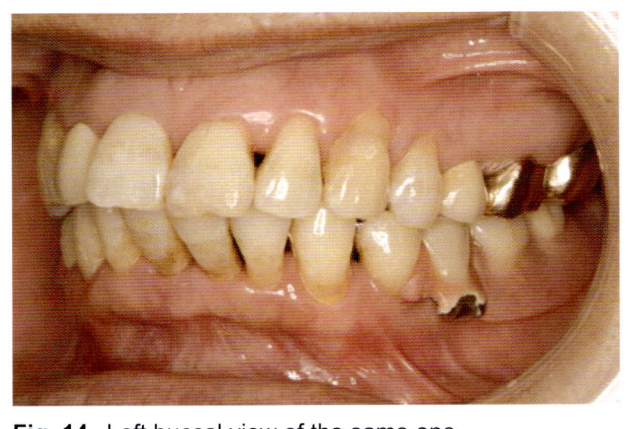

Fig. 14 Left buccal view of the same one.

Key Point !

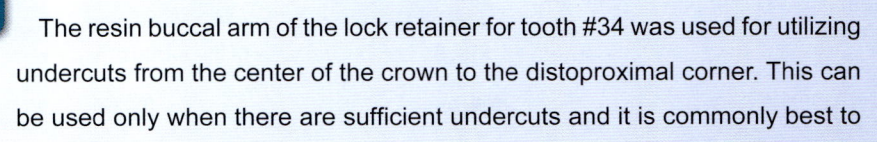

The resin buccal arm of the lock retainer for tooth #34 was used for utilizing undercuts from the center of the crown to the distoproximal corner. This can be used only when there are sufficient undercuts and it is commonly best to use a wire clasp.

3. Suginaka bolt dentures

⑨Bilateral distal extension missing case: Missing teeth #14-#17, #24-#27;
Patient: 72-year-old woman
Tooth #13: Lock retainer
Tooth #23: Akers clasp

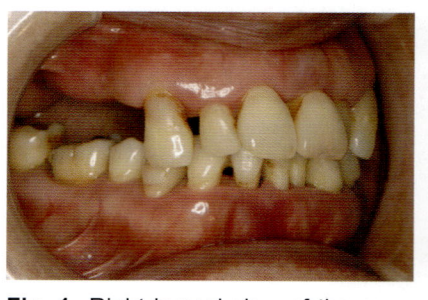

Fig. 1 Right buccal view of the case with missing teeth #14-#17, #24-#27.

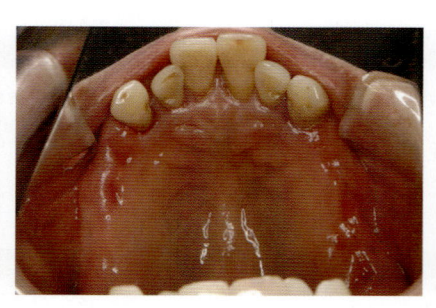

Fig. 2 Upper occlusal view of the same case.

Fig. 3 Left buccal view of the same case.

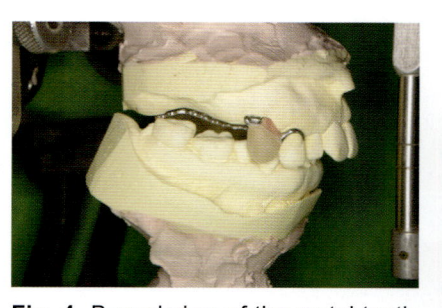

Fig. 4 Buccal view of the metal tooth covered with hybrid resin, hinge, and buccal arm placed on tooth #13.

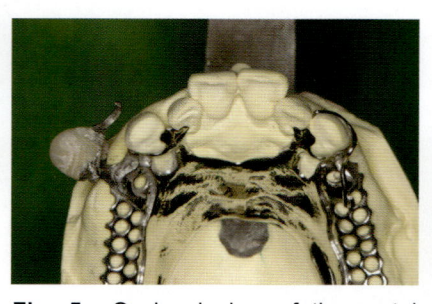

Fig. 5 Occlusal view of the metal flame with the lock retainer with the buccal arm rotating buccally for missing #14, and Akers clasps with a mesial rest placed on teeth #13, #23, respectively.

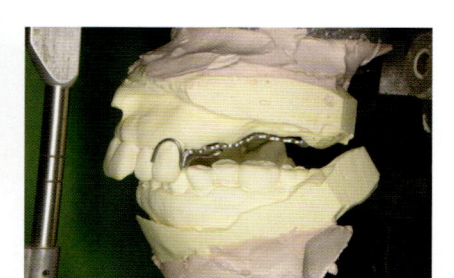

Fig. 6 Buccal view of the Akers clasp with a mesial rest place on tooth #23.

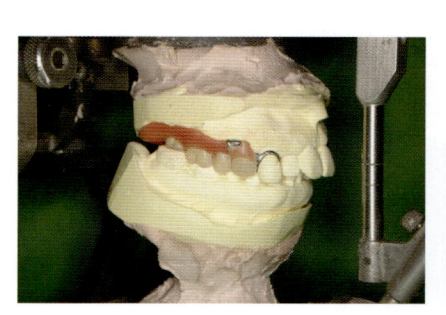

Fig. 7 Right buccal view of the wax denture after replacement of the missing teeth #14-#17, #24-#27 with the artificial teeth.

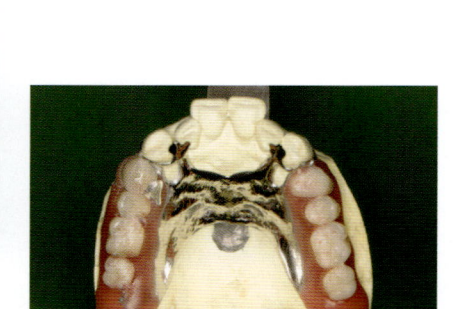

Fig. 8 Left buccal view of the same one.

Fig. 9 Occlusal view of the same one.

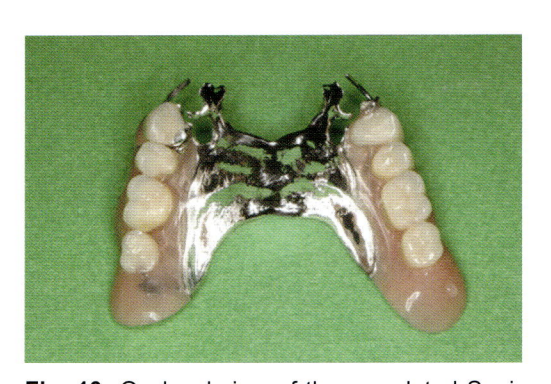

Fig. 10 Occlusal view of the completed Suginaka bolt denture for missing teeth #14-#17, #24-#27.

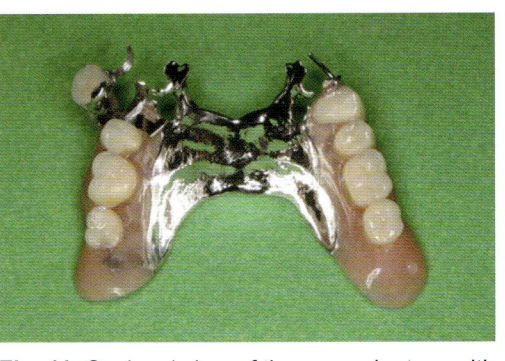

Fig. 11 Occlusal view of the same denture with the metal tooth for missing tooth #44 rotated buccally through opening the hook.

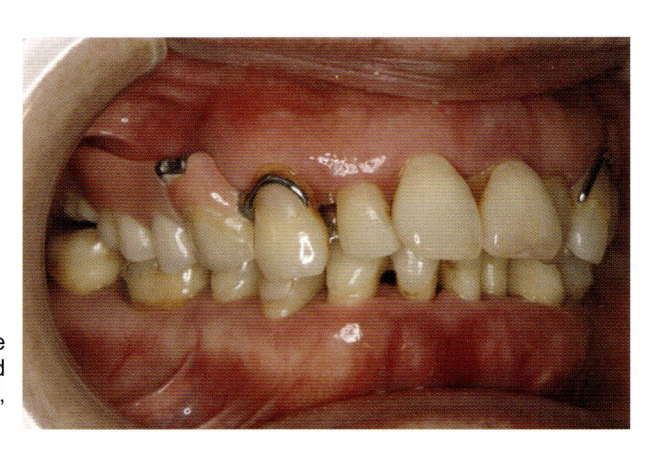

Fig.12 Right buccal view of the Suginaka bolt denture placed on the missing teeth #14-#17, #24-#27 region.

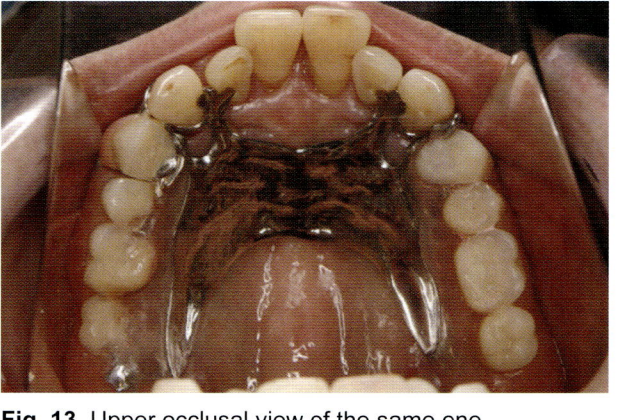

Fig. 13 Upper occlusal view of the same one.

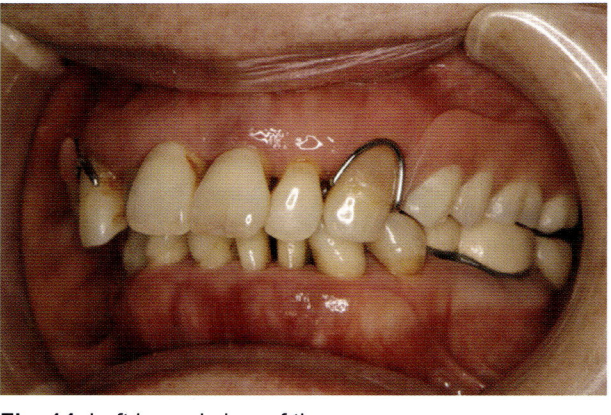

Fig. 14 Left buccal view of the same one.

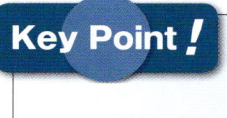
Key Point !

The denture can be inserted from direction slightly bucco-lateral to tooth #23 without the effect of the tooth #13, thus the buccal clasp for tooth #23 can be placed deeply into the cervical area. The buccal arms placed on teeth #13, #23 appears to have contact with gingiva in figures but has no contact actually. Of course, when tooth root exposure is observed, the buccal arm is never made to contact with the tooth root.

3. Suginaka bolt dentures

⑩Unilateral distal extension missing case with tooth bounded missing:
Missing teeth #34-#36, #45-#47; Patient: 74-year-old woman
Tooth #43: Facing crown
Tooth #44: 4/5 outer crown-type double crown (facing-type inner crown with a plate projection)
Tooth #33: Lock retainer
Tooth #37: Rest

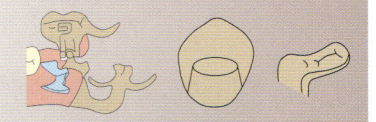

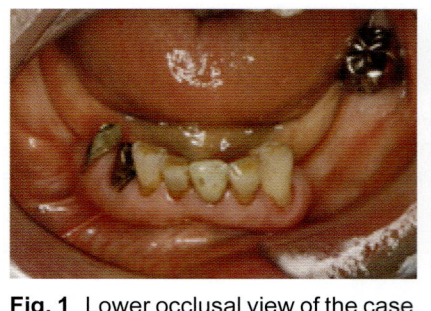

Fig. 1 Lower occlusal view of the case with missing teeth #34-#36, #45-#47.

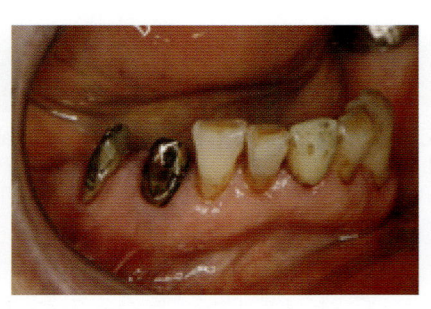

Fig. 2 Buccal view of the case with fall-out of crown restorations for teeth #43, #44.

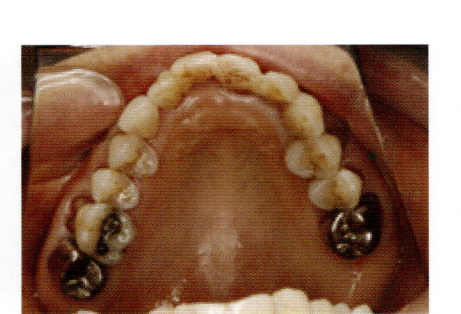

Fig. 3 Upper occlusal view of the same case.

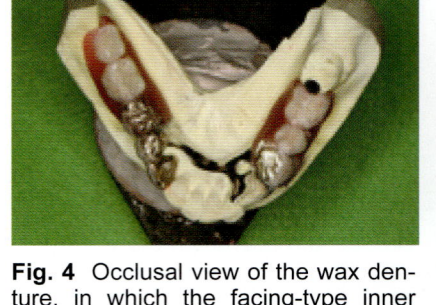

Fig. 4 Occlusal view of the wax denture, in which the facing-type inner crown with a plate projection for tooth #44 was connected to the resin facing crown for tooth #43, the 4/5 crown-type outer crown was placed on the tooth #44, the lock retainer was placed on tooth #33, and the missing teeth #35-#36, #45-#47 were replaced with the artificial teeth.

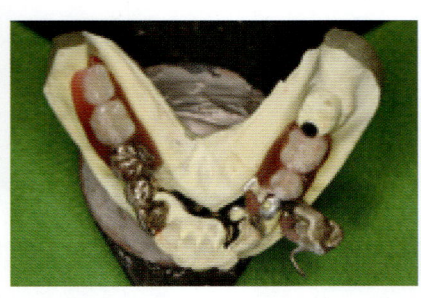

Fig. 5 Occlusal view of the wax denture with the metal tooth for missing tooth #34 rotated buccally through opening the hook.

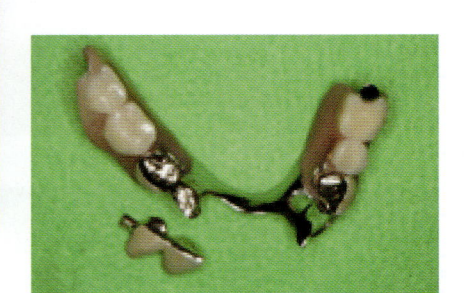

Fig. 6 Completed facing crowns for #43-#44 connected and Suginaka bolt denture for missing teeth #35-#36, #45-#47.

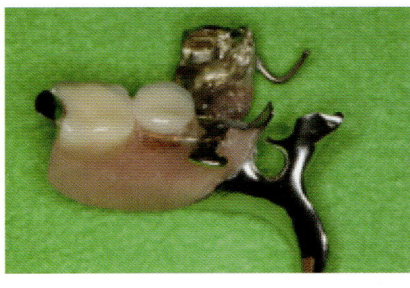

Fig. 7 Right lingual view of the completed denture with the metal tooth for missing tooth #34 rotated buccally in Fig. 6.

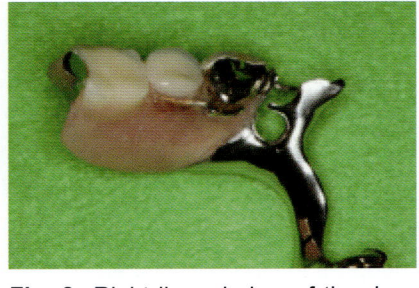

Fig. 8 Right lingual view of the denture with the metal tooth for missing tooth #34 replaced to the original position through closing the hook.

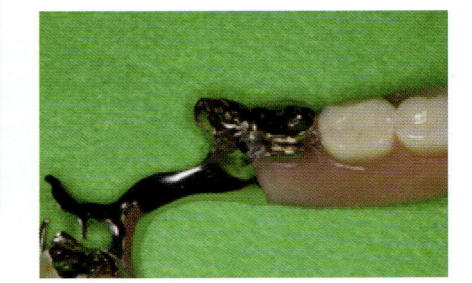

Fig. 9 Lingual view of the 4/5 crown-type outer crown for tooth #44 and Suginaka bolt attachment.

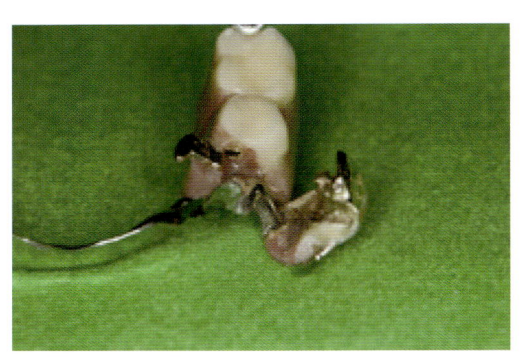

Fig. 10 Frontal view of the Suginaka bolt denture with the metal tooth for missing tooth #34 rotated buccally.

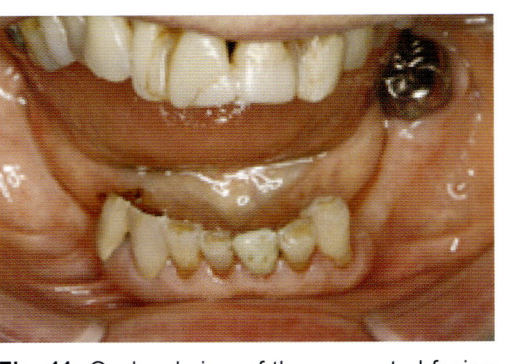

Fig. 11 Occlusal view of the connected facing crowns placed on teeth #43-#44.

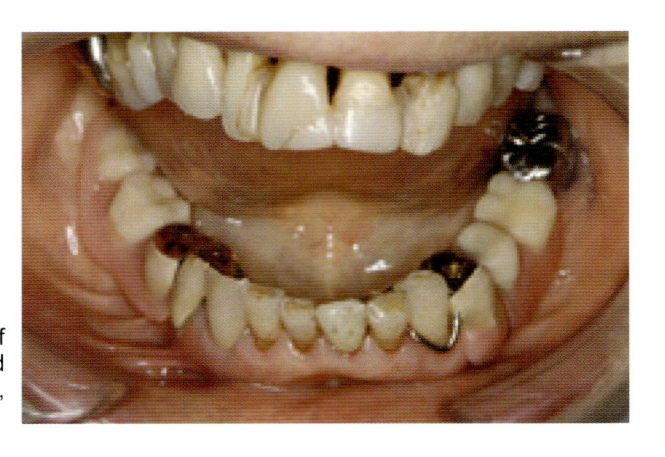

Fig. 12 Lower occlusal view of the Suginaka bolt denture placed on the missing teeth #35-#36, #45-#47 region.

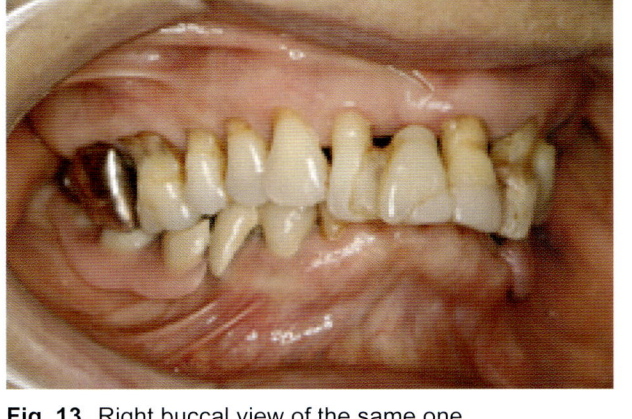

Fig. 13 Right buccal view of the same one.

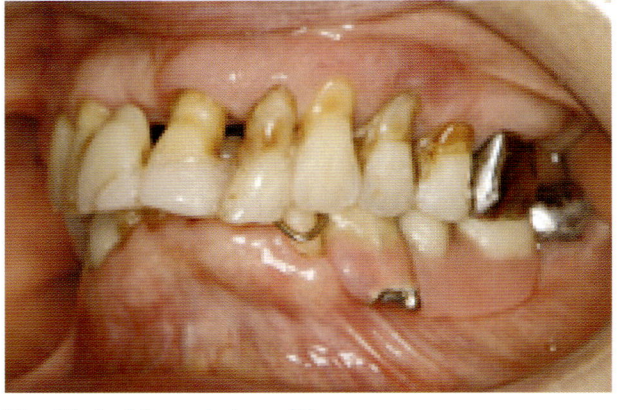

Fig. 14 Left buccal view of the same one.

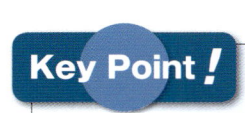
Key Point !

In case, there was no other choice but to make the mesial rest seat for tooth #33 as smaller because of the relationship between the path of insertion of the denture and the direction of tooth eruption. However, a incisal rest should have be placed to ensure stronger support.

Chapter **8**

Features of Suginaka bolt dentures

The locking mechanism has a great advantage without exerting any frictional force on the abutment tooth during denture insertion/removal. While the original bolt precision retainer uses retention produced by the latch effect, that means the retentive projection gets in touch with the mucosa and the tissue surface of the denture base and the lever is tightly-fitted into the slit prepared in the retentive projection, the functional pressure from the denture base are directly-transmitted to the abutment tooth, resulting in overloading the abutment tooth in free end dentures. In addition, for this purpose it needs precision instruments including a special bolt milling machine, resulting in complex and cumbersome laboratory procedures and high cost. The new Suginaka bolt system was designed to facilitate laboratory operations and simplify laboratory processes and clinical handling.

The Suginaka bolt is a simple device consisting of a housing, in which an easily retractable lever is placed in advance. It is placed in a denture base without soldering and brought into contact with a projection on an abutment tooth or a slit provided in a plate projection for obtaining retention through the latch effect. Consequently, this makes laboratory procedures dramatically easy and get a serious cost reduction. Moreover, the Suginaka bolt is little damaged, because of a simple mechanism and can be reused when the denture is refabricated.

For providing latch effect-derived retention, Suginaka bolt-combined retainers include two types of attachment denture and lock denture types available. The former is the type of locking the Suginaka bolt in a retentive projection attached to the proximal surface of the restoration on the abutment tooth. As the attachment type-Suginaka bolt denture is designed to keep the retentive projection contact with the denture base, the retentive section of the Suginaka bolt is to get away from the retentive projection during denture function. This differs significantly from precision retainers, which means that no occlusal forces from the denture base are transferred to the abutment tooth through the Suginaka bolt and retentive projection.

Because the Suginaka bolt has only retentive function, the retainer must has both support and bracing functions. Therefore, the Suginaka bolt is incorporated into a clasp or Cone-crown-telescope with the exception of only retentive function, which can be used as a retainer.

In this way, friction and retention developing during denture function or denture insertion/removal exert no adverse effect on the abutment tooth and various clasps are made easy to use, the applicability of the clasp can be further extended as results. Also, problems with frictional problem between the inner and outer crowns can be minimized with good oral feeling, functionality, and denture stability as with Cone-telescopic crowns by incorporating the Suginaka bolt into the loosely-fitted Cone-telescopic crown without creating surface friction between the outer and inner crowns. Although the frequency of root fracture can be considerably reduced by loosely fitting, still, it happens occasionally. In case of short-span denture bases and distal extension dentures with poor residual ridge mucosa, the use of a retainer with great connecting rigidity involves the risk of root fracture, but splinting of abutment teeth can avoid its risk. Even if the connecting rigidity of the retainer is lowered, with weaker bracing effect, retention of the Suginaka bolt is not affected at all.

The Suginaka bolt lock retainer is based on a RPPA clasp with the wider bracing surface. Bracing provided by both proximal surfaces of the abutment tooth diminishes mesiodistal rotation and mobility of the denture base. However, because the RPPA clasp is too strong in connecting rigidity, denture insertion/removal is difficult and excessive lateral forces are applied to the abutment tooth during denture removal. A decrease in bracing area for reducing this burden on the abutment tooth leads to an increase in mesiodistal rotation of the denture proportionally. Thus, adding a lingual arm, which is not provided for a RPPA clasp, to the lock retainer with a buccal arm for placing both arms within the deep undercut area allows diminution of mesiodistal rotation and mobility of the denture base. Also, as bracing provided by the buccal and lingual arms placed on the cervical surface of the abutment tooth is close to the center of buccolingual rotation of the denture, its rotational load applied to the abutment tooth can be reduced. In addition, bracing provided by 4 surfaces consisting of both proximal surfaces and the buccolingual cervical surfaces of the abutment tooth resists horizontal movement of the denture by bodily movement of the abutment tooth. However, to minimize such denture mobility, it is important to place an adequate occlusal rest on the abutment tooth.

However, how to provide bracing by 4 surfaces of the abutment tooth makes denture insertion/removal difficult. Thus, the buccal arm is joined to the metal tooth with the denture base that turns around the hinge. The denture can be removed through opening the hook of the Suginaka bolt attachment for locking and retaining the metal tooth in place in the denture base to separate the buccal arm that provide latch effect-derived retention from deep undercuts of the abutment tooth. When the unilateral distal extension missing is restored unilaterally, both buccal and lingual arms can be placed in the deep undercut area below the survey line on the abutment tooth, while the bilateral distal extension missing is restored, the lingual arm has to be placed on the survey line.

Since the buccal arm with latch effect-derived retentive function create no friction, there is no load exerted on the abutment tooth both on denture function and denture insertion/removal. In other words, the Suginaka bolt lock retainer allows application to both a normal and restored teeth and use of the residual teeth as it is.

As the retentive mechanism for retainers used in the Suginaka bolt dentures whether the attachment type or lock retainer type is based on the latch principle, no frictional force is not only created during both denture function and denture insertion/removal, but also no detachment force during denture insertion/removal. The Suginaka bolt system is an independent retentive mechanism and unaffected by the support and bracing mechanisms of the retainer or has no effect on those. Thus, the Suginaka bolt retainer allows use of support and bracing functions for the conditions of the abutment tooth and residual ridge mucosa.

However, it is very difficult that the patient inserts or removes the Suginaka bolt denture, particularly the Suginaka bolt lock denture. Therefore, for unilateral distal extension partial dentures restored unilaterally, it is important to provide a temporary base for them and practice on models before becoming capable of easily inserting/removing the Suginaka bolt denture. In addition, it should be remembered that it may take a long time to be accustomed use to inserting/removing procedures.

Reference

1) Rehm H, Körber KH, Körber E. Biophysikalisher Beitrag zur Problematik starr abgestützter Freiendprothesen. Dtsch Zahnärztl Z 1962 17: 963-974.

2) Preiskel HW. Precision Attachments in Dentistry, 3rd ed., Henry Kimpton London: 1969.

3) Böttger H. Das Teleskopsystem in der Zahnärztlichen Prothetik, Johann Anbrosius Barth Leipzig: 1969.

4) Mizukawa K. Swing Lock Attachment—The Theory and the Technical Practice—, Morita Osaka: 1976. [in Japanese]

5) Sekine H. The Partial Denture and the Load Reduction of the Retainer. In: Obana J, Sekine H, Matsuo E, Mitani H, editors. Practice in Partial Denture, p155-173, Ishiyaku publishers Tokyo: 1977. [in Japanese]

6) Tsuru H, Matsuo E, editors. The Partial Denture using the Milling Technique 1. Practice in Prosthodontics / extra issue 1979. [in Japanese]

7) Tsuru H, Matsuo E, editors. The Partial Denture by the Milling Technique 2. Practice in Prosthodontics / extra issue 1980. [in Japanese]

8) Sekine H, Kishi M. Dynamics and Partial Denture. In: Ai M, Kaneko K, editors. Partial Denture, Japan Dental Review / extra issue 1981 p37-53. [in Japanese]

9) Körber KH. Zahnärztliche Prothetik Band Ⅱ: Behandlungsplanung, Kronenzahnersatz, Brückenzahnersatz, Partielle Prothesen, Vollprothesen, Georg Thieme Stuttgart: 1975.

10) Kuroda M. Konuskrone, Ishiyaku publishers Tokyo: 1985. [in Japanese]

11) Kaneko K, Miyaji T, editors, Cone-Crown Telescope Now, Gnosis Tokyo: 1986. [in Japanese]

12) Goto T. Practice in Cone-Crown Telescope, Quintessence Publishing Tokyo: 1986. [in Japanese]

13) Inaba S, Igarashi Y, editors, Contemporary Telescopic System. —Practice and Technology in Konusukrone, Resilienz and Riegel—. QDT extra issue 1987. [in Japanese]

14) Goto T, Miyata T, editors, Planning Guidelines of the Partial Denture based on the rigid support. Practice in Prosthodontics / extra issue 1987. [in Japanese]

15) Körber, KH. Konuskronen Teleskope, Einführung in Klinik und Technik, Alfred Hüthig Heidelberg: 1973.

16) Gründler H. Die Riegel, Ein Befestigungssystem für den herausnehmbaren Zahnersatz, Quintessenz Verlags Berlin: 1984.

17) Goto T. Treatment Planning and Designing in Removable Partial Denture. Ishiyaku publishers Tokyo: 1995. [in Japanese]

18) Igarashi Y, Goto T. Ten-year Follow-up Study of Conical Crown-Retained Dentures. Int J Prosthodont 1997 10: 149-155.

19) Aoki T, Ohno J, Onodera Y, editors, The Milling, Basis and Practice in the Milling Technique. The Journal of Dental Technology / extra issue 1996. [in Japanese]

20) Ogata A, Igarashi Y, Shibano J, et al. In vivo Assessment of Occlusal Stress Distribution in Free-end Saddle Removable Partial Dentures Part 1. Stress Distribution in Various Removable Partial Dentures. J Jpn Prosthodont Soc 1997 41: 423-428. [in Japanese]

21) Ogata A. In vivo Assessment of Occlusal Stress Distribution in Free-end Saddle Removable Partial Dentures Part 2. Connecting Rigidity Affecting the Stress Distribution in Free-end Saddle Removable Partial Dentures. J Jpn Prosthodont Soc 1998 42: 393-401. [in Japanese]

22) Nokubi T, Miyaji T, Tsutsumi T, editors, Chairside & Laboside Designing / Structuring for Partial Denture Construction. The Journal of Dental Technology / extra issue 2000. [in Japanese]

23) Ai M, Igarashi Y, Hirai T, et al. Standard Partial Prosthodontics, Gakken Shoin Tokyo: 2001. [in Japanese]

24) Koide K, Hoshi H. editors, Fandamentals of Clasp Denture Design. Practice in Prosthodontics / extra issue 2002. [in Japanese]

25) Tanaka K. The Story of the Friction, Japan Standard Association Tokyo: 2004. [in Japanese]

26) Nokubi T, Inoue H, Hosoi N, Igarashi Y, editors, Partial Denture Technique, 4th ed., Ishiyaku publishers

Tokyo: 2006. [in Japanese]

27) Nokubi T, Igarashi Y. Contemporary Partial Denture —Clinical Guideline in Prosthodont of Missing teeth—, Quintessence Publishing Tokyo: 2008. [in Japanese]

Suginaka Bolt-related literature (literature published by author)

1) Design of a retainer for protecting abutment tooth for Cone-telescopic crowns. Dental Outlook 1994 83: 1377-1388. [in Japanese]
2) Removable partial denture for molar missing teeth with a prefabricated bolt-type retainer with easier lab ratory procedures. Journal of Dental Techniques 2000 28: 524-532. [in Japanese]
3) Design of bolt-type retainer that allows easier laboratory procedures. JNADT 2000 21: 39-43. [in Japanese]
4) Clinical report of Suginaka Bolt® partial denture for unilateral distal extension missing case—Missing teeth #25-#27—. JNADT 2000 23: 114-117. [in Japanese]
5) Advantages of a New Type of bolt Attachment. Prosthodont Res Pract 2002 2: 94-99.
6) Suginaka Bolt® RPD for tooth bounded missing case with missing premolars. JNADT 2003 24: 152-156. [in Japanese]
7) Suginaka Bolt® clasp denture for bilateral distal extension missing case. JNADT 2004 25: 114-119. [in Japanese]
8) Selection Criteria for Retainers in Suginaka Bolt® Dentures. Prosthodont Res Pract 2004 3: 98-107.
9) Suginaka Bolt Lock Denture Eliminates the Need for a Retentive Projection. J Jpn Prosthodont Soc 2008 52: 550-554.